WITHDRAWN
UTSA LIBRARIES

EVIDENCE-BASED
OUTCOME RESEARCH

EVIDENCE-BASED OUTCOME RESEARCH

A PRACTICAL GUIDE TO CONDUCTING
RANDOMIZED CONTROLLED TRIALS
FOR PSYCHOSOCIAL INTERVENTIONS

EDITED BY
ARTHUR M. NEZU & CHRISTINE MAGUTH NEZU

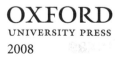

OXFORD
UNIVERSITY PRESS
2008

OXFORD
UNIVERSITY PRESS

Oxford University Press, Inc., publishes works that further
Oxford University's objective of excellence
in research, scholarship, and education.

Oxford   New York
Auckland   Cape Town   Dar es Salaam   Hong Kong   Karachi
Kuala Lumpur   Madrid   Melbourne   Mexico City   Nairobi
New Delhi   Shanghai   Taipei   Toronto

With offices in
Argentina   Austria   Brazil   Chile   Czech Republic   France   Greece
Guatemala   Hungary   Italy   Japan   Poland   Portugal   Singapore
South Korea   Switzerland   Thailand   Turkey   Ukraine   Vietnam

Copyright © 2008 by Oxford University Press, Inc.

Published by Oxford University Press, Inc.
198 Madison Avenue, New York, New York 10016

www.oup.com

Oxford is a registered trademark of Oxford University Press

All rights reserved. No part of this publication may be reproduced,
stored in a retrieval system, or transmitted, in any form or by any means,
electronic, mechanical, photocopying, recording, or otherwise,
without the prior permission of Oxford University Press.

Library of Congress Cataloging-in-Publication Data
Evidence-based outcome research : a practical guide to conducting randomized controlled trials for
psychosocial interventions / edited by Arthur M. Nezu and Christine Maguth Nezu.
     p. ; cm.
Includes bibliographical references and index.
ISBN 978-0-19-530463-3
1. Evidence-based psychiatry.   2. Psychiatry—Research—Methodology.   3. Psychotherapy—Research—
Methodology.   4. Clinical trials.   I. Nezu, Arthur M.   II. Nezu, Christine M.
[DNLM: 1. Psychotherapy—methods.   2. Evidence-Based Medicine.   3. Randomized Controlled Trials—
methods.   4. Treatment Outcome.   WM 420 E9223 2007]
RC455.2.E94E94 2007
616.89—dc22   2007009365

9 8 7 6 5 4 3 2 1
Printed in the United States of America
on acid-free paper

Library
University of Texas
at San Antonio

To all who have volunteered as participants in RCTs around the world

PREFACE

W e provide psychosocial treatments, whether to address a mental health (e.g., major depression, obsessive-compulsive disorder, generalized anxiety) or health (e.g., obesity, stress related to having the diagnosis of cancer, chronic back pain) problem, with the hope, assumption, and intent that such treatments will "work." However, how can we be sure that such inferences are correct? Whereas the provision of "psychotherapeutic techniques" can be traced back to various ancient civilizations, such as the Chinese and Greeks, it has only been within the past century that the scientific study of such questions has prevailed (see Chapter 1, Table 1.1, for a brief overview of the early history of this endeavor). The basic question—"Does this form of psychotherapy work?"—essentially has been asked and answered using the *randomized controlled trial* (RCT) during the past five to six decades and is generally thought of as the "gold standard" with regard to questions of treatment *efficacy*.

More recently, psychotherapy outcome research has embraced additional questions, such as "Can this therapy approach that has been found to be efficacious in the controlled setting also be effective in the real world of clinical settings?" (Lochman & Wells, 2003; Seligman, 1995). In addition to such *effectiveness studies,* another important question has arisen—"Is this particular intervention working for this particular patient?" This last inquiry has been represented by a research approach labeled "patient-focused research" (Howard, Moras, Brill, Martinovich, & Lutz, 1996; Lambert, Hansen, & Finch, 2001). Collectively, these three research strategies can be very powerful in providing information about the scientific standing of psychotherapy in general, and specific interventions in particular. Moreover, they can offer one means by which to enhance progress in improving the quality and success of psychosocial interventions.

This book focuses primarily on RCTs—what they are and how to carry them out, although much of what is contained has significant implications for all types of psychotherapy outcome research. In developing this idea, we especially wanted to create a book that provides for a practical guide to conducting RCTs. With the increased scientific and economic interest in identifying empirically supported treatments (ESTs; e.g., American Psychological Association, 2006), the need to conduct scientifically sound RCTs also grows. We should note that RCTs, as currently conducted, are not without critics, on both conceptual/methodological (e.g., Westen, Novotny, & Thompson-Brenner, 2004) and clinical (e.g., Levant, 2004) grounds. We should also note that we are not advocating that RCTs can answer all clinical questions relevant to providing the best treatments for all our patients; rather, it is the best approach to date that can provide for an important basis on which additional questions can be asked and more empirically informed clinical decisions can be made (Nezu, Nezu, & Cos, 2007; Nezu, Nezu, & Lombardo, 2004). In that light, we wish to provide for a detailed, cutting-edge, and practical guide to devising and implementing such investigations.

With this goal in mind, we asked leading researchers and statisticians across disciplines to contribute to this practical guide. Whereas multiple sources exist regarding the conceptual and theoretical underpinnings of much of the advice offered in this book, they are scattered across journals, and few (if any) compendiums are available that provide for practical advice by leading (and successful) investigators in one location. The book includes five sections, loosely presented in the order in which investigators devise an RCT (i.e., conceptual issues, assessment issues, methodological and design issues, data analysis issues, and special topics). As such, this book can serve as a useful "how-to guide" for the beginning outcome researcher or student, as well as a meaningful "encyclopedic" sourcebook for experienced investigators searching for cutting-edge ideas.

We wish to thank all the chapter authors for their important contributions and the simultaneous education we received as a function of reviewing each chapter. For her support, patience, and expert shepherding, we extend our deep gratitude to Mariclaire Cloutier at Oxford University Press.

■ References

American Psychological Association (2006). Evidenced-based practice in psychology. *American Psychologist, 61*, 271–285.

Howard, K. I., Moras, K., Brill, P. L., Martinovich, Z., & Lutz, W. (1996). Efficacy, effectiveness, and patient progress. *American Psychologist, 51*, 1059–1064.

Lambert, M. J., Hansen, N. B., & Finch, A. E. (2001). Patient-focused research: Using patient outcome data to enhance treatment effects. *Journal of Consulting and Clinical Psychology, 69*, 159–172.

Levant, R. F. (2004). The empirically validated treatments movement: A practitioner/educator perspective. *Clinical Psychology: Science and Practice, 11*, 219–224.

Lochman, J. E., & Wells, K. C. (2003). Effectiveness of the Coping Power Program and of classroom intervention with aggressive children: Outcomes at a 1-year follow-up. *Behavior Therapy, 34,* 493–515.

Nezu, A. M., Nezu, C. M., & Cos, T. A. (2007). Case formulation for the behavioral and cognitive therapies: A problem-solving perspective. In T. D. Eells (Ed.), *Handbook of psychotherapy case formulation* (2nd ed., pp. 349–378). New York: Guilford.

Nezu, A. M., Nezu, C. M., & Lombardo, E. R. (2004). *Cognitive-behavioral case formulation and treatment design: A problem-solving approach.* New York: Springer.

Seligman, M. E. P. (1995). The effectiveness of psychotherapy: The Consumer Reports study. *American Psychologist, 50,* 965–974.

Westen, D., Novotny, C. M., & Thompson-Brenner, H. (2004). The empirical status of empirically supported psychotherapies: Assumptions, findings, and reporting in controlled clinical trials. *Psychological Bulletin, 130,* 631–663.

CONTENTS

ABOUT THE EDITORS

Arthur M. Nezu, PhD, ABPP

Dr. Nezu is currently Professor of Psychology, Professor of Medicine, and Professor of Community Health and Prevention at Drexel University in Philadelphia. Among his multiple previous administrative positions, he served as Senior Associate Dean for Research at the Medical College of Pennsylvania/Hahnemann University. He has conducted multiple randomized controlled trials and has contributed to over 175 professional and scientific publications. Several of his works have been translated into various foreign languages, including Japanese, Spanish, Dutch, French, and Italian. His research has been funded by university, state, and federal agencies, including the National Cancer Institute and Veterans Administration. Dr. Nezu is a member of eight editorial boards of scientific and professional journals in psychology, and he is a standing member of the Interventions Research Review Committee of the National Institute of Mental Health. An award-winning psychologist, he was previously President of the Association for Advancement of Behavior Therapy, the Behavioral Psychology Specialty Council, the World Congress of Behavioral and Cognitive Therapies, and the American Board of Cognitive and Behavioral Psychology. He is a fellow of the American Psychological Association, the Association for Psychological Science, the Society for Behavior Medicine, the Academy of Cognitive Therapy, and the Academy of Cognitive and Behavioral Psychology. Dr. Nezu was awarded the diplomate in Cognitive and Behavioral Psychology from the American Board of Professional Psychology, currently serves as a trustee of that board, has an active private practice, and is conducting outcome studies in behavioral medicine.

Christine Maguth Nezu, PhD, ABPP

Dr. Maguth Nezu is currently Professor of Psychology, Associate Professor of Medicine, and Director of the Masters Programs in Psychology at Drexel University in Philadelphia. She previously served as Associate Provost for Research and Scientific Integrity Officer for the Medical College of Pennsylvania/Hahnemann University. She is the co-author or editor of over 100 scholarly publications, including 15 books. Her publications cover a wide range of topics in mental health and behavioral medicine, many of which have been translated into a variety of foreign languages. Dr. Maguth Nezu is currently the President-Elect of the American Board of Professional Psychology, on the board of directors for the American Board of Cognitive and Behavioral Psychology, and on the board of directors for the American Academy of Cognitive and Behavioral Psychology. She is the recipient of numerous grant awards supporting her research and program development, particularly in the area of clinical interventions, from a variety of agencies, including the National Cancer Institute, the Philadelphia Office of Behavioral Health and Mental Retardation, and the National Institute of Justice. She serves on the editorial boards of several leading psychology and health journals, has served as a grant reviewer for the Department of Education and the National Institutes of Health, and frequently provides workshops on clinical interventions, both nationally and internationally. She holds a diplomate in Cognitive and Behavioral Psychology from the American Board of Professional Psychology, has an active private practice, and is interested in the treatment of depression in medical patients, as well as individuals with personality disorders.

About the Contributors

Stephanie Bauer received her PhD in psychology from the University of Tübingen in Germany. She is currently Research Fellow at the Center for Psychotherapy Research at the University Hospital of Heidelberg. Her main research field is the development and evaluation of IT-based tools (e.g., Internet chat, text messaging) for service optimization for patients with mental disorders.

Judith S. Beck, PhD, is the Director of the Beck Institute for Cognitive Therapy, Clinical Associate Professor of Psychology in Psychiatry at the University of Pennsylvania, and President of the Academy of Cognitive Therapy. She is the author of *Cognitive Therapy: Basics and Beyond, Cognitive Therapy for Challenging Problems, The Oxford Textbook of Psychotherapy, Cognitive Therapy of Personality Disorders,* and *The Beck Diet Solution.*

Juan Botella is Professor at the Autonoma University of Madrid. He has published several papers and books on research methods. His research activity involves many fields of psychology but focus mostly on selective attention and the problem of binding and formation of illusory conjunctions. Other research areas cover mathematical models of psychological processes and psychological assessment.

C. Hendricks Brown is Professor of Epidemiology and Biostatistics at the College of Public Health, University of South Florida. He also holds adjunct professor positions in the Department of Biostatistics and the Department of Mental Health at the Johns Hopkins Bloomberg School of Public Health, and is Senior Research Scholar at the American Institutes for Research. He designs randomized field trials to prevent aggression, drug abuse, and suicide.

LeeAnn Cardaciotto is Visiting Assistant Professor in the Department of Psychology at the University of Delaware. She received her PhD in clinical psychology from Drexel University and completed a postdoctoral fellowship at the University of Delaware. Her research interests include the study of emotion regulation, mindfulness, and acceptance in the context of treatments for depression and anxiety disorders.

Kathleen M. Carroll, PhD, is Professor of Psychiatry at the Yale University School of Medicine. The author of more than 200 journal articles, chapters, and books, Dr. Carroll currently holds both K05 (Senior Scientist) and MERIT awards from the National Institute on Drug Abuse (NIDA). She received the Distinguished Scientific Contributions to Education and Training Award from Division 50 of the American Psychological Association.

Tracy E. Costigan, PhD, is a Principal Research Scientist at the American Institute for Research in Washington, DC, and holds an adjunct faculty appointment in the Department of Psychology at Drexel University. Her work focuses on experimental design, methodology, and evaluation in the areas of pediatric school psychology, teacher education, and workforce issues. The goal of these projects is to assure implementation of effective programming, including accountability and continuous improvement.

Geoff Cumming, DPhil, has taught research methods and statistics in the School of Psychological Science at La Trobe University for more than 30 years. His main current research is in the area of statistical cognition. Exploratory Software for Confidence Intervals (ESCI; http://www.latrobe.edu.au/psy/esci) is his interactive graphical software that runs under Microsoft Excel, and which is intended to support better understanding of sampling, confidence intervals, meta-analysis, and other statistical techniques and their use by researchers and students.

Karina W. Davidson, PhD, is the Codirector of the Center for Behavioral Cardiovascular Health at Columbia College of Physicians and Surgeons in New York. Her program of research focuses on psychosocial interventions for patients with cardiovascular disease. She has a multisite, multiproject NIH contract exploring the etiology, course, and treatment of depressive symptoms in patients with acute coronary syndromes. She formed and was the Chair of the Evidence-Based Behavioral-Medicine Committee. She is now Convenor of the Cochrane Behavioral Medicine Field.

David DeMatteo, JD, PhD, is an Assistant Professor in the Drexel University Department of Psychology, and Codirector of the JD/PhD Program in Law and Psychology offered by Drexel University and Villanova University School of

Law. His teaching interests include research methods, statistics, psychopharmacology, substance abuse, and courses integrating law and psychology. He is the coauthor of *Essentials of Research Design and Methodology* (Wiley).

Sopagna Eap, MS, is a doctoral student in clinical psychology at the University of Oregon. Her research interests address issues related to the conceptualization, assessment, and treatment of mental health for ethnic minorities.

Diane L. Fairclough, PhD, is Professor in the Department of Preventive Medicine and Biometrics of the Colorado Health Outcomes Program at the University of Colorado Health Sciences Center. Her interests include design and analysis of longitudinal studies with missing data due to disease morbidity or mortality, and the psychosocial issues of survivors of childhood and adult cancer. Among her many publications is the recent book *Design and Analysis of Quality of Life Studies in Clinical Trials.*

Cathy Faulkner has a doctorate in clinical psychology from La Trobe University. Her research interests are evidence-based practice, progress in clinical psychology, and improvement in the statistical techniques used by clinical researchers. She currently works as a clinical psychologist in an innovative practice, predominantly treating clients with depression, anxiety, and complex trauma reactions.

Rocío Fernández-Ballesteros is Professor at the Autonoma University of Madrid, where she teaches psychological assessment and evaluation. She is author of 20 books and more than 250 articles on assessment, evaluation, and aging. One of her research programs involves self-report and response distortions. She has contributed to the development of evaluation systems for several international and national intervention programs.

David S. Festinger, PhD, is a senior scientist in the Section on Law and Ethics at the Treatment Research Institute and Adjunct Assistant Professor of Psychiatry at the University of Pennsylvania School of Medicine. His research focuses on examining the active mechanisms of drug courts and major ethical dilemmas in research. He has authored numerous scientific articles and chapters and is a coauthor of *Essentials of Research Design and Methodology* (Wiley).

Fiona Fidler is a Postdoctoral Fellow in the School of Psychological Science at La Trobe University in Australia. She has an undergraduate degree in psychology and a PhD in philosophy of science. Her postgraduate research explored resistance to statistical and methodological change in psychology, medicine, and ecology. Her main current research is in the field of statistical cognition (i.e., human cognition of statistical ideas).

Michele Galietta, PhD, is Associate Professor of Psychology at the John Jay College of Criminal Justice, City University of New York. She is Codirector of the forensic psychology doctoral program and Director of clinical training. She teaches ethics and specializes in ethical issues surrounding research and treatment of prisoners. She has also done research on the ethical issues surrounding research with individuals at the end of life. She has served on the APA Committee on Professional Practice and Standards.

Joan S. Grant, DSN, RN, CS, is a Professor in the University of Alabama at Birmingham School of Nursing. Her research program primarily relates to developing social problem-solving telehealth interventions to assist family members in managing caregiving problems in the home and other settings.

Gordon C. Nagayama Hall, PhD, is Professor of Psychology at the University of Oregon. He is currently investigating the effectiveness with Asian Americans of treatments that are empirically supported for other groups. He is also interested in behavioral genomics approaches to genetic and cultural factors implicated in antisocial behavior. He was previously President of the Society for the Psychological Study of Ethnic Minority Issues and is currently editor of *Cultural Diversity and Ethnic Minority Psychology,* as well as Associate Editor of the *Journal of Consulting and Clinical Psychology.*

Nathan B. Hansen received a PhD in clinical psychology from Brigham Young University. He currently is an Assistant Professor of Psychology in the Division of Prevention and Community Research of the Department of Psychiatry at Yale University School of Medicine, where his clinical and research work focuses on developing interventions to decrease the impact of sexual trauma and interpersonal violence on health-risk behavior, particularly substance abuse and HIV risk behavior.

Adele M. Hayes is Associate Professor and Director of Clinical Psychology in the Department of Psychology at the University of Delaware. She completed her PhD in clinical psychology at the State University of New York at Stony Brook and her postdoctoral fellowship at Duke University Medical Center. Her research focuses on the process of change in psychosocial treatments (particularly depression and personality disorders) and on developing new methods to identify mechanisms of change in clinical trials. Her work has been supported by grants from NIMH.

Stephen N. Haynes received his PhD from the University of Colorado at Boulder. He is currently Professor and Chair of the Department of Psychology, University of Hawaii at Manoa. He has published multiple articles and books in the areas of behavioral assessment, psychometrics, case formulation, and health psychology and is the former editor of the journal *Psychological Assessment*.

Louis M. Hsu is Professor Emeritus, Fairleigh Dickinson University, Department of Psychology. He received his PhD in psychometrics from Fordham University. His publications include articles in *Psychological Methods,* the *Journal of Consulting and Clinical Psychology, Multivariate Behavioral Research, Psychological Assessment, Structural Equation Modeling, Psychological Bulletin, Journal of Applied Psychology, Journal of Abnormal Psychology,* and *Journal of Counseling Psychology,* and in nineteen other refereed journals, and chapters in nine books.

Irene Belle Janis is a doctoral candidate in the Department of Psychology at Harvard University. She received her AB in psychology from Harvard University. She is interested broadly in decision making and impulsiveness, and her research focuses primarily on the role of decision making, impulsiveness, and delay of gratification in self-injurious thoughts and behaviors.

Joseph Keawe'aimoku Kaholokula is at the Department of Native Hawaiian Health, John A. Burns School of Medicine, University of Hawaii. He received his PhD in psychology from the Clinical Studies Program at the University of Hawaii. His clinical and research interests are in the prevention and management of chronic medical conditions, culturally informed behavioral assessments, and the effects of acculturation on mental and physical health among Asian and Pacific Islander populations.

Duck-Hee Kang, RN, PhD, FAAN, is Professor and Marie L. O'Koren Endowed Chair at the University of Alabama at Birmingham School of Nursing. Her program of research primarily addresses the impact of stress, social support, and other psychosocial factors on immune responses and health outcomes. Most recently, she examined the impact of a cognitive-behavioral modification program and exercise training on psychosocial well-being, immune responses, and clinical symptoms in breast cancer patients.

Kimberly T. Kendziora, Principal Research Analyst at the American Institutes for Research, works in the broad areas of child mental health and school-based initiatives for students at risk of school failure. She directs evaluations of a school-based mental health initiative in the Bronx, the Alaska Initiative for Community Engagement, and the Iowa Learning Supports initiative and is working on efficient measures of the conditions for learning in schools. These projects advance understanding of how schools can support all children's academic, social, and emotional development.

Michael J. Lambert, PhD, is a Professor and holds an Endowed Chair in Psychology at Brigham Young University, teaching in the Clinical Psychology Program. He has been in private practice as a psychotherapist throughout his career. His research spans 35 years and has emphasized psychotherapy outcome, process, and the measurement of change. He has edited, authored, or coauthored 9 academic research-based books and 40 book chapters, while publishing more than 150 scientific articles on treatment outcome.

Jean-Philippe Laurenceau is Associate Professor in the Department of Psychology at the University of Delaware. He completed a BA cum laude in psychology from Cornell University and received his PhD from the Pennsylvania State University. His research interests include intimacy processes in close relationships, evaluation of interventions targeting the prevention of marital dysfunction, and applications of modern methods for the analysis of change. His research is supported by grants from the NIMH.

Elizabeth Mostofsky, BA, is completing her MPH at the Columbia University Mailman School of Public Health in the epidemiology track. She is currently a Clinical Coordinator in the Center for Behavioral Cardiovascular Health at Columbia University.

Cory F. Newman, PhD, ABPP, is Director of the Center for Cognitive Therapy and Associate Professor of Psychiatry at the hospital of the University of Pennsylvania School of Medicine. He is a Diplomate of the American Board of Professional Psychology and a Founding Fellow of the Academy of Cognitive Therapy. He is an international lecturer and has been a protocol therapist and supervisor on a number of large-scale randomized controlled trials. He has authored dozens of articles and chapters on cognitive therapy and has coauthored four books, including *Bipolar Disorder: A Cognitive Therapy Approach.*

Matthew K. Nock, PhD, is Assistant Professor and Director of the Laboratory for Clinical and Developmental Research in the Department of Psychology at Harvard University. He received his MS, MPhil, and PhD in psychology from Yale University. At Harvard, he teaches courses on statistics, clinical research methods, and self-injurious behaviors. His research focuses primarily on the etiology, assessment, and treatment of self-injurious and aggressive behaviors.

James L. Raper, DSN, CRNP, JD, is Associate Professor of Medicine at the University of Alabama at Birmingham School of Medicine. His research interests include psychosocial issues and behavioral interventions to promote secondary prevention of HIV in men who have sex with men and the treatment programs for substance abuse in HIV.

Robert Rosenthal, PhD, is Distinguished Professor at the University of California at Riverside and Edgar Pierce Professor of Psychology, Emeritus, at Harvard University. His research has centered on the role of the self-fulfilling prophecy in everyday life and in laboratory situations. He also has strong interests in sources of artifact in behavioral research and in various quantitative procedures. He has written extensively on these topics, as well as on experimental design and data analysis in many books and articles.

Ralph L. Rosnow, PhD, is Thaddeus Bolton Professor Emeritus at Temple University, where he taught in the Department of Psychology and headed the graduate program in social and organizational psychology. He has also taught at Boston University and Harvard University and was a visiting professor at the London School of Economics. His research has centered on how people make sense of their experiential world. His many books and articles have also examined methodological, statistical, and philosophical issues.

Bruce J. Rounsaville, MD, is Professor of Psychiatry at the Yale University School of Medicine and Director of the U.S. Veterans Administration New England Mental Illness Research Education and Clinical Center. Since he joined the Yale faculty, Dr. Rounsaville has focused his clinical research career on the diagnosis and treatment of patients with alcohol and drug dependence. He has contributed extensively to the psychiatric treatment research literature in more than 300 articles and 6 books.

Olle Jane Z. Sahler, MD, is Professor of Pediatrics, Psychiatry, Medical Humanities, and Oncology at the University of Rochester School of Medicine and Dentistry. She was the Principal Investigator of the Sibling Adaptation to Childhood Cancer epidemiological study (1987–1995), and since then has led the Psychosocial Adaptation to Childhood Cancer Research Collaboration, which has conducted a series of multisite randomized clinical trials of problem-solving skills training for mothers of newly diagnosed pediatric cancer patients.

Barbara Stanley, PhD, is Professor of Psychology at John Jay College of the City University of New York and Director of the Suicide Intervention Center at the New York State Psychiatric Institute at Columbia University College of Physicians and Surgeons. She is currently a member of an APA presidential task force on IRBs and social science research and editor in chief of the *Archives of Suicide Research*. She has written extensively on ethical issues in research, particularly competency of research participants, suicidal behavior, self-injury, aggressive behavior, and borderline personality disorder. She is the former Chair of the APA Research Ethics Committee and the founder of ARENA, the membership arm of PRIM&R, a national organization for promotion of ethical research practices.

Judith K. Stuhr, PhD, is a co-owner of Millennium Park Psychological Associates, LLC, which specializes in health psychology in downtown Chicago. She is affiliated with Rush University Medical Center, where she conducts an outpatient clinic in primary care and participates in training primary care residents. She earned her doctorate in clinical psychology from the University of Alabama and completed both her residency and fellowship in health psychology at Rush University Medical Center.

Kimberlee J. Trudeau, PhD, is Research Scientist at Inflexxion, Inc., in Newton, Massachusetts, where she designs and tests on-line health interventions. She was previously Administrator of the Cochrane Behavioral Medicine Field at Mount Sinai School of Medicine. She was trained in social psychology specializing in health-related research. Her doctoral work was on the promotion of patient empathy as part of nursing education.

Michael T. Weaver, PhD, RN, FAAN, is Professor and Senior Scientist in the University of Alabama at Birmingham School of Nursing. His research focuses on health promotion in various populations (e.g., cardiovascular, family). In examining psychosocial variables, he applies various statistical analyses, including those that allow individualized estimation of across-time changes to examine trajectories of change in these populations.

Michelle M. Wedig is a doctoral candidate in the Department of Psychology at Harvard University. She received her BS from Tufts University and subsequently worked in the Psychiatric Neuroimaging Research Program at Massachusetts General Hospital. At Harvard, her primary research focus is on difficulties in emotion regulation and the role this plays in self-injurious behaviors. Additional areas of interest include the definition, assessment, function, and treatment of all intentional self-injurious behaviors.

Thomas A. Widiger, PhD, is Professor of Psychology at the University of Kentucky. He is currently Associate Editor for the *Journal of Abnormal Psychology, Journal of Personality and Social Psychology, Annual Review of Clinical Psychology,* and *Journal of Personality Disorders.* He has published extensively in the areas of personality and personality disorder, both with respect to assessment and diagnosis.

Rand R. Wilcox, PhD, Professor of Psychology at the University of Southern California, has published 7 books and more than 250 articles, most of which address statistical issues. His primary research interests deal with robust inferential methods, which cover such topics as ANOVA, regression, rank-based methods, and multivariate techniques, including outlier detection methods. He is an Associate Editor of *Computational Statistics and Data Analysis, Communications in*

Statistics, and *Psychometrika* and serves on the editorial board of four other journals. He is the recipient of the T. L. Saaty Award.

Dawn T. Yoshioka is a graduate student in the experimental psychopathology program at the University of Hawaii at Manoa. Her areas of interest include research, neuropsychology, assessment, integrated health care, and cultural issues in psychology.

SECTION I

CONCEPTUAL ISSUES

1. The "Devil Is in the Details"

Recognizing and Dealing With Threats to

Validity in Randomized Controlled Trials

Arthur M. Nezu and Christine Maguth Nezu

During the past half century, the randomized controlled trial (RCT) has come to represent the "gold standard" method for evaluating the efficacy of a psychosocial intervention (see Table 1.1 for a brief history of the RCT). The purpose of this chapter is to delineate an important set of principles related to the valid conduct of the RCT, that is, minimizing threats to validity. We view such principles as providing a conceptual framework within which a researcher can ultimately develop a sound outcome investigation. By adequately recognizing and understanding those factors that can limit the validity of one's inferences and conclusions, the outcome researcher is better prepared to think of conceptual, methodological, statistical, ethical, and practical issues that help to overcome such threats. At the end of the day, we all want consumers of our research, whether journal or grant reviewers, clinicians or other researchers, and especially our patients, to feel confident that our conclusions are sound, reasonable, and based on the best science available to us. By minimizing the influence of such threats, we can get closer to such a goal.

■ Threats to Validity

A major objective of an RCT is to provide reliable and valid evidence that a given treatment had a given effect. Sample statements reflecting such a goal might include the following: Treatment A "caused" a decrease in depressive symptoms; Treatment B "caused" an increase in self-reported self-confidence; a patient's gender moderated (i.e., "caused" a differential effect regarding) the efficacy of Treatment C; and Treatment D "caused" a decrease in anxiety symptoms because it initially "caused" an increase in patients' ability to tolerate frustration and worry, which led to (i.e., "caused") a decrease in anxiety. In other

3

TABLE 1.1
Early History of the Randomized Controlled Trial

- According to Streiner (as reported in Tansella, 2002), the "first" RCT was described in the biblical book of Daniel (1:11–20), whereby two groups of people (i.e., Jews and Babylonians) were evaluated with regard to the effects of two 10-day diets (note that randomization did not actually occur).
- The first instance of random allocation of patients to experimental and control conditions is believed to have been conducted by James Lind, a naval surgeon, in Edinburgh in 1747 (Tansella, 2002). The basic research question asked was whether the consumption of lemons and oranges prevented the development of scurvy.
- It is believed that the use of a placebo control was first applied in 1954 by a professor of anesthesia at Harvard—H. K. Beecher, who previously observed during World War II that distilled water was very effective in the treatment of pain and shock when morphine was unavailable (Tansella, 2002).
- The origin of the RCT in medicine is generally attributed in the literature to A. B. Hill, a professor of biostatistics, who chaired the 1948 Medical Research Council trial evaluating the use of streptomycin for the treatment of pulmonary tuberculosis, although other examples can be found to predate Hill's pioneering work, setting the stage for such groundbreaking studies to be conducted (Doll, 1998; Tansella, 2002; Vandenbroucke, 1987).
- The first controlled clinical trial in psychiatry was published by Davies and Shepherd (1955) in the *Lancet*. They described a double-blind investigation comparing reserpine with placebo in the treatment of 54 patients suffering from anxiety and depression.
- The continued spread of RCT usage since then appeared to be largely a function of peer pressure within the field of medicine. According to Vandenbroucke (1987), physicians in favor of controlled trials "wanted comparability of treatment groups, for which they preferred some form of stratified randomization. Peer pressure was used to challenge claims of benefits of treatment which were not validated by comparisons with some form of control group" (p. 987).
- The use of statistical approaches to help interpret results from RCTs can be traced back to Sir Ronald Fisher of England, who literally split plots of land in order to (statistically) analyze the differential effects of various fertilizers (hence the birth of the nomenclature of a "split-plot" design").
- William Gosset, a statistician working in Ireland for the Guinness brewery, applied his statistical knowledge both in the brewery and on the farm regarding the selection of the best yielding varieties of barley. With the help of Karl Pearson (of Pearson's *r* fame) and Fisher, Gosset published several statistical papers in the early 1900s. Because the brewery prohibited employees from publishing, he used the pseudonym "Student" (hence, Student's *t* test).
- The first application of statistics in a treatment context can be attributed to William Cobbett (Tansella, 2002). Cobbett, a farmer, politician, and journalist, in calculating the mortality rate in Philadelphia in 1800, argued that the treatment of yellow fever by bloodletting and purgatives was not only ineffective but likely quite dangerous.

words, RCTs should be able to help us determine the presence and strength of a causal relationship between a given treatment and a given outcome.

What is a causal relationship? The philosopher John Stuart Mill provides a very useful answer in his treatise entitled *A System of Logic* (1859). As Shadish, Cook, and Campbell (2002) note, Mill's explication indicated that "a causal relationship exists if (1) the cause preceded the effect, (2) the cause was related to the effect, and (3) we can find no plausible alternative explanation for the effect other than the cause" (p. 6). In essence, RCTs should be designed to set the stage for ensuring that each of these three characteristics is present in order to be able to make valid conclusions based on the resulting findings.

The first condition appears rather easy to demonstrate (although it can be deceptive unless one addresses the issue of a given research participant's prior treatment history), whereas for the second two, it is a bit more difficult to ensure that they are being met. As such, the principal investigator (PI) of a given RCT needs to extend his or her efforts toward developing a protocol that allows one to state with confidence that any conclusions cited are based on meeting these three causal assumptions. For the remainder of this chapter, we describe a set of challenges or obstacles to achieving this goal that a PI is always confronted with when designing and implementing an RCT—that is, "threats to validity."

Types of Validity and Their Threats

Validity, with regard to an RCT, involves the degree to which one's conclusions are sound, correct, or veridical with regard to causal statements such as those noted earlier. Campbell (1957) first made a distinction between *internal validity* and *external validity* regarding experimental investigations in general, defining the former as whether a given stimulus made a significant difference in a given situation, and the latter as the degree to which such an effect can be generalized to other populations, settings, and variables (see also Campbell & Stanley, 1963). Cook and Campbell (1979) extended these concepts to include two additional types of validity—*statistical conclusion validity,* which focuses on the appropriate use of various statistical analytic procedures to determine the actual covarying relationship between a given *independent variable* (IV) and a given *dependent variable* (DV), and *construct validity,* which addresses the generalizability of a given operational definition to a cause-effect construct. More important, these authors (see also Shadish et al., 2002) identified specific concerns that serve to threaten or limit the strength or soundness of one's inference or interpretation of a given cause-and-effect statement. As such, knowledge of these threats helps the PI to develop an RCT in such a way as to minimize the influence of such limitations in order to increase the validity of the overall investigation.

In teaching graduate students these threats, we often make the point that even though a good understanding of the basic principles underlying the concepts of the various forms of validity, as well as their threats, can substantially foster the methodological soundness of a particular treatment study, it is especially important to remember that "the devil is in the details." In other words, the actual application and implementation of these principles often involves substantially more thought than "we need to include a control group and randomly assign patients." Increasingly complex questions are being asked by psychotherapy researchers, and the task of designing methodologically sound studies is becoming increasingly more difficult and sophisticated. In applying such principles, the need to address a plethora of details is imperative. Given this context, the remaining chapters in this volume are geared to teach the reader how to address such details when applying these principles across varying research questions and settings.

Internal Validity

With regard to outcome studies, this form of validity refers to the types of inferences or conclusions one can make regarding the degree to which a given treatment condition actually had a given effect. Shadish et al. (2002) identify the following as areas in which a threat to internal validity can emerge: temporal precedence, participant selection, history, maturation, statistical regression, participant attrition, and assessment (testing and instrumentation). It should be noted that not only can each serve individually as a threat, but that at times, such threats can be additive or interactive.

TEMPORAL PRECEDENCE

As noted earlier, the first condition that needs to be met in terms of establishing a causal relationship involves temporal precedence, in other words, the cause (e.g., psychotherapy) needs to occur *prior* to the effect (e.g., outcome). At first glance, this appears to be an irrelevant concern with regard to this threat's impact on the directionality of psychotherapy outcome—of course, the outcome always is measured *after* the treatment is implemented. However, consider the situation where the PI is interested in assessing the effects of stress management training on reducing symptoms of fibromyalgia. One concern, in order to address this threat, would involve better assessing a given participant's *previous* experience with stress management training. Having participated in such a treatment regimen 15 years prior for test anxiety during college may have little impact on the present RCT. However, unless this PI has an exclusion criteria of the presence of *recent* stress management training (or psychotherapy in general depending on the specific research questions being asked) for treating the fibromyalgia, it is possible that latent effects of the prior therapy involvement may have led to reduced symptoms, which actually *precede* the current RCT.

SELECTION

This threat to internal validity involves the existence of significant and systematic differences between groups in the RCT *before* treatment begins. Having prior differences exist between experimental groups regarding various participant characteristics (e.g., gender, age, socioeconomic status, ethnicity) can "muddy the waters" with regard to valid interpretations of cause-effect relationships concerning the impact of treatment. For example, consider an RCT where the PI is interested in evaluating the effects of a new psychosocial intervention for training spousal caregivers of cancer patients in coping skills. The effects of this new therapy approach is slated to be compared with a waiting-list control (WLC) condition. In addition, as is often the case, more than one research site is required in order to maximize statistical power (i.e., increase the sample size). If the PI inadvertently, due to convenience's sake, chooses to conduct the therapy at Hospital A and has the control condition at Hospital B, then he or she is not adequately controlling for this particular threat. In other words, at the end of the study, if the treated participants are found to cope better than the WLC individuals, the conclusion that this PI has identified an effective intervention is compromised due to the interference of potential *preexisting* differences between Hospitals A and B. Such divarications might involve substantial differences in socioeconomic status, leading to possible preexisting differences regarding health knowledge, as well as financial and personal resources. Whereas random assignment to condition is considered a crucially important ingredient in any RCT for a variety of reasons, its use in this case especially reduces the potential negative impact of this threat to validity.

HISTORY

This refers to any event, other than the differing treatment conditions, that occurs in or out of the study and that provides for a reasonable alternative explanation of why a given treatment worked or did not work. For example, in an RCT addressing the efficacy of an intervention for the treatment of test anxiety, such an event might involve the occurrence of final exams. Consider the situation where treated subjects are provided therapy during a time period that includes such tests, whereas the wait-list control participants are evaluated pre-post fashion *after* such an event. If the actual results indicate no difference at posttreatment between the experimental and control conditions, one explanation that can be invoked suggests that the treatment under investigation is actually not effective.

However, because a significant historical event was not controlled for, it is also possible that treated subjects experienced a major upsurge in anxiety as a function of taking final exams and, therefore, led to poorer outcome than if the study had been conducted at another time.

Controlling for this threat to validity suggests either that the experience of all participants needs to be as similar as possible, whether internal (e.g., inadvertent hospital strike) or external (e.g., severe weather storm) to the study, or that the research design or subsequent statistical analysis is able to actually separate out such differences.

MATURATION

This threat to internal validity involves the potential problem whereby various processes that are *internal* to study participants, similar to problems due to history, can lead to problems in separating out alternative interpretations of the results of the RCT. Such processes occur over time, are not the focus of the study, and can include natural growth or deterioration concerning such factors as age, intelligence, physical strength, or interest in continuing to participate in the outcome investigation. Consider the RCT where the PI is interested in evaluating a program that teaches adopted children aged 5 to 10 years old coping skills to order to enhance adaptation to the adopting family and situation. If at the end of a 10-week program, a group of children are found to be happier, less anxious, and receiving better reports from their teachers at school, it is certainly possible that the intervention was an efficacious one. However, besides not having a baseline condition against which to compare such changes, it is highly possible that, over time, such changes occur naturally for the children without the aid of a formal program.

Whereas controlling for concerns due to maturational issues involves consideration of a multitude of factors (e.g., homogeneity among participants regarding age, intellectual level), it particularly invokes the need to have adequate control groups to minimize this threat to internal validity.

REGRESSION TO THE MEAN

This refers to the general tendency for someone who receives an extreme score (either very high or very low) on a measure at a given testing to receive a score on a subsequent testing that is closer to the distribution mean. In other words, the second score is less extreme. If this threat is not accounted for, then reductions in high scores (e.g., high depression scores) or improvements in low scores from baseline to posttreatment cannot necessarily be interpreted as a direct impact of efficacious treatment. Rather, such changes can simply be due to statistical regression. In addition, the practice of depending solely on psychometric assessments to identify psychopathology, such as high scores on a self-report measure of anxiety, may also be questionable, because such scores may hypothetically regress toward the mean and no longer be in the range of the desired cutoff criterion. For example, in a previous study we conducted (Nezu & Perri, 1989) with clinically depressed adults, a high score on a self-report measure of depression was used to identify an initial pool of depressed individuals. However, due to this regression threat (as well as the variability of depression scores per se), a second testing 2 weeks later was also administered. Only those individuals who *continued* to report high levels of depressive symptomatology at this second point were asked to undergo a formal diagnostic assessment interview.

Adequately addressing this threat also entails choosing dependent measures that are represented by adequate to high levels of test–retest reliability, as well as including adequate control groups (e.g., no-treatment control at a minimum) to be able to parse out the effects due to treatment versus the effects due to regression (i.e., changes in the DVs over time for treated individuals should be significantly greater than for those in the control group that may be related to the regression effect).

ATTRITION

This issue involves significant or differential loss of participants over time. According to Kazdin (2003), large numbers of individuals tend to drop out of therapy at an early stage of treatment, indicating that PIs of RCTs are potentially likely to experience substantial attrition. People leave a treatment study for a variety of reasons—travel difficulties, lack of progress, change of job, boredom, death, and disappointment with the study. Even if such dropout rates are similar across experimental and control conditions, if the overall dropout rate is high, then the issue of potential differences between those who stayed and those who left can emerge. For example, it is possible that the participants who left a study were, in fact, more severely impaired, and therefore dropped out of the study due to lack of substantial immediate treatment gains. As such, those who stayed are not likely to be equivalent to the initially recruited sample of patients. Moreover, even if the baseline–posttreatment changes on various dependent measures are large, it is possible that the treatment has such an effect only for mildly impaired individuals, rather than for the entire diagnostic category under study.

Differential attrition across conditions serves to undermine the PI's ability to validly interpret the results of an RCT. Perhaps larger numbers of individuals in one treatment condition left before the study ended as a result of boredom, higher potential for negative iatrogenic effects, or higher costs, rendering any differences between the effects of the two treatment conditions identified difficult to interpret. As such, a significant responsibility of the PI prior to implementing an RCT is to predict the likely impact that various treatment and control conditions might have on attrition rates. For example, if the individual who is suffering significantly is randomly assigned to a no-treatment control condition, it is possible that he or she may opt out early (i.e., not to complete the posttreatment assessment protocol) in order to seek treatment elsewhere. Therefore, choice and design of appropriate control conditions can impact across a variety of threat issues (e.g., history, maturation), including the one involving participant attrition.

TESTING AND INSTRUMENTATION

This class of threats involves the potential inadvertent unwanted effects due to collecting data from study participants. Testing threats refer to whether the simple act of taking a test can impact subsequent performance on a second (or third) administration of the same test. For example, in most RCTs, pre-post measurement is routinely conducted. However, any changes that occur from the first to the second administration may be a function of an efficacious treatment protocol; however, they can also be the result of practice effects or familiarity with the testing procedure. Various major tests have been developed to include alternative forms in order to prevent practice effects. Psychotherapy researchers should consider using such measures if concerns about testing effects arise. In addition, the inclusion of a control condition (e.g., no-treatment control at a minimum) that separates the influence of treatment versus testing becomes imperative to guard against this threat to internal validity.

Measuring instruments or procedures can also change over time. Various psychophysiological measurement systems, for example, may need to be recalibrated (i.e., brought back to baseline) after each use in order to be reliable across assessment points. Individuals who collect data from study participants can also change over time (e.g., become more competent with practice or more bored across multiple assignments). Actual changes in participants' scores on a dependent variable may be more a function of such instrumentation threats, rather than the effects of a given therapeutic procedure. Kazdin (2003) further points to the issue of changing response shifts among subjects, which are changes in a person's internal standards of measurement. For example, although a given testing protocol may remain exactly the same, a given participant may react to it differently as a function of such response shifts (e.g., change in values, perspectives, attitudes) that may or may not be directly related to the intended effects of treatment.

Collectively, these threats require the PI to be vigilant not only with regard to initial choices of the dependent variables but also in terms of how these measures may or may not be reliably administered to, and interpreted by, study participants.

External Validity

External validity focuses on the types of interpretations related to the extent to which the results of an RCT can be generalized beyond the conditions of the specific study to other individuals, settings, and outcomes. The process and duration of such generalization can be very diverse, including generalizing from the specifics of a given study to larger populations, from the experimental group to a single person, from one variable to another at a similar level, as well as to differing groups, and to the universal population of interest (Shadish et al., 2002). Important threats to external validity to control for in clinical investigations include sample characteristics, setting characteristics, and effects due to testing (see also Kazdin, 2003).

SAMPLE CHARACTERISTICS

This issue entails the degree to which one is able to generalize from the sample included in a given RCT to other individuals who vary across certain demographic characteristics, such as age, sexual identity, gender, ethnic background, and socioeconomic background. A major goal of an RCT is to produce evidence that can provide for statements that are more representative of general principles (e.g., Treatment X reliably reduces anxiety symptoms for adults), rather than being specific only to a given RCT (e.g., where it was conducted, who specifically served as participants, therapists, assessors, recruiters). As such, research personnel and patient participants should not be highly unique such that one is unable to generalize to other patients, therapists, and so forth (unless that is the specific research question being asked). Neither should they be significantly different than the group to which one wishes to generalize. An example of the former involves including only therapists who have 30 or more years of experience, whereas an instance of the latter is to focus on treating depression among a college student sample (out of convenience) when one is really interested in generalizing to the "universe of clinically depressed adults."

The need to adequately control for this threat to external validity can also be seen in the formal policy statement of the National Institutes of Health (NIH) with regard to the inclusion of women and minorities as subjects in clinical research (NIH, 2001). Specifically, NIH requires that women and members of minority groups be included in all NIH-funded clinical research, unless a clear and compelling rationale justifies that such inclusion is inappropriate with regard to the health of the study participants or the purpose of the research (e.g., the research focuses exclusively on heart disease among men). In other words, in order to be able to adequately generalize to relevant populations (e.g., adults), the PI needs to be inclusive across gender and ethnicity.

SETTING CHARACTERISTICS

This issue addresses one's ability to generalize beyond the specific aspects or stimuli of a given investigation. Such factors can include the physical setting, research personnel, therapists, and assessors. A significant discrepancy regarding such characteristics, for example, between the "laboratory-like" setting in a large university–based medical school setting as compared with a "real-life" clinic, potentially limits the external validity of the RCT. When one is concerned about external validity issues, it becomes important to consider how all elements of the investigation can potentially deviate from those characteristics that one uses to generalize in order to then modify them. For example, it is important to conduct the RCT in a physical environment that is perceived as reasonably professional, no more (e.g., a very expensive setting) and no less (e.g., a "dirty" basement area).

EFFECTS DUE TO TESTING

An inherent component of an RCT is multiple assessments, both across conditions and over time. One threat to external validity involves the potential for study participants to react differently than they otherwise would as a function of knowing that they are being assessed. This may manifest itself in particular with regard to self-report biases (e.g., putting oneself in a more favorable light). As such, the PI may need to consider including multiple measures of a given construct (e.g., depression) that are less obtrusive and reactive, for example, ratings by collaterals (e.g., spousal ratings of depressive behavior).

Another threat to external validity involving assessment issues concerns *pretest sensitization*, which is the possibility that an individual may respond differentially to subsequent treatment (e.g., more amenable) as a function of the administration of baseline testing (Kazdin, 2003). If somehow pretesting can affect subsequent reactions to a psychosocial intervention, one's ability to generalize outside of the RCT where individuals are usually *not* pretested becomes limited. Therefore, choices regarding individual DVs, as well as the design of the overall assessment protocol, should take such concerns into consideration.

A final threat to external validity regarding assessment issues involves the actual timing of the testing. One temporal dimension in outcome research that becomes of potential concern involves the length of time between posttreatment and follow-up evaluations. Often tradition suggests including either a 3-month or 6-month follow-up testing point. However, depending on several factors (e.g., normal fluctuations in a given behavior or disorder, presence of a lengthy cumulative impact), the possibility exists that had testing occurred at 4 months, for example, rather than at 3 months, results might have been substantially different. A second temporal dimension involves the time of day (or day of the week) of a given test administration. It is unlikely that the average PI would schedule testing sessions at 4:00 A.M., which would obviously impact on the generalizability of the responses, but if a given target problem or disorder can fluctuate over the course of a day (e.g., glucose levels), for example, the PI needs to be aware that timing of testing is one of those "devil-like details" to be concerned about.

Construct Validity

This type of validity focuses on the ability to infer or generalize from specific aspects of a given investigation to the higher order constructs of interest. In other words, do the operational definitions (e.g., self-report measure) of a given construct (e.g., depression) truly represent that construct? According to Shadish et al. (2002), some important threats to construct validity entail the following: inadequate explication of constructs, confounding constructs, single definitions, participant reactivity, experimenter expectancies, and treatment diffusion.

INADEQUATE EXPLICATION OF CONSTRUCTS

This issue focuses on the situation in which the construct of interest is not adequately described or detailed operationally. For example, a typical operational definition of a given intervention is a detailed therapy manual. If the manual does not adequately contain all the important ingredients (or actually contains elements *not* considered conceptually as part of the therapy under investigation), then it may inadvertently limit one's ability to generalize to the construct that the given treatment is supposed to represent. This concern is unrelated to outcome—in other words, the treatment could produce significant reductions in the hypothesized targets. However, the issue is whether one can validly claim that it was the treatment that was responsible for the outcome. A common example is the inappropriate use of the term *cognitive-behavioral therapy* (CBT). Perusal of the outcome literature indicates, for instance, that CBT in one study can specifically refer to the use of cognitive restructuring and behavioral activation to treat depression, whereas in another RCT, it might refer to a combined package of exposure to a feared stimulus plus response prevention to treat a complex phobia. In this case, the construct "label" is identified at too general a level (i.e., it is better to refer to these interventions by their specific names) (see Mark, 2000).

This threat can also take the form of confusing a construct as a whole with varying levels of the construct. With regard to an RCT, it becomes important to ensure that the treatment under investigation actually represents the construct as originally conceptualized, rather than a "diluted" or partial form of that construct. For example, consider the situation where the PI is interested in evaluating the differential efficacy of Treatment A, which he or she developed, versus Treatment B, which is the current standard treatment. If Treatment B is implemented in a "less-than-optimal" manner (e.g., lower "dosage" than originally recommended), then the comparison is actually between nonequivalent conditions. If Treatment A fares better than Treatment B, the conclusion that Treatment B is less efficacious (as compared with "a truncated version of Treatment B is less efficacious") is flawed.

CONFOUNDING CONSTRUCTS

This threat is invoked when the PI inadvertently confuses constructs. For example, an investigator focusing on various ethnic minority populations may confuse the construct of "ethnicity" in interpreting results of a study with the construct of "socioeconomic status" (SES). In other words, a given minority group included in a study may represent more validly the construct of lower SES rather than one representing their ethnic background. This is not a simple matter of semantics—rather, the operational definition of the construct is inaccurately explained.

SINGULAR DEFINITIONS

This issue refers to the frequent use of only one operational definition of a construct under study, in terms of both the operation (i.e., mono-operation bias) and the method (monomethod bias). In the first case, the primary concern is that single-operation research limits one's ability to generalize to the overall construct of interest. For example, in the RCT where only one therapist is engaged to conduct the treatment of interest, the threat to construct validity comes in the form of being able to determine whether any effects (i.e., significant treatment gains or lack thereof) are generalizable to "therapists in general" or if the effects are due to the unique characteristics of the single therapist (e.g., extremely competent, highly charismatic). This suggests that it would be important to include multiple therapists conducting the same treatment as a means of enhancing construct validity.

The monomethod bias can occur if a given construct is defined only by a single method. An example would involve using only a self-report procedure to assess the construct of a particular disorder. In measuring anxiety, for instance, it would be important to include several different methods, beyond self-report, such as clinician ratings, behavior observed in simulated role-plays, physiological assessments, and evaluations provided by significant others.

PARTICIPANT REACTIVITY

This threat to construct validity involves multiple ways in which study participants can react to aspects of the RCT that are unintended and not part of the actual investigation. One example involves the reactions of individuals in control conditions if they respond to the idea of not being in the "favored" condition. Obviously, PIs need to adhere to ethical considerations regarding the overall informed consent procedure. As such, it is highly likely that a potential participant knows that, for example, "a fifty-fifty chance exists that you will be assigned to one of two experimental conditions, one of which involves meeting with a counselor for 10 one-hour weekly sessions. The second condition involves completing a series of inventories on two differing occasions that are separated by 10 weeks." Therefore, the control participant, after learning that he or she is in the condition that does not involve any treatment, may react negatively, feeling demoralized and disappointed, or respond more favorably, feeling motivated to get better on his or her own efforts, attempting to "compensate" for lack of treatment. In other words, the actual results obtained at posttreatment assessment may not necessarily reflect "no treatment"; rather, they may reflect changes due to reactions of the control subjects. This suggests that the choice of a control condition against which to compare the effects of treatment conditions is very important in terms of minimizing the threats to construct validity of such unwanted responses.

Another situation involving unintended participant reactions entails various demand characteristics of the investigation. Primary among these are expectations and increased motivation due to simply being in a treatment study. Such outcomes, if not controlled for, can limit construct validity because it is unknown whether a given treatment was efficacious (i.e., was due to the hypothesized "active treatment ingredients") or whether the significant improvement was due to the *placebo* effect. As such, the need to include adequate control groups becomes especially important to be able to parse out such effects, often referred to as *common* or *nonspecific* psychotherapy factors (e.g., simple contact with a therapist, belief that one will get better, being convinced by the treatment rationale, increased hope because one is about to receive treatment). The trick here is to ensure that any "attention-placebo" condition is constructed such that it is perceived by study participants as potentially valuable, rather than as the "less desirable" treatment group.

EXPERIMENTER EXPECTANCIES

This issue concerns the effects of an experimenter's unintentional biases. In most RCTs, it is likely that the PI has an a priori hypothesis, for example, that Treatment A will fare better than Treatment B. In describing the study, training the therapists, or debriefing study participants, such "biases" may be inadvertently conveyed. As such, differential subject responses may result, some in the form of being consistent with the hypothesis, whereas others can be in the opposite direction. Controlling for such expectancies might include such strategies as limiting contact between the PI and study patients, "blinding" research personnel as much as possible (e.g., assessors do not know which condition a given patient is assigned to), requesting all research personnel involved to be "on guard" in order to minimize the impact of such an influence, and including treatment integrity protocols to be able to assess the presence of such biases with regard to how the differing treatments are actually implemented.

TREATMENT DIFFUSION

This threat refers to the situation where various components of a given treatment can be accidentally provided to a control condition. This can easily occur when a new psychosocial treatment is being compared with "treatment as usual" (TAU), where the TAU condition involves meeting with various professionals. For example, consider the RCT where the PI is interested in evaluating the effects of a multicomponent stress management intervention for the treatment of cancer pain among oncology outpatients. It is typical that cancer patients see a variety of health professionals during their cancer treatment, including physicians, nurses, physical therapists, social work staff, and clergy. For both ethical and practical purposes, it is unreasonable to limit access to such clinical resources as a requirement for study participation. As a research strategy, the stress management protocol should be viewed as an addition to TAU, whereby the specific research question becomes, What is the efficacy of this stress management intervention in reducing cancer pain *above and beyond that related to TAU?*

Relevant to this discussion, further consider the "good intentions" of a particular health care provider who learns of an ongoing RCT, investigates and is impressed by the rationale of the included stress management procedures, and therefore decides to offer certain training exercises to individuals in the TAU condition unbeknownst to the PI and research staff. At the end of the clinical trial, it is possible that participants in *both* conditions improve significantly as a function of stress management training. In all likelihood, the PI is likely to be "scratching his or her head," not knowing why persons in the TAU condition actually got substantially much better than usual.

In consulting with PIs on conducting RCTs, we have additionally advised them to ensure that even the smallest potential for such threats needs to be identified. For example, it is not uncommon for patients to talk with each other in waiting rooms. Imagine the situation where a person in Treatment A stays a bit later than usual waiting for her spouse to pick her up and meets another patient, who is assigned to Treatment B, who comes to the waiting room several minutes early for her appointment. This can certainly lead to "diffusion of treatment" if they talk about their experiences and learn what types of services each other receives. As such, we advise PIs to even focus on such small details as appropriate appointment scheduling.

Statistical Conclusion Validity

This form of validity refers to those aspects of the quantitative evaluation that can affect the conclusions one reaches about the presence and strength of cause-effect relationships between treatment and outcome. Important threats to this type of validity can include low statistical power, family-wise error rates, unreliable measures, unreliability of treatment implementation, and subject heterogeneity (Shadish et al., 2002).

LOW STATISTICAL POWER

Statistical power is usually defined as the ability to detect an effect when, in fact, it does "truly exist in nature" (i.e., the probability that a test will reject the null hypothesis when it is false). Power varies as a function of the alpha level (i.e., Type I error rate), the number of participants included in a study, and the actual effect size. The convention of null hypothesis testing approaches to statistical analysis suggests that a minimal level of power should be set at .80 (i.e., 1—a Type II error rate, or β, of .20), whereas α is set at .05. Assuming that the alpha level remains constant (or no higher than .05), smaller effect sizes and/or lower numbers of subjects lead to lower levels of power. In part due to the low number of study participants across conditions, Kazdin and Bass (1989) found that most psychotherapy studies were represented by low power. More recently, Maxwell (2004) found that "underpowered" studies continued to be rampant in the psychological literature. Strategies to increase power include increasing sample size, increasing the strength of the contrast (i.e., include more robust treatments), varying the alpha level when appropriate, using one-tailed tests of significance if appropriate, and decreasing error within the study as much as possible by minimizing unwanted variability (Kazdin, 2003; see also Shadish et al., 2002).

FAMILY-WISE ERROR RATES

This threat involves the difference in alpha levels between single versus multiple analyses. For example, the probability of making a Type I error associated with a single test (i.e., .05) increases to .143 when conducting three separate tests. What becomes important when conducting statistical analyses is to control for the threat due to multiple analyses by using more conservative test procedures, such as the Bonferroni correction, whereby the conventional alpha criterion of .05 is divided by the number of tests conducted within a set (or family), and then this corrected alpha is used as the criterion in all individual tests.

UNRELIABLE MEASURES

If variables are assessed in an unreliable fashion, then inferences about their covariation can be inaccurate. Unreliability in general leads to attenuated associations between two variables, as well as increased variability, which can further lead to reduced power.

UNRELIABILITY OF TREATMENT IMPLEMENTATION

This threat occurs when a given treatment is variably implemented across differing participants (e.g., therapists conducting treatment differentially as a function of differing patients' age, gender, or ethnic background), settings (e.g., therapists at one site perform less effectively than at other study sites), or therapists (e.g., therapists become more competent over time with practice across the length of an RCT; they can also become bored and less attentive as time goes on). Effective selection, training, and supervision (peer or otherwise) of therapists may help attenuate this threat. Assessing therapists' competent adherence to the protocols across therapists, by including a formal treatment integrity system, can also help address this threat.

SUBJECT HETEROGENEITY

In general, the more homogeneous the study participants, the less will be the variability (i.e., standard deviations) regarding that factor. Subject heterogeneity can serve to hide the true nature of the relationship between treatment and outcome. Controlling for such concerns involves establishing appropriate inclusion and exclusion criteria to enhance the homogeneity of the participant sample, as well as using various blocking or matching strategies when randomly assigning to differing conditions. For example, with regard to the latter point, rather than relying exclusively on a random numbers table to assign individuals to two conditions and hope that they are equivalent with regard to gender makeup, it would be important to use a blocking strategy to minimize subject heterogeneity.

■ Summary

In this chapter, we defined four types of validity that are the foundation underlying our ability to make veridical inferences about our data from an RCT—internal validity, external validity, construct validity, and statistical conclusion validity. For each type, we further identified various threats that can limit the veracity of our inferences. Each threat represents a situation whereby, if not properly addressed, our confidence about making cause-effect statements can be attenuated. Table 1.2 provides a list of these threats as applied to RCTs, as well as a list of potential remedies. It should be underscored that such a list is not exhaustive; rather, the psychotherapy outcome researcher needs to put on his or her "empirically informed thinking cap" when devising and implementing an RCT in order to adequately overcome such threats, as each new study is likely to have unique challenges as new questions arise.

TABLE 1.2
Threats to Validity and Possible Solutions

Threat	Brief description of threat	Potential remedies
Internal validity		
Temporal precedence	Ambiguity regarding "which comes first."	• Exclude subjects with recent prior psychotherapy experience if relevant to current research question.
Selection	Existence of significant differences between groups prior to random selection.	• Carefully select subjects knowing their backgrounds. • Randomly assign to condition by blocking on relevant demographic characteristics (e.g., gender, age, ethnicity). • Statistically analyze impact of systematic prior differences.
History	Presence of an event that occurs during the course of the study that can provide for an alternative explanation of the results.	• Ensure that the experiences of all participants across conditions are equivalent during implementation of RCT. • Randomly assign participants to conditions. • Statistically analyze impact if event does occur.
Maturation	Presence of various "natural growth" processes internal to subjects that may be responsible for change.	• Select subjects carefully with this threat in mind. • Randomly assign participants to conditions. • Include adequate control conditions.

continued

TABLE 1.2 (*continued*)

Threat	Brief description of threat	Potential remedies
Regression to the mean	General tendency of extreme scores to regress to distribution mean.	• Ensure that all DVs have strong test-retest reliability. • Include multitrait-multimethod approach to screening and selecting subjects (i.e., do not rely on single measure to "diagnose" caseness). • Include adequate control groups.
Attrition	Significant and/or differential loss of participants over time.	• Foster motivation for continued participation. • Ensure that treatment condition(s) do not radically differ from control conditions regarding attrition-related factors (e.g., amount of attention provided to controls). • Consider alternative control condition instead of the "no-treatment" control.
Testing and instrumentation	Untoward effects emanating from assessment issues.	• Choose testing protocols that have minimal effects on subsequent performance. • Conduct quality-control checks on instruments (e.g., continued calibration) and assessment procedures (e.g., rater drift). • Include adequate control conditions to assess impact of testing.

External validity

Sample characteristics — Limited ability to generalize to other individuals.

- Ensure that study sample includes adequate representation across important subject characteristics (e.g., gender, SES, ethnicity, comorbidity).

Setting characteristics — Limited ability to generalize to other settings.

- Ensure that all aspects of the study (e.g., physical setting, therapists, research assistants) represent "universal" variables of interest.

Testing effects — Reactions of participants due to (a) awareness that they are being tested, (b) pretest sensitization, or (c) timing of testing.

- Include additional measures beyond self-report inventories to control for self-report biases.
- Consider using unobtrusive measures.
- Time assessments in clinically meaningful ways (e.g., length of follow-up should be based on understanding of course of disease rather than convenience).

Construct validity

Inadequate explication of constructs — Constructs of interest are not operationally defined well or adequately.

- Be specific in describing all constructs (e.g., avoid jargon and ambiguous labels).
- Ensure that all operational definitions of constructs adequately represent the entire construct of interest.

Confounding constructs — Constructs are confused with others.

- Ensure that the construct of interest truly is the correct construct that you want to investigate.

continued

TABLE 1.2 (*continued*)

Threat	Brief description of threat	Potential remedies
Singular definitions	Using only one operation or method to define a construct.	• Use multitrait–multimethod approach when operationally defining all constructs (e.g., use more than one therapist).
Participant reactivity	Unwanted reactions of subjects.	• Choose control groups that will minimize this threat (e.g., a no-treatment control can lead to subject demoralization or compensation). • Include adequate attention-placebo control conditions that are likely to be perceived as potentially effective. • Include "manipulation checks" to assess whether participants across conditions rated the conditions (and therapists) equivalently.
Experimenter expectancies	Effects of an experimenter's unintentional biases.	• "Blind" all research personnel as much as ethically possible. • Request that all research personnel be "on guard." • Include treatment integrity protocol to analyze such effects.
Treatment diffusion	Aspects of one condition are inadvertently provided to a control or other condition.	• Use different therapists to implement differing conditions. • "Blind" all assessors, research personnel, etc., as much as possible to study hypotheses.

Statistical conclusion validity

		• Conduct treatment integrity assessment to evaluate the presence of this threat. • Keep subjects in differing conditions separate.
Low statistical power	Low power limits one's ability to detect differences when they do exist.	• Have adequate number of subjects. • Include robust treatments. • Decrease variability in implementing RCT.
Family-wise error	Conducting multiple statistical tests.	• Be conservative in the number of tests conducted. • Use Bonferroni correction when conducting multiple tests.
Unreliable measures	Use of unreliable assessment procedures and tests.	• Only use reliable tests; strong test-retest reliability is important for repeated measures assessments.
Unreliability of treatment implementation	RCT is variably implemented across subjects, conditions, or settings.	• Select, train, and supervise therapists, assessors, and research assistants with goal of ensuring consistent and reliable performance. • Use detailed but flexible training, therapy, and assessment manuals as guides. • Include treatment integrity protocol as major guide to guard against this threat.
Subject heterogeneity	Increased heterogeneity leads to increased unwanted variability.	• Delineate and adhere to appropriate inclusion and exclusion criteria regarding subject selection. • Randomly assign to conditions using methods (e.g., blocking) that adequately distribute variability across conditions.

■ References

Campbell, D. T. (1957). Factors relevant to the validity of experiments in social settings. *Psychological Bulletin, 54,* 297–312.

Campbell, D. T., & Stanley, J. C. (1963). *Experimental and quasi-experimental designs for research.* Chicago: Rand McNally.

Cook, T. T., & Campbell, D. T. (1979). *Quasi-experimentation: Design and analysis issues for field settings.* Chicago: Rand McNally.

Davies, D. L., & Shepherd, M. (1955). Reserpine in the treatment of anxious and depressed patients. *Lancet, 266,* 117–120.

Doll, R. (1998). Controlled trials: The 1948 watershed. *British Medical Journal, 317,* 1217–1220.

Kazdin, A. E. (2003). *Research designs in clinical psychology* (4th ed.). Boston: Allyn & Bacon.

Kazdin, A. E., & Bass, D. (1989). Power to detect differences between alternative treatments in comparative psychotherapy outcome research. *Journal of Consulting and Clinical Psychology, 57,* 138–147.

Mark, M. M. (2000). Realism, validity, and the experimenting society. In L. Bickman (ed.), *Validity and social experimentation: Donald Campbell's legacy* (Vol. 1, pp. 141–166). Thousand Oaks, CA: Sage.

Maxwell, S. E. (2004). The persistence of underpowered studies in psychological research: Causes, consequences, and remedies. *Psychological Methods, 9,* 147–163.

National Institutes of Health. (2001). *NIH policy and guidelines on the inclusion of women and minorities as subjects in clinical research—amended, October, 2001.* Retrieved January 19, 2007, from http://grants.nih. Gov/grants/funding/women_min/women_min.htm

Nezu, A. M., & Perri, M. G. (1989). Problem-solving therapy for unipolar depression: An initial dismantling investigation. *Journal of Consulting and Clinical Psychology, 57,* 408–413.

Shadish, W. R., Cook, T. D., & Campbell, D. T. (2002). *Experimental and quasi-experimental designs for generalized causal inference.* Boston: Houghton Mifflin.

Tansella, M. (2002). The scientific evaluation of mental health treatments: An historical perspective. *Evidence-Based Mental Health, 5,* 4–5.

Vandenbroucke, J. P. (1987). A short note on the history of the randomized controlled trial. *Journal of Chronic Disease, 40,* 985–987.

2. Explanation of the CONSORT Statement With Application to Psychosocial Interventions

Kimberlee J. Trudeau, Elizabeth Mostofsky, Judith K. Stuhr, and Karina W. Davidson

The acronym CONSORT stands for Consolidated Standards of Reporting Trials. Just as the randomized controlled trial (RCT) is the gold standard in research methodology for testing the efficacy of a treatment, the CONSORT Statement is recognized as the gold standard of RCT reporting in medicine. More than 70 journal editors endorsed it internationally by 1997 (Moher, 1998)—and almost 200 editors by 2005, including editors of psychology journals such as *Health Psychology* and *Journal of Pediatric Psychology*. In addition, the American Psychological Association's Publications and Communications Board adopted the principles of the CONSORT guidelines in April 2003 and now requires relevant journals (e.g., *Journal of Consulting and Clinical Psychology*) to use such guidelines (Dittman, 2004). Despite this widespread endorsement, a review of author guidelines for 167 top medical journals indicated that only 16% of these journals referred authors to the most recent CONSORT guidelines. Therefore, authors should check the CONSORT Web site (http://www.consort-statement.org) for the most up-to-date information on CONSORT when reporting a clinical trial (Altman for the CONSORT Group, 2005).

Although CONSORT was originally developed to aid researchers in reporting RCTs clearly and comprehensively, it can also be a helpful tool in the design and conduct of RCTs (Altman, 1996). In this chapter, we describe the history of CONSORT, its application to psychological intervention research using a specific example, and how it has evolved based on feedback. A table of additional methodological checklists (e.g., CLEAR NPT for evaluating quality of nonpharmacological trials; Boutron et al., 2005) and resources (RE-AIM Framework for evaluating effectiveness of trials; Glasgow, Vogt, & Boles, 1999) that may be useful in psychological intervention research is included as Table 2.1.

TABLE 2.1
Additional Methodological Checklists in Alphabetical Order

Acronym	Name	Author	Citation	Web site (if available)
CHERRIES	**Che**cklist for **Re**porting **R**esults of Internet **E**-Surveys	Eysenbach G.	J Med Internet Res. 2004 Sep 29;6(3):e34.	None known
CLEAR NPT	Checklist to assess quality of RCT of **N**onpharma-cological **T**reatment	Boutron I, Moher D, Tugwell P, Giraudeau B, Poiraudeau S, Nizard R, Ravaud P.	J Clin Epidemiol. 2005 Dec;58 (12):1233–40. Epub 2005 Oct 13.	None known
MOOSE	**M**eta-analysis **O**f **O**bservational **S**tudies in **E**pidemiology	Stroup DF, Berlin JA, Morton SC, Olkin I, Williamson GD, Rennie D, Moher D, Becker BJ, Sipe TA, Thacker SB.	JAMA 2000 Apr 19;283(15): 2008–2012.	Stroup et al. (2000) article can be found at www.consort-statement.org/ Initiatives/ MOOSE/moose. .pdf
QUOROM	**Qu**ality **o**f **R**eporting **o**f **M**eta-analyses	Moher D, Cook DJ, Eastwood S, Olkin I, Rennie D, Stroup DF.	Lancet 1999 Nov 27;354 (9193): 1896–1900.	http://www .consort-statement.org/ QUOROM.pdf
RE-AIM	**R**each, **E**fficacy/ Effectiveness, **A**doption, **I**mplemen-tation, **M**aintenance	Glasgow RE, Vogt TM, Boles SM.	Am J Public Health 1999 Sep;89(9): 1322–1327.	http://www. re-aim.org/ 2003/ck_ccs.html
STARD	**STA**ndards for **R**eporting of **D**iagnostic Accuracy	Bossuyt PM, Reitsma JB, Bruns DE, Gatsonis CA, Glasziou PP, Irwig LM,	Clin Chem. 2003 Jan; 49(1):7–18.	http://www. consort-statement .org/newstard.htm

continued

TABLE 2.1 (*continued*)

Acronym	Name	Author	Citation	Web site (if available)
		Moher D, Rennie D, de Vet HC, Lijmer JG; Standards for Reporting of Diagnostic Accuracy.		
STROBE	**ST**rength-ening the **R**eporting of **OB**ser-vational studies in **E**pidemiology	Erik von Elm MD MSc et al.	None known	http://www. strobe-statement .org/
TREND	**T**ransparent **R**eporting of **E**valuations with **N**onran-domized **D**esigns	Des Jarlais DC, Lyles C, Crepaz N; TREND Group.	Am J Public Health 2004 Mar;94(3): 361–366.	www .trend-statement .org
Not applicable	Not applicable. Article title: "A scale for rating the quality of psychological trials for pain"	Yatres, SL, Morley, S, Eccleston C, de C Williams AC	Pain 2005 Oct;117(3): 314–321.	None known

■ History of CONSORT

Systematic evaluations of RCTs conducted in the middle to late 1980s indicated that the reporting of RCTs was problematic (Altman & Doré, 1990; Pocock, Hughes, & Lee, 1987), thus limiting their benefit to science and society (Free-mantle, Mason, Haines, & Eccles, 1997). Therefore, a group of 30 researchers with experience in scale design and RCTs convened in Ottawa, Ontario, to cre-ate a scale to evaluate the quality of RCTs. This Standards of Reporting Trials (SORT) group met in October 1993 and produced a list of items for reporting RCTs (SORT Group, 1994).

Five months later, in March 1994, another group, the Asilomar Working Group on Recommendations for Reporting of Clinical Trials in Biomedical Literature (1994), created guidelines for journal editors to include in the Instructions to Authors for future manuscript submissions. These recommendations were published in *Annals of Internal Medicine* in 1994.

In 1995, Drummond Rennie wrote an editorial in the *Journal of the American Medical Association (JAMA)*, recommending that these groups work together to combine their recommendations in one list. The merged group, now known as the CONSORT Group, was composed of nine members, including editors, clinical epidemiologists, and statisticians. The group convened in September 1995 in Chicago, Illinois, and composed the CONSORT Statement, which was published in *JAMA* in August 1996 (Begg et al., 1996).

■ Application of CONSORT to a Psychology RCT

The Consolidated Standards for Reporting Trials (CONSORT) Statement includes 22 items that aid in the transparent reporting of psychological research. The use of these items is demonstrated here by applying them to Dr. Judith Stuhr's dissertation research (2004) on anger intervention in hypertensive patients. In this study, Stuhr examined the efficacy of a group anger intervention for increasing the use of a constructive type of anger management (Constructive Anger Behavior–Verbal; CAB-V; Davidson, MacGregor, Stuhr, Dixon, et al., 2000; Davidson, MacGregor, Stuhr, & Gidron, 1999; Stuhr, 1999) in patients with hypertension, using a randomized, wait-list controlled design. The primary hypothesis was that anger would be reduced in the intervention group compared with the wait-list control group. Secondary hypotheses were that increases in CAB-V during anger-provoking situations would lead to subsequent decreases in the blood pressures of these hypertensive patients. In the following, each CONSORT item is listed, followed by an explanation of that item and a description of how Stuhr should report her study to be consistent with the CONSORT Statement.

Item 1: How participants were allocated to interventions (e.g., random allocation, randomized, or randomly assigned). This information is expected to be included in the title and abstract.

Stuhr should entitle her manuscript for submission as she did her dissertation study to highlight that it was an RCT, that is, "Randomized Controlled Constructive Anger Intervention for Medicated Hypertensives." The abstract should also indicate that patients were matched and randomized. Not only does the inclusion of these design details help to present the study clearly, but it also ensures that this citation will be among the records produced by a search of randomized controlled trials. This is important because systematic reviews and meta-analyses rely on searches for studies that note the specific study design.

Item 2: Scientific background and explanation of rationale. This information should be reported in the Introduction section of an article.

The purpose and rationale of the research study should explain the importance of the study based on previous findings, or lack thereof, and the plausibility of exposing people to any potential risks. In the write-up of her study for publication, Stuhr should explain the theoretical reasoning behind her study and cite the relevant findings on anger, including a description of the previous research on this topic (i.e., the efficacy of psychosocial interventions for hypertensive patients). She should also justify why this topic (specifically, CAB-V-based anger management clinical trial with medicated hypertensive patients) necessitates further study.

Information regarding items 3 through 12 should be reported in the Methods section of the report.

Item 3: Eligibility criteria for participants and the settings and locations where the data were collected.

To fully assess the generalizability of the results, the study sample characteristics should be described in detail. Additionally, the author should describe the location where the data were collected because this may indicate characteristics related to the study results. To address this item, Stuhr should report that hypertension patients on medication with low CAB-V scores were enrolled from a Medicaid medical center, a "Good Samaritan" (uninsured) medical center, and two private internal medicine offices in Tuscaloosa, Alabama. She should also provide details on all the inclusion and exclusion criteria that were used to determine patient eligibility.

Item 4: Precise details of the interventions intended for each group and how and when they were actually administered.

The details of the various intervention sessions should be provided so that the treatment can be properly replicated in future studies and compared with previous methods. Because this is sometimes difficult to do in psychology research, the manner in which a therapy manual or training can be obtained should be provided. In addition, clear explanations ease the process of generating evidence-based guidelines for psychological interventions. Compensation and other potential simultaneous treatments (e.g., pharmacological) in the study should be noted. For her study, Stuhr should present a synopsis of the therapy protocol and provide the locations of the therapy manual and any training that might be available.

Item 5: Specific objectives and hypotheses.

The objectives and hypotheses should be described explicitly to ensure that other researchers fully understand the goals of the study. Therefore, Stuhr should report the objectives and hypotheses for her dissertation: The primary focus was to test if an intervention would improve constructive anger verbal expression in hypertensive patients and, secondarily, to determine if increasing CAB-V reduces diastolic blood pressure. She should also describe the proposed secondary analyses such as whether there is a dose-response relationship between CAB-V and diastolic blood pressure.

Item 6: (a) Clearly defined primary and secondary outcome measures and, (b) when applicable, any methods used to enhance the quality of measurements (e.g., multiple observations, training of assessors).

Outcomes in an RCT should be articulated as primary outcomes, the main effects under study, and secondary outcomes, the additional measures that are hypothesized to be affected by the intervention. The rationale for using particular outcome measures should be provided. For instance, in the Stuhr study, the primary outcome was changes in CAB-V scores, and the secondary outcomes were diastolic blood pressure changes, quality-of-life changes, and depression changes. She should report the methods used to ensure the accuracy of the outcome measurements, that is, the CAB-V coders were masked to treatment status, a blood pressure machine was used to reduce operator bias for blood pressure assessment, the 1997 Joint National Commission (JNC-VI) criteria were used for obtaining blood pressure readings, the data entry clerk was masked to treatment status, and the CAB-V coders were trained and tested for interrater reliability.

Item 7: (a) How sample size was determined and, (b) when applicable, explanation of any interim analyses and stopping rules.

These details are necessary to properly evaluate the validity of study findings. Before recruiting participants, the researcher must indicate the expected sample size for the alpha level to be used for inferential statistics, and the power to detect the expected difference between the control and treated arms for the primary outcome. Sample size determination is necessary so that the reader can understand the effect size that was expected. This information should be reported for Stuhr's study as it was in her dissertation; in addition, details of stopping rules or interim analyses, if any, should be provided. Although it was not a factor in Stuhr's study, authors must note when a study has been prematurely terminated due to unexpectedly large benefit, unexpected harm, or futility.

Item 8: Method used to generate the random allocation sequence, including details of any restriction (e.g., blocking, stratification).

Any methods used to control the randomization procedure, such as matching and clustering on a certain characteristic, should be noted so that the reader can understand how participants were randomized. Stuhr should report that the randomization procedure in her study involved matching participants on CAB-V scores (within 3 points) and on diastolic blood pressure levels (with 5 mmHg). Unmatched but eligible patients remained in the screening pool until a match was found. To report the randomization procedure by CONSORT standards, Stuhr should describe it in detail: (a) Matched pairs of patients were given identification numbers, and those numbers were written on separate pieces of paper (one per pair); (b) these pieces of paper, once folded, were all put into a jar together; (c) then the pieces of paper were drawn individually from the jar. The matched patients represented by the identification number on the first (third, fifth, etc.) piece of paper selected from the jar were put into the treatment group. The matched patients represented by the identification number of the second (fourth, sixth, etc.) piece of paper selected from the jar were put into the control condition.

Item 9: Method used to implement the random allocation sequence (e.g., numbered containers or central telephone), clarifying whether the sequence was concealed until interventions were assigned.

Details regarding the allocation process, and actions taken to assure that there are no biases in allocation should be described. For Stuhr's study, she should report that no preexisting sequence existed, so concealment could not be accomplished (a limitation of this study). One jar with preprinted identification numbers enclosed was used for the randomization procedure.

Item 10: Who generated the allocation sequence, who enrolled participants, and who assigned participants to their groups.

By describing the roles of the study staff, the integrity of the research process can be evaluated. For our example, Stuhr should report that there was no sequence generated and that she, the principal investigator, enrolled and assigned participants herself—a possible bias in this particular trial.

Item 11: Whether or not participants, those administering the interventions, and those assessing the outcomes were blinded to (i.e., unaware of) group assignment. If done, how the success of blinding (i.e., keeping staff unaware of group assignment) was evaluated.

While a study may be designed with the full intention of keeping as many staff as possible unaware of a participant's group assignment, occasionally an assignment may be discovered accidentally. For instance, in a pharmacological study, though a researcher may be unaware of which participants are in the medication arm, the lab results may hint at which medication is in use by the report of certain side effects, such as sexual dysfunction. From this hint, the assessment staff members might think they know the participant's group assignment, thus potentially biasing the subsequent assessment. Therefore, in pharmacological studies it would be preferable for a different person to administer the assessment measures, so that the person who is aware of the lab results does not bias the results. In her write-up, Stuhr should note that the one staff member who coded the CAB-V measure was unaware of treatment status, as were the CAB-V interviewers. Participants were obviously aware of whether or not they received therapy. Before assessments, participants were reminded to conceal their assignment from the CAB-V interviewer. Assessors of blood pressure and CAB-V and the data entry clerk were unaware of participants' group assignment. Stuhr should mention that one patient revealed her or his assignment on video, and no check of staff awareness of group assignment was conducted after the assessment data were collected.

Item 12: (a) Statistical methods used to compare groups for primary outcome(s); (b) methods for additional analyses, such as subgroup analyses and adjusted analyses.

By providing the details of the statistical analysis, the study results can be replicated and utilized more efficiently for a meta-analysis, an important resource in conducting evidence-based medicine.

Stuhr should report the analyses that she used to test her hypotheses about preintervention (Assessment 1) to the 2-month follow-up (Assessment 4) comparisons, including *t* tests (e.g., on demographic and clinical factors) and repeated measures of ANOVA using the calculation of change scores on the four dependent measures (i.e., CAB-V scores, Quality of Life Inventory scores, Beck Depression Inventory–II scores, and resting diastolic blood pressure measures). She should also note that no subgroup analyses were performed.

The information for items 13 through 19 should be reported in the Results section of the article.

Item 13: Flow of participants through each stage (a diagram is strongly recommended). Specifically, for each group report the numbers of participants randomly assigned, receiving intended treatment, completing the study protocol, and analyzed for the primary outcome. Describe protocol deviations from study as planned, together with reasons.

The flowchart provides a clear portrayal of the flow of participants over the duration of the study procedure. By providing information regarding those who drop out of the study or are disqualified, readers gain a greater understanding of the logistical complexities, potential arising biases, and issues to be addressed in future similar studies. In Stuhr's study, one patient became blind from required surgery, one patient missed one group and was rescheduled for individual appointment, and one cotherapist missed one session (see Figure 2.1).

Item 14: Dates defining the periods of recruitment and follow-up.

By reporting this detail, researchers incorporate their findings into a larger social-cultural context, such as the introduction of a new clinical care

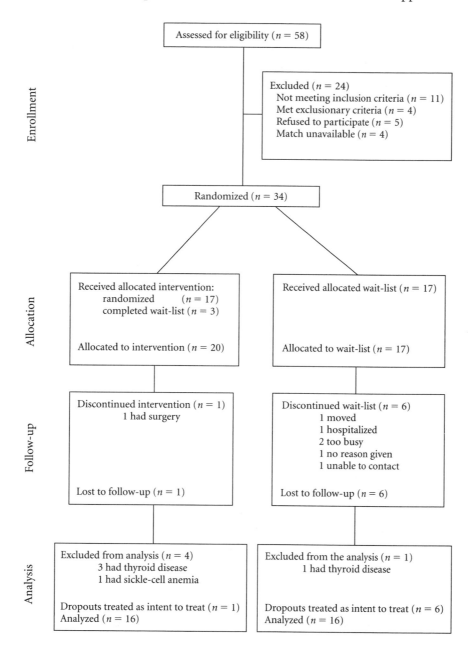

FIGURE 2.1. Flow diagram of participant progress through the phases of the randomized trial.

regimen for hypertension, or a change in reimbursement, that may limit the usefulness of the trial results. The dates of data collection are valuable for designing other studies and combining findings from previous research. For Stuhr's study, data collection occurred between August 2000 and August 2001.

Item 15: Baseline demographic and clinical characteristics of each group.

The value of RCTs rests on the assumption that all groups are equivalent at the beginning of the study. Thus, researchers must demonstrate how the groups are comparable on the baseline characteristics. As presented in her dissertation, Stuhr should provide a table of two groups with all the pretest variables included. Demographics for her sample are included in Table 2.2. Other baseline characteristics are included in Table 2.3.

Item 16: Number of participants (denominator) in each group included in each analysis and whether the analysis was by "intention to treat." State the results in absolute numbers when feasible.

Authors should describe the criteria for inclusion in the statistical analyses, preferably in absolute numbers. Once again, these values are needed for meta-analyses. In Stuhr's study, analyses used a modified intention to treat (i.e., included all participants randomized to treatment group, not just those who received treatment, but excluded those found to have comorbid disease, postrandomization). The type of intention-to-treat analysis that is conducted is more easily determined when the CONSORT is followed for reporting of a trial; the Stuhr modification of intention-to-treat analysis will be evident both in the flowchart and in the absolute numbers reported for the outcome analyses.

Item 17: For each primary and secondary outcome, a summary of results for each group and the estimated effect size and its precision (e.g., 95% confidence interval).

Well-designed tables help readers detect any differences in outcomes between groups in an intervention study. In addition, publication of effect sizes provides important information to subsequent reviewers of the body of literature for which one's study is a part. For Stuhr's study, effect sizes from residual gains analyses should be reported in one table, preferably with confidence intervals, although these were not presented in Dr. Stuhr's dissertation (see Table 2.4).

Item 18: Address multiplicity by reporting any other analyses performed, including subgroup analyses and adjusted analyses, indicating those that are prespecified and those that are exploratory.

Though journal editors emphasize the page limits for publications, authors should provide, at minimum, how many subgroup analyses were conducted. In Stuhr's study, she should report that there were no subgroup analyses; in addition, she should note that as the three primary analyses were conducted, familywise error rate was employed, thus reducing the likelihood of an inflated familywise alpha level.

TABLE 2.2

Demographics of the Treatment Group, the Control Group, the Overall Study Sample, and the Screening Sample

Group	Age***		Years of education		Ethnicity (%)			Marital status (%)		
	M	SD	M	SD	African American	Caucasian	Other	Single	Married	Separated, divorced, widowed
Treatment (n = 16)	50.25	11.30	13.1	3.27	62.5 (n = 10)	37.5 (n = 6)	0.0 (n = 0)	6.2 (n = 1)	43.8 (n = 7)	50.0 (n = 8)
Control (n = 16)	51.50	9.45	14.0	2.57	43.7 (n = 7)	56.3 (n = 9)	0.0 (n = 0)	12.5 (n = 2)	31.3 (n = 5)	56.2 (n = 9)
Study sample (N = 30)[a]	50.80	10.47	13.1	3.18	53.3 (n = 16)	46.7 (n = 14)	0.0 (n = 0)	10.0 (n = 3)	40.0 (n = 12)	50.0 (n = 15)
Screening sample (N = 24)	38.29	11.25	13.6	1.82	54.2 (n = 13)	45.8 (n = 11)	0.0 (n = 0)	4.2 (n = 1)	8.3 (n = 2)	8.3 (n = 2)

Note. Nineteen participants were missing marital status data from the screening sample. The independent samples *t*-test results reported were with equal variances assumed.
[a] Study sample of 30 includes only once the two participants in both the control and treatment groups.
*** *p* < .001.

TABLE 2.3

One-Way ANOVA of Baseline Measures: CAB-V, Resting DBP, BDI-II, and QOLI

| | Group | | | | One-way ANOVA | | |
| | Treatment ($n = 16$) | | Control ($n = 16$) | | | | |
Measure	M	SD	M	SD	df	F	p
CAB-V	15.31	3.10	15.56	2.25	(1,30)	0.07	.80
Resting DBP	80.97	10.00	80.88	8.65	(1,30)	0.001	.98
BDI	16.80	12.02	12.00	12.13	(1,30)	0.31	.58
QOLI	2.19	1.22	2.43	1.20	(1,30)	1.26	.27

Note. CAB-V = Constructive Anger Behavior–Verbal; resting DBP = resting diastolic blood pressure; BDI-II = Beck Depression Inventory, Second Edition; QOLI = Quality of Life Inventory. Multivariate results also revealed no significant difference ($F(4, 27) = .30, p = .87$).

Item 19: All important adverse events or side effects in each intervention group.

Provision of this information is necessary for the reader to assess the risks of the evaluated interventions. Although many believe that psychological interventions can cause no harm, evidence should be presented to support this sentiment. In a CONSORT write-up of Stuhr's study, she should report that no adverse events were found except for emergency eye surgery, and this was judged to be non-treatment-related.

The information for items 20 through 22 should be reported in the Comments/Discussion section of an article.

TABLE 2.4

Residual Gains Score Analyses for the CAB-V, Resting DBP, QOLI, and BDI-II Completed by Treatment Group

Measures	Residual gains score[a] (R^2 change)
CAB-V	.13*
Resting DBP	.05
QOLI	.04
BDI-II	.05

Note. CAB-V = Constructive Anger Behavior–Verbal; resting DBP = resting diastolic blood pressure; QOLI = Quality of Life Inventory; BDI-II = Beck Depression Inventory, Second Edition.
[a]The residual gains score was obtained from the R^2 change from the regression analysis.
*$p = .05$.

Item 20: Interpretation of the results, taking into account study hypotheses, sources of potential bias or imprecision, and the dangers associated with multiplicity of analyses and outcomes.

The researchers' experience in carrying out the study leads to further research questions and provides insight into the logistical complexities of the proposed intervention. When potential biases and risks are presented, others can attempt to reduce these barriers in future studies by designing research that addresses these concerns. For example, Stuhr should discuss issues of selection bias and the narrow range of socioeconomic status and explain that she also recognized the statistical problem of multiple analyses.

Item 21: Generalizability (external validity) of the trial findings.

Because the eligibility criteria, study setting, timing, and aspects of participation in the RCT all influence the characteristics of the sample, even statistically significant findings may not be indicative of interventions ready for large-scale application. Therefore, issues of generalizability should be fully discussed. As provided in her dissertation, Stuhr should explain how the recruitment locations and the low socioeconomic status, mostly minority, patient sample impacted the interpretation/generalizability of the results of the study.

Item 22: General interpretation of the results in the context of current evidence.

Authors should summarize the study results, taking into account the risks and benefits involved. For example, Stuhr should note that there was low power to find blood pressure outcomes.

■ Additional CONSORT Items

In addition to the CONSORT Statement items described previously, there are five more items that relate specifically to RCTs in psychology and in behavioral medicine (Davidson et al., 2003). These items were developed and proposed by members of the Evidence-Based Behavioral Medicine (EBBM) Committee of the Society for Behavioral Medicine because psychological and behavioral medicine research have additional methodological vulnerabilities that one is unlikely to encounter in an active drug-versus-placebo study—such as treatment fidelity and treatment allegiance. These additional items are described in detail below while applied to Stuhr's dissertation as an example of proper reporting.

EBBM Recommended Item—No. 23: Training of treatment provider(s) should be reported.

The usefulness of a proposed intervention must take into account the amount of training necessary to administer such a treatment. For example, Stuhr should report that the therapists who conducted the support groups in her study were master's-level clinical psychology graduate students who had specific training in how to conduct group therapy and how to implement the anger management treatment according to the study treatment manual.

EBBM Recommended Item—No. 24: Supervision of treatment provider(s).

Supervision can help ensure therapist competence at providing the intervention as it was originally designed over the duration of the trial. In addition, if a therapist without regular supervision drifts from the intended intervention protocol, then it would be impossible to replicate the study using other therapists. Stuhr should report that throughout the interventions, the therapists participated in weekly hour-long supervision sessions with licensed clinical psychology faculty.

EBBM Recommended Item—No. 25: Treatment allegiance should be recorded and reported.

Subtle changes in the way a treatment is described or delivered can occur with allegiance effects. Recording therapist allegiance or preference for differing treatment arms allows this effect to be detected. By measuring the adherence to the proposed treatment, researchers can evaluate whether a lack of effect was due to a suboptimal treatment intervention or whether it was simply due to the fact that the treatment arm did not receive the proper "dose" of the treatment under study. Because Stuhr did not record treatment allegiance in her study, she should state that clearly in the manuscript she submits for publication.

EBBM Recommended Item—No. 26: A detailed description of the manner of testing, and success of, treatment fidelity should be included.

Although this description may be brief, it helps confirm that the quality of the treatment administration remained consistent throughout the study. Stuhr should report that she recorded all the sessions and randomly had them rated 0 to 6 for three components of the therapy intervention using a 10-question measure to determine how well the therapists adhered to the treatment manual. The raters scored therapy sessions on general interview procedures (agenda setting, eliciting patient feedback, pacing, and efficient use of time), interpersonal effectiveness (empathic skills, interpersonal skills, professionalism), and specific cognitive-behavioral techniques (use of guided discovery, focus on key cognitions, application of behavioral techniques, and use of homework). A score of 45 or higher indicated that the treatment was delivered in the intended manner.

EBBM Recommended Item—No. 27: Treatment adherence should also be monitored and reported.

Patients can receive the treatment appropriately but not enact it in any way. Thus, it is important to test that the recommendations of a treatment are followed or adhered to by the patient. In this way, the research hypotheses can be tested properly, and potential findings can be replicated appropriately. Stuhr should report that the participants' weekly homework logs were assessed for their adherence to treatment recommendations.

In addition to the EBBM recommended items described above, Nezu and Nezu (2005) suggested that a discussion of adherence within study reports should include a comment on therapist competence. Stuhr should report that therapist competence was evaluated using the 7-item Therapist and Treatment Evaluation, an instrument developed by Dawn Wilson from other intervention research questionnaires (Cragan & Deffenbacher, 1984; Deffenbacher, 1994; Hazaleus & Deffenbacher, 1986).

This presentation of Dr. Stuhr's study as an example of how psychosocial intervention trials can be written in compliance with the CONSORT reporting items should give you a sense of the strengths and limitations of her study and facilitate your ability to judge the biases and strengths of this particular trial. Our discussion continues with a description of how CONSORT has changed since its inception.

■ CONSORT: An Evolving Resource

The CONSORT Group appreciates that the CONSORT Statement is an evolving document. Thirteen members met in May 1999 to revise the statement and published the revised recommendations in 2001 (Moher Schulz, & Altman for the CONSORT Group, 2001). Changes to the original CONSORT Statement included numbering the items in the checklist, separation of some items, and a revised flow diagram. The revision of the flow diagram was influenced by a report by CONSORT members that found that the use of flow diagrams improved transparency of reporting (Egger, Jüni, & Bartlett for the CONSORT Group, 2001). Detailed explanations of the new CONSORT items, including the new flow diagram, and evidence for the inclusion of each item can be found in Altman et al. (2001). This article is an excellent resource for investigators who want to use CONSORT when designing, reporting, and/or reviewing RCTs.

Since the 2001 revisions, the CONSORT Statement has been extended for use in various ways. As mentioned earlier, the Evidence-Based Behavioral Medicine Committee proposed five additional behavioral medicine–related items (Davidson et al., 2003). In addition, 15 of the 22 items have been augmented for application to trials in which a group of individuals (e.g., a family) instead of an individual is randomized to the treatment condition (e.g., a dietary intervention), known as *cluster randomized trials* (Campbell, Elbourne, & Altman for the CONSORT Group, 2004). The CONSORT Statement has also been augmented with 10 additional items to foster enhanced reporting of harms (Ioannidis et al. for the CONSORT Group, 2004).

CONSORT creators also respond to criticism of their tool. For example, Fergusson, Glass, Waring, and Shapiro (2004) suggested that CONSORT should require that all authors of RCT reports include an assessment of the success of keeping investigators unaware of each participant's group assignment in their studies.

In response, the CONSORT Group described the methodological complexity of applying this recommendation to all RCTs, accompanied by the reminder that: "CONSORT is a set of reporting recommendations—it does not make statements on how trials should be done, but asks that what was done should be fully and accurately reported" (Altman, Schulz, & Moher, 2004, p. 1135).[1]

■ Applying CONSORT to Psychological Research

In 2001, the Evidence-Based Behavioral Medicine Committee, initiated by the Society of Behavioral Medicine (http://www.sbm.org/ebbm/), endorsed the CONSORT Statement as a valuable tool in reporting behavioral medicine research. Therefore, the committee adopted the CONSORT Statement to address its mandate of creating guidelines for evidence-based behavioral medicine. The EBBM Committee has been committed to introducing the CONSORT guidelines to our colleagues in the field of behavioral medicine, health psychology, and psychosomatic medicine.

This introduction by the EBBM Committee took the following forms: (a) "A CONSORT Primer" published in a society newsletter (*Outlook* of the Society of Behavioral Medicine), which was an evaluation of a brief report of an RCT published in *Health Psychology* to show how CONSORT items could be applied to a behavioral medicine study (Trudeau & Davidson for the Evidence-Based Behavioral Medicine Committee, 2001–2002; available at www.sbm.org/ebbm/); (b) a detailed description of CONSORT items as applied to behavioral medicine research, in general, with the addition of 5 items specific to behavioral medicine, which was published in *Annals of Behavioral Medicine* (Davidson et al., 2003; also available at www.sbm.org/ebbm/); (c) correspondence to psychology journals (e.g., *Health Psychology*), including editorials (e.g., Kaplan, Trudeau, & Davidson, 2004; *Annals of Behavioral Medicine*), recommending the adoption of CONSORT in their peer review process; and (d) an invited symposium that was presented at the Society of Behavioral Medicine meeting in March 2002 (Davidson et al., 2002; this chapter is loosely based on the presentation given by Davidson and Trudeau during that symposium).

■ Research on Effects of CONSORT Adoption

Since the publication of the CONSORT Statement, several studies have been conducted to evaluate the effects of this tool on reporting trials. For example, a

---

1. Following the popularity of CONSORT, many checklists have been devised to improve reporting. Examples include TREND, MOOSE, QUORUM[0], etc. Citations for these checklists are presented in Table 2.1.

review of the reporting of details included in CONSORT before (1994) versus after (1998) publication of CONSORT (1996) in the four general medical journals (*Journal of the American Medical Association, British Medical Journal, Lancet, New England Journal of Medicine*) indicated that more CONSORT-related details were reported post-CONSORT. Reporting was particularly improved in the three journals that had adopted CONSORT in comparison to the journal that had not (Moher, Jones, & Lepage for the CONSORT Group, 2001). Similar results were found in a subsequent study of 26 medical journals, including 10 that promoted CONSORT and 16 that did not (Devereaux, Manns, Ghali, Quan, & Guyatt, 2002). Both of these studies concluded that despite journal endorsement of the CONSORT Statement, there is still insufficient reporting of methodological details (e.g., masking—staff's unawareness of participants' group assignment). This finding was echoed in a review of more recent RCT reports published between July 2002 and June 2003 in the five highest impact medical journals, leading its authors to recommend that CONSORT guidelines be adopted and enforced by journal editors (Mills, Wu, Gagnier, & Devereaux, 2005).

Although reporting of some study details (such as masking) has not significantly improved after the publication of CONSORT, the use of "randomized" in the title or abstract as dictated by Item 1 of CONSORT appears to have improved from pre- (68%) to post (85%)-CONSORT; this improvement facilitates the searching of RCTs for conducting systematic reviews of the literature (Royle & Waugh, 2005).

■ Summary

In this chapter, we described the inception, evolution, and evaluation of the CONSORT Statement in medical and psychological research, accompanied by a demonstration of how to apply it using the unpublished dissertation of Judith Stuhr. Methodological reporting is correlated with methodological quality (Huwlier-Müntener, Jüni, Junker, & Egger, 2002); therefore, for research on the efficacy of psychological interventions to achieve credibility and ascend to usual practice, it is important to incorporate the CONSORT Statement for designing and reporting intervention research in psychology.

■ Acknowledgments

This work was supported by NIH contract N01HC25197 and grants HL44058, HL076857, and NLM00–158/LTN.

■ References

Altman, D. G. (1996). Better reporting of randomised controlled trials: The CONSORT Statement. *British Medical Journal, 313,* 570–571.

Altman, D. G., for the CONSORT Group. (2005). Endorsement of the CONSORT statement by high impact medical journals: Survey of instructions for authors. *British Medical Journal, 330,* 1056–1057.

Altman, D. G., & Doré, C. J. (1990). Randomization and baseline comparisons in clinical trials. *Lancet, 335,* 149–153.

Altman, D. G., Schulz, K. F., & Moher, D. (2004). Turning a blind eye: Testing the success of blinding and the CONSORT statement. *British Medical Journal, 328,* 1135.

Altman, D. G., Schulz, K. F., Moher, D., Egger, M., Davidoff, F., Elbourne, D., et al., for the CONSORT Group (2001). The revised CONSORT Statement for reporting randomized trials: Exploration and elaboration. *Annals of Internal Medicine, 134,* 663–694.

Asilomar Working Group on Recommendations for Reporting of Clinical Trials in Biomedical Literature. (1994). Call for comments on a proposal to improve reporting of clinical trials in the biomedical literature: A position paper. *Annals of Internal Medicine, 121,* 894–895.

Begg, C. B., Cho, M. K., Eastwood S., Horton, R., Moher, D., Olkin, I., et al. (1996). Improving the quality of reporting of randomized controlled trials: The CONSORT statement. *Journal of the American Medical Association, 276,* 637–639.

Boutron, I., Moher, D., Tugwell, P, Giraudeau, B., Poiraudeau, S., Nizard, R. M., et al. (2005). A checklist to evaluate a report of a nonpharmacological trial (CLEAR NPT) was developed using consensus. *Journal of Clinical Epidemiology, 58,* 1233–1240.

Campbell, M. K., Elbourne, D. R., & Altman, D. G., for the CONSORT Group. (2004). CONSORT Statement: Extension to cluster randomized trials. *British Medical Journal, 328,* 702–708.

Cragan, M. K., & Deffenbacher, J. L. (1984). Anxiety management training and relaxation as self-control in the treatment of generalized anxiety in medical outpatients. *Journal of Counseling Psychology, 31,* 123–131.

Davidson, K. W., Goldstein, M., Kaplan, R. M., Kaufmann, P. G., Knatterud, G. L., Orleans, C. T., et al. (2003). Evidence-based behavioral medicine: What is it, and how do we achieve it? *Annals of Behavioral Medicine, 26,* 161–171.

Davidson, K., MacGregor, M., Stuhr, J., Dixon, K., & MacLean, D. (2000). Constructive anger verbal behaviors predict blood pressure in a population-based sample. *Health Psychology, 19,* 55–64.

Davidson, K., MacGregor, M., Stuhr, J., & Gidron, Y. (1999). Increasing constructive anger verbal behavior decreases resting blood pressure: A secondary analysis of a randomized controlled hostility intervention. *International Journal of Behavioral Medicine, 6,* 268–278.

Davidson, K. W., Orleans, C. T., Whitlock, E., Spring, B., Trudeau, K., & Pagoto, S. (2002, March). *Designing, reviewing, and using Evidence-Based Behavioral*

Medicine (EBBM). Postconference seminar presented at the annual meeting of the Society of Behavioral Medicine, Washington, DC.

Deffenbacher, J. L. (1994). Anger reduction: Issues, assessment, and intervention strategies. In A. W. Siegman & T. W. Smith (Eds.), *Anger, hostility, and the heart* (pp. 239–269). Hillsdale, NJ: Erlbaum.

Devereaux, P. J., Manns, B. J., Ghali, W. A., Quan, H., & Guyatt, G. H. (2002). The reporting of methodological factors in randomized controlled trials and the association with a journal policy to promote adherence to the Consolidated Standards of Reporting Trials (CONSORT) checklist. *Controlled Clinical Trials, 23,* 380–388.

Dittman, M. (2004). Guidelines seek to prevent bias in reporting of randomized trials. *APA Monitor on Psychology, 35*(8), 20.

Egger, M., Jüni, P., & Bartlett, C., for the CONSORT Group. (2001). Value of flow diagrams in reports of randomized controlled trials. *Journal of the American Medical Association, 285,* 1996–1999.

Fergusson, D., Glass, K. C., Waring, D., & Shapiro, S. (2004). Turning a blind eye: The success of blinding reported in a random sample of randomized, placebo controlled trials. *British Medical Journal, 328,* 432–434.

Freemantle, N., Mason, J. M., Haines, A., & Eccles, M. P. (1997). CONSORT: An important step toward evidence-based health care. *Annals of Internal Medicine, 126,* 81–83.

Glasgow, R. E., Vogt, T. M., & Boles, S. M. (1999). Evaluating the public health impact of health promotion interventions: The RE-AIM framework. *American Journal of Public Health, 89,* 1322–1327.

Hazaleus, S. L., & Deffenbacher, J. L. (1986). Relaxation and cognitive treatments of anger. *Journal of Consulting and Clinical Psychology, 54,* 222–226.

Huwlier-Müntener, K., Jüni, P., Junker, C., & Egger, M. (2002). Quality of reporting of randomized trials as a measure of methodologic quality. *Journal of the American Medical Association, 287,* 2801–2804.

Ioannidis, J. P. A., Evans, S. J. W., Gøtzsche, P. C., O'Neill, R. T., Altman, D. G., Schulz, K., et al., for the CONSORT Group (2004). Better reporting of harms in randomized trials: An extension of the CONSORT Statement. *Annals of Internal Medicine, 141,* 781–788.

Joint National Committee of Prevention, Development, Evaluation, and Treatment of High Blood Pressure, VI. (1997). *Sixth report* (NIH Publication No. 98–4080). Washington, DC: U.S. Government Printing Office.

Kaplan, R. M., Trudeau, K. J., & Davidson, K. W. (2004). Editorial: New policy on reports of randomized clinical trials. *Annals of Behavioral Medicine, 27,* 81.

Mills, E. J., Wu, P., Gagnier, J., & Devereaux, P. J. (2005). The quality of randomized trial reporting in leading medical journals since the revised CONSORT statement. *Contemporary Clinical Trials, 26,* 480–487.

Moher, D. (1998). CONSORT: An evolving tool to help improve the quality of reports of randomized controlled trials. *Journal of the American Medical Association, 279,* 1489–1491.

Moher, D., Jones, A., & Lepage, L., for the CONSORT Group. (2001). Use of the CONSORT Statement and quality of reports of randomized trials: A comparative before-and-after evaluation. *Journal of the American Medical Association, 285,* 1992–1995.

Moher, D., Schulz, K. F., & Altman, D. G., for the CONSORT Group. (2001). The CONSORT Statement: Revised recommendations for improving the quality of reports. *Journal of the American Medical Association, 285,* 1987–1991.

Nezu, A. M., & Nezu, C. M. (2005). Comments on "Evidence-based behavioral medicine: What is it and how do we achieve it?": The interventionist does not always equal the intervention—The role of therapist competence. *Annals of Behavioral Medicine, 29,* 80.

Pocock, S. J., Hughes, M. D., & Lee, R. J. (1987). Statistical problems in the reporting of clinical trials. *New England Journal of Medicine, 317,* 426–432.

Rennie, D. (1995). Reporting randomized controlled trials: An experiment and a call for responses from readers. *Journal of the American Medical Association, 273,* 1054–1055.

Royle, P., & Waugh, N. (2005). A simplified search strategy for identifying randomized controlled trials for systematic reviews of health care interventions: A comparison with more exhaustive strategies. *BMC Medical Research Methodology, 5,* 23.

Standards of Reporting Trials Group. (1994). A proposal for structured reporting of randomized controlled trials. *Journal of the American Medical Association, 272,* 1926–1931.

Stuhr, J. K. (1999). *Constructive anger behavior and blood pressure in African Americans and Caucasians.* Unpublished master's thesis, University of Alabama, Tuscaloosa.

Stuhr, J. (2004). Randomized controlled anger intervention for hypertensives. *Dissertation Abstracts International—B, 64*(08), 4066.

Trudeau, K. J., & Davidson, K., for the Evidence-Based Behavioral Medicine Committee. (2001–2002). A CONSORT Primer. *Outlook: A Quarterly Newsletter of the Society of Behavioral Medicine,* 5–8.

SECTION II

ASSESSMENT ISSUES

3. CLINICAL INTERVIEWS

Thomas A. Widiger

It is an accepted principle in psychological assessment that the optimal approach is to use multiple methods of assessment (Campbell & Fiske, 1959; Eid & Diener, 2006), including specifically the assessment of treatment outcome (Behar & Borkovec, 2003; Lambert & Hawkins, 2004). Any reliance on one specific method will be subject to the inevitable limitations and systematic biases of that method. The use of multiple methods seems to invariably indicate the presence of at least some unique validity of each particular approach. Nevertheless, this chapter focuses on one particular method of assessment: the interview. The interview method has perhaps a unique distinction in psychological assessment. The clinical interview is the preferred method of assessment in general clinical practice (Watkins, Campbell, Nieberding, & Hallmark, 1995) and in clinical research (Rogers, 2001, 2003; Zimmerman, 2003), although the preferred outcome measure in treatment research is generally a self-report inventory (Ogles, Lambert, & Fields, 2002), and the typical method of interviewing in general clinical practice and clinical research can be quite different.

The purpose of this chapter is to discuss assessment issues in the administration of clinical interviews for evidence-based outcome research. The chapter begins with a general discussion of the advantages and limitations of three fundamental forms of clinical interviewing: unstructured, semistructured, and structured. The chapter concludes with a discussion of issues for future research, including reliability, validity, normative data, and validity scales. Individual interview instruments are cited for illustrative purposes, but a systematic or comprehensive review of clinical interview schedules is not provided. These are available in a number of other sources (e.g., Barbour & Davison, 2004; Ogles et al., 2002; Summerfeldt & Antony, 2002; Rogers, 2001; Rush et al., 2000).

■ Format

Clinical interviews will, of course, vary with regard to quite a few considerations, including the domain of functioning that is being assessed, time frame that is being covered, population that is being interviewed, and functional purpose of the assessment (Craig, 2003, 2005). A fundamental methodological distinction is the extent to which the interview is structured. Most readers of this chapter will be concerned primarily with the application of interviews for the development of empirically validated treatments and, as such, will likely be well familiar with or at least favorable toward structured interviews. However, it is still useful and important to consider the strengths and limitations of this methodology and the precise reasons for which structured interviews are generally preferred.

Degree of Structure

An unstructured interview is one in which the clinician (or whoever is conducting the interview) is free to assess whatever clinical constructs he or she considers to be relevant or informative. Even if the constructs that are to be assessed have been explicitly identified, an unstructured interviewer will assess these constructs using whatever questions or observations he or she considers to be most useful. Unstructured interviews are then quite idiosyncratic to the person conducting the interview. This is described most favorably by Shedler (2002) when he explains how the administration of the Shedler and Westen Assessment Procedure–200 (Westen & Shedler, 1999) relies on "the empathically attuned and dynamically sophisticated clinician given free rein to practice his or her craft" (Shedler, 2002, p. 433).

In stark contrast, fully structured interviews provide a systematically guided assessment through standardizing the questions used by the interviewer, the sequencing of these questions, and the scoring of the responses (Rogers, 2001). Examples of fully structured interviews are the Diagnostic Interview Schedule (DIS; Compton & Cottler, 2004; Robins, Helzer, Croughan, & Ratcliff, 1981) and the Alcohol Use Disorder and Associated Disabilities Interview Schedule—*DSM-IV* version (AUDADIS-IV; Grant et al., 2003). Semistructured interviews deviate somewhat from this fully structured format. Structured interview questions are typically phrased in such a manner that the scoring will be unambiguous (e.g., questions that can be answered by a "yes" or "no"). In contrast, semistructured interviews will often include quite open-ended questions, the responses to which will be idiosyncratic to the respondent and can be complex in content. Semistructured interviews do provide a standard set of questions that generally must be administered, along with explicit rules for scoring responses. However, semistructured interviews will often encourage the provision of follow-up queries that can be worded in a manner that is idiosyncratic to the interviewer, they might allow for the exclusion of questions when an interviewer considers them to be unnecessary to provide a confident assessment, and they often allow, at times even require, the scoring of items on the basis of the interviewer's interpretation of a respondent's verbal answers, as well as observation of the respondent's behavior.

Some of the questions used in semistructured interviews might even be best described as probes whose purpose it is to elicit behavior that is then observed by the interviewer to determine if a clinical feature is present. For example, one of the features of narcissistic personality disorder is a grandiose sense of self-importance. Most clinicians would not assess this feature through a direct inquiry as to its presence because it is unlikely that a narcissistic person would be so forthright as to acknowledge its presence (Westen, 1997; Widiger & Samuel, 2005). Therefore, the Personality Disorder Interview–IV (PDI-IV; Widiger, Mangine, Corbitt, Ellis, & Thomas, 1995) uses such probes as asking persons if they have any special talents or abilities, what are their future goals, and how they would evaluate their achievements. The purpose of these probes is to provide a situational context in which it is likely that the diagnostic criterion will be manifested and its presence can then be observed by the interviewer.

Examples of semistructured interviews include the Anxiety Disorders Interview Schedule for *DSM-IV* (ADIS-IV; Di Nardo, Brown, & Barlow, 1994; Grisham, Brown, & Campbell, 2004), the Structured Clinical Interview for *DSM-IV* Axis I Disorders (SCID-I; First & Gibbon, 2004), the Schedule for Affective Disorders and Schizophrenia (SADS; Spitzer & Endicott, 1978), and the International Personality Disorder Examination (IPDE; Loranger, 1999). There is, of course, considerable variation among these semistructured interviews in the extent to which they deviate from a fully structured interview. For example, comparing just the five personality disorder semistructured interviews, the Diagnostic Interview for Personality Disorders (DIPD; Zanarini, Frankenburg, Chauncey, & Gunderson, 1987) is probably the most structured in its format, whereas the PDI-IV (Widiger et al., 1995) is probably the least structured (Widiger, 2002).

There are quite a few structured and semistructured interviews (Rogers, 2001; Rush et al., 2000; Summerfeldt & Antony, 2002), many of which include modifications for the assessment of change in functioning that would facilitate their application to studies of treatment outcome. For example, most structured and semistructured interviews include methods for obtaining precise dating of the symptomatology or, at least, only minor modifications would be necessary to make the instrument optimally suitable for assessing changes in symptom status. Any such modification (if necessary) can become problematic for instruments that are assessing disorders that, by definition, are chronic, such as the personality disorders (Widiger & Samuel, 2005). An innovation of the semistructured DIPD (Zanarini et al., 1997) is the development of a monthly "follow-along" assessment of personality disorder symptoms, as well as an exploration of various durations in time that might be useful for determining if and when a personality disorder has gone into remission (Gunderson et al., 2000).

A model for and frequently used interview for tracking symptom change over time is the Longitudinal Interval Follow-Up Evaluation (LIFE; Keller et al., 1987). The LIFE tracks the course of symptoms by assessing in an ongoing fashion the onset, severity, and absence of symptoms on a week-to-week or month-to-month schedule. Assessments can also be anchored by memorable dates for the patient (e.g., holidays, school or work schedule changes). This systematic follow-along assessment facilitates substantially the effort to define explicitly and document empirically specific symptom reduction, remission, and absence. A recent illustration of the application of the LIFE is provided by Birmaher et al. (2006), who studied the clinical course of bipolar spectrum disorders in children and adolescents.

Strengths and Limitations of Degree of Structure

An unstructured interview is the preferred method in clinical practice (Watkins et al. 1995; Westen, 1997). Unstructured clinical interviews are substantially more flexible than alternative methods. Interviewers can alter the focus, the depth, or even the style of an interview to be optimally responsive to the particular demands, interests, or needs of the respondent (Craig, 2003, 2005). Most omnibus self-report inventories attempt to cover virtually all domains of psychopathology but must then compromise or limit the assessment of particular areas of functioning in order to cover the broad range. An interviewer has the unique advantage of being able to virtually abandon a focus of inquiry during the course of an assessment to spend more time and effort focusing on a particularly significant or complex concern.

Structured and semistructured interviews are the preferred method for clinical research (Antony & Rowa, 2005; Joiner, Walker, Pettit, Perez, & Cukrowicz, 2005; Rogers, 2003; Zimmerman, 2003). Studies of unstructured clinical assessments have repeatedly indicated that because these interviews are idiosyncratic in approach and focus, they are prone to yielding unreliable and even biased results and at times fail to provide comprehensive assessments (Garb, 2005; Segal & Coolidge, 2003; Wood, Garb, Lilienfeld, & Nezworski, 2002). Because the unstructured interviewers will often focus the interview on matters of specific concern (to the interviewer and/or the interviewee) that arise during the course of the interview, they can fail to provide a systematically comprehensive assessment and might even miss important symptoms and features (Zimmerman & Mattia, 1999). Semistructured interviews provide specific, carefully selected questions, the application of which increases the likelihood that assessments will be systematic, reasonably comprehensive, and consistent across interviewers. In addition, the manuals that accompany a semistructured interview will often provide a considerable amount of helpful information for understanding the constructs that are being assessed, for interpreting vague or inconsistent symptomatology, and for resolving diagnostic ambiguities (e.g., Loranger, 1999; Widiger et al., 1995).

The advantages of more structured interviews are so evident that consideration is even being given to their explicit inclusion with diagnostic criteria sets for the next edition of the American Psychiatric Association's (APA) diagnostic manual (Widiger & Clark, 2000). A significant achievement of the third edition of the APA's *Diagnostic and Statistical Manual of Mental Disorders* (*DSM-III*; APA, 1980) was the inclusion of relatively more specific and explicit diagnostic criteria that contributed to a marked improvement in the reliability of clinical assessments (Nathan & Langenbucher, 1999). However, "although diagnostic criteria are the framework for any clinical or epidemiological assessment, no assessment of clinical status is independent of the reliability and validity of the methods used to determine the presence of a diagnosis" (Regier et al., 1998, p. 114). It is apparent that unreliable clinical assessments can still occur despite the presence of specific and explicit criteria sets if clinicians are not in fact conducting systematic assessments of these diagnostic criteria (Kirk & Kutchins, 1992).

Researchers would be hard-pressed to get their findings published if they failed to document that their assessments were based upon a systematic, replicable, and objective method, yet no such requirements are currently provided for clinical diagnosis, with the notable exception of mental retardation and learning disorders. Included within the diagnostic criteria sets for these disorders is the documentation of the administration of a structured assessment. Few clinicians would attempt to diagnose mental retardation in the absence of a structured test, yet it is common to diagnose schizophrenia, major depressive disorder, or antisocial personality disorder in the absence of a structured assessment (Watkins et al., 1995). A recommendation of the APA and National Institute of Mental Health DSM-V Nomenclature Work Group is to incorporate more structured assessments into the *DSM-V* criterion sets for other disorders to ensure that they also are being assessed systematically. "At present, results of psychological testing are not included in *DSM-IV* diagnostic criteria, with the exception of IQ testing and academic skills . . . [and] this exception points the way for research that could lead to incorporation of psychological test results as diagnostic criteria for other disorders" (Rounsaville et al., 2002, p. 24).

Structured interviews, however, are not without their own notable disadvantages. Structured interviews typically require considerably more time than is reasonably available to a practicing clinician (Antony & Rowa, 2005; Widiger & Samuel, 2005). In addition, the systematic coverage of a wide range of symptoms and features that are not of immediate concern to the patient can interfere with the establishment of rapport (Craig, 2003, 2005; Westen, 1997). Time and rapport might not be as serious a problem for the researcher relative to the practicing clinician. Researchers can at times obtain the commitment of a person to complete literally hours of assessment, much of which can even be tedious. An advantage of an interview relative to a self-report inventory is the ability to use the direct contact with the respondent to help engage him or her in the process of assessment, even one that can take hours. This is a luxury that is simply not feasible for the practicing clinician.

An advantage of semi-semistructured interviews, relative to a self-report inventory (or to a fully structured interview that does not even allow for follow-up queries), is the ability to ask follow-up questions to ensure that the respondent understands the question and to clarify the respondent's answer.

A common technique for doing so is to ask the respondent to provide examples for or details concerning any symptom he or she endorses (e.g., suicidal gesture or drug use) to ensure that the respondent is applying a clinically meaningful threshold for the presence of that symptom. However, to the extent that an interview uses follow-up queries or probes, the need for professional expertise or training in the administration and scoring of the interview does increase.

A significant advantage of fully structured interviews, relative to a semistructured interview, is that they can be so straightforward they can be administered and scored reliably by laypersons. This facilitates substantially the ability to conduct studies that sample large numbers of participants. For example, the National Epidemiologic Survey on Alcohol and Related Conditions (NESARC) consisted of face-to-face interviews of a nationally representative sample of 43,093 respondents (Grant et al., 2004). The data collection was provided by 1,800 lay interviewers from the U.S. Census Bureau.

An issue that is not fully resolved is the extent to which an optimally valid assessment can in fact be obtained with a fully structured interview administered by a layperson. A fully structured interview is essentially equivalent to an oral administration of a self-report inventory. To the extent that this is in fact true, the need for or benefit of having a person, even a layperson, administer the interview might not always be clear. Lay interviewers administering fully structured interviews do probably provide an important function in developing a respondent's motivation to answer all the questions in a faithful and sincere manner, as well as helping the respondent clarify the meaning of questions. These can be important advantages relative to a self-report inventory. Nevertheless, the reason that semistructured (and structured) interviews are preferred over self-report inventories in psychiatric research is the opportunity to have the interviewer impact the assessment rather than relying solely on the respondent's opinions or beliefs, which are often not particularly trustworthy when assessing substance use or psychotic, personality, and other mental disorders (Rogers, 2001; Segal & Coolidge, 2003; Widiger & Samuel, 2005). However, to the extent that an interview is preferred over a self-report inventory, one might question why a structured interview is preferred over an unstructured interview.

It is apparent, though, that as the structure of the assessment increases, convergent validity coefficients increase as well (Widiger, 2002). The preference of researchers for semistructured interviews could then be analogous to the preference of clinicians for unstructured interviews. Semistructured interviews are preferred over self-report inventories because they provide the interviewer the opportunity to have a direct, personal impact on the assessment; follow-up queries can be provided, and inadequacies in self-insight and awareness can be addressed (Rogers, 2001; Segal & Coolidge, 2003). However, the opportunity of the interviewer to personally impact the assessment might also contribute to less reliable and ultimately less valid assessments (comparable to the lower reliability obtained with unstructured interviews relative to semistructured interviews). The findings obtained with self-report inventories are more likely to replicate across research sites than the findings obtained with semistructured interviews simply because there is little to no room for interrater disagreement in the administration and scoring of a self-report inventory. Given the considerable expense of administering structured and semistructured interviews, additional research on the relative validity of interview and inventory methods of assessment is perhaps warranted.

■ Issues

The preference of researchers for structured and semistructured interviews over unstructured inventories and self-report inventories is defensible and well reasoned. Nevertheless, there are a number of issues that should be addressed in future research and considered in treatment outcome studies to be more confident that the method is in fact producing the optimally valid results. Considered in the following will be matters of reliability, validity, norms, and validity scales.

Reliability

Reliability is essentially the extent to which an assessment is free from measurement error. An estimate of reliability is generally obtained by varying a nonsubstantive aspect of the measurement process to evaluate its impact on the consistency of the obtained score. There are four widely used methods for assessing reliability: test-retest stability, internal consistency coefficients, alternative forms, and scorer reliability (Morey, 2003). Scoring reliability is generally very high, if not maximal, for self-report inventories, although even here some unreliability can occur (e.g., errors resulting from flaws in computer scanning). According to Morey (2003), "As the 2000 U.S. presidential election revealed, use of automated scoring systems will not necessarily result in perfect scorer reliability; thus, even with these systems, scorer reliability should be assessed if a high degree of precision is critical" (p. 400).

Scoring reliability is centrally important when interview methods are used. The typical statistic that is used is the kappa coefficient, a derivation of an intraclass correlation coefficient that adjusts the simple percentage of agreement to account for the probability of chance agreement. The predominant method for determining scoring reliability is through the alternate coding of a joint or videotaped interview (Rogers, 2001; Segal & Coolidge, 2003).

There are many studies to indicate that good to excellent interrater reliability is obtained when semistructured interviews are used (Rogers, 2001, 2003; Segal & Coolidge, 2003). Nevertheless, it is also worth noting that the reliability data that are reported in many of these studies have been confined to the agreement in the coding of respondents' answers to interview questions. For fully structured interviews, this evaluation is comparable to determining whether a self-report inventory has been reliably administered and scored across research settings. As the structure of an interview increases, the reliability of response coding can be no more demanding than obtaining agreement as to whether respondents said "yes" or "no" in response to a straightforward question. Answering this reliability question is perhaps trivial, or at least it is not answering the more important or fundamental concern with respect to reliability, particularly if a semistructured interview is used (Clark & Harrison, 2001). Of greater importance to the replicability of clinical and research assessments would be studies addressing whether semistructured interviews are administered reliably (Segal & Coolidge, 2003). For example, are the questions being administered by different interviewers in a consistent manner? Are some interviewers providing substantially more follow-up queries than other interviewers? Do patients respond to the same open-ended questions in a consistent manner over time? These questions are best answered through reliability studies that involve the independent administrations of the same interview to the same person by different people at different (but reasonably close) times. Sophisticated reliability studies are being conducted (e.g., Brown, Di Nardo, Lehman, & Campbell, 2001; Trull, 2001; Zanarini & Frankenburg, 2001), but further research is perhaps needed on the agreement between independent administrations of the same interview to the same patient.

Validity

The failure of a study to confirm the validity of a construct can be the result of an invalid research design or an invalid assessment of the respective construct, instead of any invalidity of the construct itself (Cronbach & Meehl, 1955). Similarly, empirical support for a theoretical construct depends as much on the validity of the research design and construct assessment as it does on the actual validity of the construct. Much of the research that informs our knowledge of psychopathology and its treatment has relied on assessments provided by structured or semistructured interviews. Assuming that this knowledge is indeed valid, this extensive research then provides considerable empirical support for the validity of structured and semistructured interviews (Summerfeldt & Antony, 2002; Widiger & Samuel, 2005).

CONCURRENT VALIDITY

Nevertheless, it is perhaps still worth noting that there are surprisingly few studies assessing the convergent or concurrent validity of alternative interview schedules (Widiger, 2002). There are a considerable number of studies assessing the convergent validity of self-report inventories, and their convergent validity with semistructured and structured interviews, but interview schedules do appear to receive relatively less attention when it comes to validation research. The exceptions most often concern the validation of fully structured interviews (e.g., validity data concerning the AUDADIS-IV; Grant et al., 2004), in part because they are so heavily relied upon for major epidemiological information (e.g., Robins et al., 1981) and because of concerns regarding the validity of interviews administered by laypersons, but perhaps as well because they require substantially less labor and effort to research.

For example, there are currently five different personality disorder semi-structured interviews (Kaye & Shea, 2000; Rogers, 2001; Widiger, 2002). Data from these interviews have been appearing within the published literature since 1984 (Widiger et al., 1995), yet there have been only two published studies on their convergent validity, and each was confined to just two of the five interviews (i.e., O'Boyle & Self, 1990; Skodol, Oldham, Rosnick, Kellman, & Hyler, 1991). The most comprehensive study was by Skodol et al. (1991). They administered the IPDE (Loranger, 1999) and the Structured Clinical Interview for *DSM-IV* Axis II Personality Disorders (SCID-II; First, Gibbon, Spitzer, Williams, & Benjamin, 1997) to 100 inpatients of a personality disorders treatment unit. Both interviews were administered by different persons on the same day (one in the morning, the other in the afternoon) without any knowledge of the results obtained by the other interview. Order of administration was staggered. Kappa for individual diagnoses ranged from a low of .14 (schizoid) to a high of .66 (dependent), with a median kappa of .53 (borderline). The authors considered the agreement for some of the categorical diagnoses to be discouraging. Skodol and colleagues, for example, conclude: "It is fair to say that, for a number of disorders (i.e., paranoid, schizoid, schizotypal, narcissistic, and passive-aggressive) the two [interviews] studied do not operationalize the diagnoses similarly and thus yield disparate results" (1991, p. 22).

Data concerning the concurrent validity of structured and semistructured interviews are of considerable importance, given that different instruments can provide different results and our knowledge base rests so heavily on their findings. For example, Regier et al. (1998) lamented the substantial variability in findings provided by the two major epidemiological studies to date: the Epidemiologic Catchment Area (ECA) study (Robins & Regier, 1991) and the National Comorbidity Survey (NCS; Kessler et al., 1994). The ECA used the DIS (Robins et al., 1981), a structured interview administered and scored by laypersons. Subsequent to the ECA study, the DIS has undergone quite a number of modifications (Compton & Cottler, 2004), eventually becoming the University of Michigan Composite International Diagnostic Interview (UM-CIDI) when it was used in the NCS (Kessler et al., 1994). As indicated by Regier et al. (1998), "Once community-based rates of specific syndromes, defined by explicit research criteria, were shown to be obtainable, relatively small changes in diagnostic criteria (e.g., *DSM-III* to *DSM-III-R*) and methods of ascertainment (e.g., DIS to the University of Michigan [UM], Ann Arbor [CIDI]) have produced substantially different results" (p. 110). The solution proposed by Regier et al. is for researchers in the future to agree to use only one standard instrument, so that more consistent findings are obtained.

However, to the extent that different findings are being provided by different interview schedules, it would appear best to conduct methodological studies of these instruments prior to any arbitrary endorsement of and confinement to one particular interview. Variability of findings across instruments is a compelling reason for instrument research, rather than a reason for neglecting the existence of this variability through the use of only one instrument. Such research might also effectively address the fundamental differences, strengths, and limitations of structured and semistructured interviews.

OPERATIONAL DEFINITIONS

A goal of the authors of *DSM-III* was to develop operational diagnostic criteria such that they would be applied consistently across clinicians (Spitzer, Williams, & Skodol, 1980). In prior editions of the diagnostic manual, "explicit criteria [were] not provided, [and] the clinician [was] largely on his or her own in defining the content boundaries" (APA, 1980, p. 8). Ideally, at least for the authors of *DSM-III,* each symptom would be assessed by one simple, straightforward question (Spitzer, Endicott, & Robins, 1975). To the extent that clinical judgment would be required in interpreting the response to the question, unreliability in assessment was likely to occur. By the time of *DSM-IV,* however, it became evident that operational definitions of diagnostic criteria were unrealistic and may have even compromised validity (Frances, First, & Pincus, 1995).

Frances and colleagues (1995) observe that "reducing the level of clinical inference narrows the construct that the items purportedly represent" (Frances et al., 1995, p. 22). For example, in *DSM-III-R,* antisocial recklessness was operationally defined as simply "driving while intoxicated or recurrent speeding" (APA, 1987, p. 345). This operational definition of recklessness facilitated substantially the obtainment of reliable assessments. However, it is perhaps readily apparent that there are many other ways of demonstrating antisocial recklessness than simply driving while intoxicated or recurrent speeding. Antisocial recklessness would even be impossible to assess in persons who did not possess or have access to a vehicle. Therefore, the authors of *DSM-IV* expanded the criterion to more broadly reflect a more general "reckless disregard for the safety of self and others" (APA, 2000, p. 706) that would (for example) include sexual behavior (e.g., multiple and indiscriminately selected sexual partners without using protection), drug use (e.g., use of dirty needles), and parenting behavior (e.g., leaving children without adequate supervision; Frances et al., 1995; Widiger et al., 1995). The more general criterion, however, now requires a better understanding of its meaning and intention. Its assessment is not so easily conducted by one straightforward question administered by a layperson. On the other hand, to the extent that the question does require inference or judgment, variation increases across interviewers and research sites in the scoring of the responses.

It may not in fact be possible to devise diagnostic criteria so that they can be assessed by one simple question. Structured interviews will need to include multiple questions to address all the various contexts and contingencies that might arise or, instead, semistructured interviews will need to be used that rely more heavily on an informed judgment of a sufficiently well trained interviewer. For example, in *DSM-IV*, substance tolerance can be considered present if a person indicates "a need for markedly increased amounts of the substance to achieve intoxication or desired effect" (APA, 2000, p. 181). This is a reasonable operational definition of tolerance, but it is not a valid indicator in all contexts. For example, studies of alcohol use disorders among adolescents have indicated that persons who needed only low initial quantities to become intoxicated are more likely to report larger percentage increases to obtain the same effect (e.g., an increase from 2 to 5 drinks), whereas those who started off at higher levels generally report lower percentage increases (Chung, Martin, Winters, & Langenbucher, 2001). According to Chung and Martin (2005), "Thus, in rating the presence of tolerance based on a 'marked increase' as defined by *DSM*, the tolerance symptom is frequently assigned to lighter drinkers, and often is not assigned to heavier drinkers" (p. 192). In sum, operational definitions of constructs via one or two specific questions will rarely provide an entirely or always adequate assessment (Cronbach & Meehl, 1955).

Structured interviews improve reliability in the assessment of psychopathology in large part by constructing their own operational definitions of each diagnostic criterion through the specific questions that are provided. Semistructured interviews do this as well, but also by the further training of and instructions provided to the interviewers for the coding of ambiguous responses to more open-ended questions. It is not entirely clear which approach is yielding more valid data. The wording of questions "should neither be so behaviorally specific as to be cumbersome or off the point, nor so inferential as to be unreliable and subject to idiosyncratic uses" (Frances et al., 1995, p. 220). The optimal balance is not really clear.

Both methods, structured and semistructured interviews, decrease the opportunity for disagreement among interviewers in the assessment of symptoms by requiring that each interview use a particular set of questions and follow specified guidelines for the interpretation of the answers to these questions. In the end, these questions and instructions act as operational definitions of the respective diagnostic criteria. It is then possible that each interview schedule itself represents a modified version of the diagnostic manual. It then becomes useful, if not important, to determine whether alternative interviews are providing sufficiently convergent and valid assessments.

It is important to appreciate, however, that an interest in comparing interview schedules with respect to how they are operationalizing symptomatology is not a criticism of semistructured or even structured interviews. It is true that structured interviews may at times use a wording that is ineffective, if not invalid, in the effort to develop a behaviorally specific assessment that can be administered by a lay interviewer. However, the solution to this problem is not simply to convert to an unstructured interview administered by a professional clinician. The sophisticated clinician is more likely to use good clinical judgment when faced with an unanticipated situation or a problematic wording (Westen, 1997). However, the absence of structure will complicate substantially the ability to determine empirically when this "wisdom" is in fact occurring. It is at least feasible with fully structured interviews to identify the specific source of invalidity and study empirically the precise effect of alternative wording. In contrast, one might not even know the questions that were being administered within an unstructured interview.

Normative Data

A significant advantage of self-report inventories relative to semistructured interviews is the ability to administer the inventories to substantial numbers of persons at relatively little cost. As a result, manuals for self-report inventories typically report quite a bit of normative data that facilitate substantially the interpretation of test scores, as well as a considerable amount of data that lend empirical support to the validity of the instrument. In stark contrast, such information is strikingly weak, if not absent, in the manuals of many semistructured interviews (Rogers, 2001; Widiger, 2001).

It is not entirely clear why this is the case. One reason may simply be the labor-intensive nature of a semistructured interview data collection. Compelling normative data are available for structured interviews used in national and multinational epidemiological studies. The cost of a comparable administration of a semistructured interview to sufficiently large and representative samples to obtain normative data is prohibitive. However, another possible reason is the assumption that assessments provided by clinical interviews are generally accepted at face value rather than being compared with a distribution of scores obtained from a normative sample. *DSM-IV* diagnoses are not based on a deviation from a normative mean score, as is typically done with many self-report inventories (Ben-Porath, 2003). It appears to be the case that semistructured interviews are presumed to be providing a valid assessment if the respective diagnostic criteria for a disorder are systematically assessed. Much of the research concerning the etiology, pathology, and treatment of mental disorders is based on data obtained with structured or semistructured interviews. What is considered to be known about the epidemiology for most mental disorders is based largely on the findings obtained with fully structured interviews administered by laypersons (e.g., Grant et al., 2004), not the information obtained with self-report inventories.

Nevertheless, it would be useful for the test manuals of semistructured and structured interviews to provide as much normative data as is available for that instrument. For example, it would be useful for clinicians and researchers administering the SCID-I (First, Gibbon, Spitzer, & Williams, 1996) within a particular clinical setting to be able to compare the results they obtained with those typically obtained in comparable settings. One could then at least know whether the findings one has obtained deviate in any remarkable or meaningful way from the findings that would be expected to be obtained within that setting. These data are, of course, readily present for the fully structured interviews (e.g., DIS and AUDADIS-IV) that have been used in large-scale epidemiological research.

It would additionally be useful for semistructured and structured interview manuals to provide supportive validity data, including correlations with a variety of self-report inventories. Diagnoses obtained through the administration of a semistructured interview are used as the criterion with which the validity of self-report inventories and other assessment instruments are evaluated (Kaye & Shea, 2000; Zimmerman, 2003), but semistructured interviews themselves might be relying too heavily on simple face validity for their own derivation (Farmer, 2000; Segal & Coolidge, 2003). In any case, information concerning the convergent (and discriminant) validity of a structured or a semistructured interview would appear to be appropriate and useful to provide within the test manual.

Validity Scales

It is common in the administration of a self-report inventory to consider and assess for the possibility of intentional or unintentional over- or underreporting of symptoms (Ben-Porath, 2003). This should perhaps also be a concern in studies of treatment outcome, where patients (and clinicians) might be expected at times to be biased somewhat in favor of underreporting of symptoms at the end of treatment. Quite a bit of research has in fact been conducted on the assessment and impact of response styles and biases of test respondents (Berry, Baer, Rinaldo, & Wetter, 2002). Most self-report inventories administered to clinical samples include "validity" scales to assess for systematic willful or habitual distortions in self-description. In stark contrast, most semistructured and structured interviews expend little effort on addressing this concern (Rogers, 2001), and few treatment outcome studies include an assessment (via interview) of the extent to which a respondent might have been denying or understating symptomatology. Rogers (1997), however, has provided data on the use of the SADS to evaluate patients who are minimizing their reporting of symptoms, and he and his colleagues conclude: "Among diagnostic interviews, the SADS has the best developed strategies in screening for potential malingering and defensiveness" (Rogers, Jackson, & Cashel, 2004, p. 144).

There are perhaps a number of reasons that interviews (structured, semi-structured, or unstructured) do not include validity scales. One reason is that most semistructured and unstructured interviews do not rely simply on the self-report or opinions of the respondents. Many of the questions are probes that attempt to elicit the respective symptom or behavior that is being assessed. The interviewer does not simply ask the respondent if the symptom is present but may instead ask suggestive or leading questions that are attempting to elicit, provoke, or stimulate an expression of the symptom. However, structured interviews, relative to semistructured interviews, do tend to rely more heavily on a direct and obvious inquiry as to the presence of symptomatology. Interviews administered by laypersons tend not to rely on the observations of the interviewer to determine the presence of symptoms. As a result, it would not seem to be too hard to deceive a lay interviewer through symptom denial or exaggeration. Yet, there has in fact been little to no research on the susceptibility of structured or semistructured interviews to faking.

It is possible that researchers are presuming that interviewers are sufficiently skilled at detecting symptom denial or exaggeration. One major reason that interviews are preferred over self-report inventories is the ability to have someone other than the patient determine the presence or absence of the symptomatology, preferably a skilled clinician who is capable of detecting symptom denial or exaggeration. This might, however, be a somewhat idealized view of the skills of an interviewer, particularly when laypersons are employed (Rogers, 1997, 2001).

It is also possible that a lack of attention reflects an assumption that respondents are unlikely to be exaggerating or denying symptoms to any meaningful degree. However, in the absence of any research to support this assumption, it is perhaps unwise to assume that it is valid. Estimates of malingering are as high as 27% within psychiatric inpatient settings and 19% of Veterans Administration medical patient settings (Berry et al., 2002). It might be useful for future studies to estimate the prevalence of symptom denial at treatment termination.

◼ Conclusions

Clinical interviews are perhaps the generally preferred method for the assessment of psychopathology. Clinical interviews help ensure that a valid assessment is being conducted by facilitating a patient's engagement in the process of assessment, by resolving ambiguities and confusion in the wording of questions, and by addressing through follow-up queries situational or unanticipated complexities. It appears that validity of assessment generally increases as the degree of interview structure increases, although the degree of structure that is necessary to provide the optimally valid assessment is not entirely clear. Additional methodological research is necessary to determine empirically whether it is preferable to use structured or semistructured interviews, to study for the specific impact of alternative wording of structured interview questions, and to determine whether symptom denial is problematic in the assessment of treatment outcome.

■ References

American Psychiatric Association. (1980). *Diagnostic and statistical manual of mental disorders* (3rd ed.). Washington, DC: Author.

American Psychiatric Association. (1987). *Diagnostic and statistical manual of mental disorders* (3rd ed., rev.). Washington, DC: Author.

American Psychiatric Association. (2000). *Diagnostic and statistical manual of mental disorders* (4th ed., text rev.). Washington, DC: Author.

Antony, M. M., & Rowa, K. (2005). Evidence-based assessment of anxiety disorder in adults. *Psychological Assessment, 17,* 256–266.

Barbour, K. A., & Davison, G. C. (2004). Clinical interviewing. In S. N. Haynes, E. M. Heiby, & M. Hersen (Eds.), *Comprehensive handbook of psychological assessment: Vol. 3. Behavioral assessment* (pp. 181–193). New York: Wiley.

Behar, E. S., & Borkovec, T. D. (2003). Psychotherapy outcome research. In J. A. Schinka, W. F. Velicer, & I. B. Weiner (Eds.), *Handbook of psychology: Vol. 2. Research methods in psychology* (pp. 213–240). New York: Wiley.

Ben-Porath, Y. S. (2003). Assessing personality and psychopathology with self-report inventories. In J. R. Graham, J. A. Naglieri, & I. B. Weiner (Eds.), *Handbook of psychology: Vol. 10. Assessment psychology* (pp. 553–577). New York: Wiley.

Berry, T. R., Baer, R. A., Rinaldo, J. C., & Wetter, M. W. (2002). Assessment of malingering. In J. N. Butcher (Ed.), *Clinical personality assessment: Practical approaches* (2nd ed., pp. 269–302). [CITY]: Springer.

Birmaher, B., Axelson, D., Strober, M., Gill, M-K., Valeri, S., Chiappetta, L., et al. (2006). Clinical course of children and adolescents with bipolar spectrum disorders. *Archives of General Psychiatry, 63,* 175–183.

Brown, T. A., Di Nardo, P. A., Lehman, C. L., & Campbell, L. A. (2001). Reliability of *DSM-IV* anxiety and mood disorders: Implications for the classification of emotional disorders. *Journal of Abnormal Psychology, 110,* 49–58.

Campbell, D. T., & Fiske, D. W. (1959). Convergent and discriminant validation by the multitrait-multimethod matrix. *Psychological Bulletin, 56,* 81–105.

Chung, T., & Martin, C. S. (2005). What were they thinking? Adolescents' interpretations of *DSM-IV* alcohol dependence symptom queries and implications for diagnostic validity. *Drug and Alcohol Dependence, 80,* 191–200.

Chung, T., Martin, C. S., Winters, K. C., & Langenbucher, J. W. (2001). Assessment of alcohol tolerance in adolescents. *Journal of Studies on Alcohol, 62,* 687–695.

Clark, L. A., & Harrison, J. A. (2001). Assessment instruments. In W. J. Livesley (Ed.), *Handbook of personality disorders: Theory, research, and treatment* (pp. 277–306). New York: Guilford.

Compton, W. M., & Cottler, L. B. (2004). The Diagnostic Interview Schedule (DIS). In M. J. Hilsenroth, D. L. Segal, & M. Hersen (Eds.), *Comprehensive handbook of psychological assessment: Vol. 2. Personality assessment* (pp. 153–162). New York: Wiley.

Craig, R. J. (2003). Assessing personality and psychopathology with interviews. In J. R. Graham, J. A. Naglieri, & I. B. Weiner (Eds.), *Handbook of psychology: Vol. 10. Assessment psychology* (pp. 487–508). New York: Wiley.

Craig, R. J. (Ed.). (2005). *Clinical and diagnostic interviewing* (2nd ed.). New York: Aronson.

Cronbach, L. J., & Meehl, P. E. (1955). Construct validity in psychological tests. *Psychological Bulletin, 52,* 281–302.

Di Nardo, P. A., Brown, T. A., & Barlow, D. H. (1994). *Anxiety Disorders Interview Schedule for DSM-IV: Lifetime version (ADIS-IV-L).* San Antonio, TX: Psychological Corporation.

Eid, M., & Diener, E. (2006). Introduction: The need for multimethod measurement in psychology. In M. Eid & E. Diener (Eds.), *Handbook of multimethod measurement in psychology* (pp. 3–8). Washington, DC: American Psychological Association.

Farmer, R. F. (2000). Issues in the assessment and conceptualization of personality disorders. *Clinical Psychology Review, 20,* 823–852.

First, M., & Gibbon, M. (2004). The Structured Clinical Interview for *DSM-IV* Axis I Disorders (SCID-I) and the Structured Clinical Interview for *DSM-IV* Axis II Disorders (SCID-II). In M. J. Hilsenroth, D. L. Segal, & M. Hersen (Eds.), *Comprehensive handbook of psychological assessment: Vol. 2. Personality assessment* (pp. 134–143). New York: Wiley.

First, M., Gibbon, M., Spitzer, R. L., Williams, J. B.W., & Benjamin, L. S. (1997). *User's guide for the Structured Clinical Interview for DSM-IV Axis II Personality Disorders.* Washington, DC: American Psychiatric Press.

First, M. B., Gibbon, M., Spitzer, R. L., & Williams, J. B.W. (1996). *User's guide for the Structured Clinical Interview for DSM-IV Axis I Disorders-Research Version (SCID-I).* Washington, DC: American Psychiatric Press.

Frances, A. J., First, M. B., & Pincus, H. A. (1995). *DSM-IV guidebook.* Washington, DC: American Psychiatric Press.

Garb, H. (2005). Clinical judgment and decision making. *Annual Review of Clinical Psychology, 1,* 67–89.

Grant, B. F., Dawson, D. A., Stinson, F. S., Chou, P. S., Kay, W., & Pickering, R. (2003). The Alcohol Use Disorder and Associated Disabilities Interview Schedule–IV (AUDADIS-IV): Reliability of alcohol consumption, tobacco use, family history of depression and psychiatric diagnostic modules in a general population sample. *Drug and Alcohol Dependence, 71,* 7–16.

Grant, B. F., Stinson, F. S., Dawson, D. A., Chou, S. P., Ruan, W. J., & Pickering, R. P. (2004). Co-occurrence of 12-month alcohol and drug use disorders and personality disorders in the United States: Results from the National Epidemiologic Survey on Alcohol and Related Conditions. *Archives of General Psychiatry, 61,* 361–368.

Grisham, J. R.,. Brown, T. A., & Campbell, L. A. (2004). The Anxiety Disorder Interview Schedule for *DSM-IV* (ADIS-IV). In M. J. Hilsenroth, D. L. Segal, & M. Hersen (Eds.), *Comprehensive handbook of psychological assessment: Vol. 2. Personality assessment* (pp. 163–177). New York: Wiley.

Gunderson, J. G., Shea, M. T., Skodol, A. E., McGlashan, T. H., Morey, L. C., Stout, R. L., et al. (2000). The Collaborative Longitudinal Personality Disorders Study, I: Development, aims, design, and sample characteristics. *Journal of Personality Disorders, 14,* 300–315.

Joiner, T. E., Walker, R. L., Pettit, J. W., Perez, M., & Cukrowicz, K. C. (2005). Evidence-based assessment of depression in adults. *Psychological Assessment, 17,* 267–277.

Kaye, A. L., & Shea, M. T. (2000). Personality disorders, personality traits, and defense mechanisms measures. In A. John Rush, American Psychiatric Association, and Task Force on the Handbook of Psychiatric Measures, eds., *Handbook of psychiatric measures* (pp. 713–749). Washington, DC: American Psychiatric Association.

Keller, M., Lavori, P., Friedman, B., Nielsen, E., Endicott, J., & McDonald-Scott, P. (1987). The Longitudinal Interval Follow-Up Evaluation: A comprehensive method for assessing outcome in prospective longitudinal studies. *Archives of General Psychiatry, 44,* 540–548.

Kessler, R. C., McGonagle, K. A., Zhao, S., Nelson, C. B., Hughes, M., Eshleman, S., et al. (1994). Lifetime and 12-month prevalence of *DSM-III-R* psychiatric disorders in the United States: Results from the National Comorbidity Survey. *Archives of General Psychiatry, 51,* 8–19.

Kirk, S. A., & Kutchins, H. (1992). *The selling of DSM: The rhetoric of science in psychiatry.* New York: Aldine de Gruyter.

Lambert, M. J., & Hawkins, E. J. (2004). Use of psychological tests for assessing treatment outcomes. In M. E. Maruish (Ed.), *The use of psychological testing for treatment planning and outcome assessment: Vol. 1. General considerations* (3rd ed., pp. 171–195). Mahwah, NJ: Erlbaum.

Loranger, A. W. (1999). *International Personality Disorder Examination (IPDE).* Odessa, FL: Psychological Assessment Resources.

Morey, L. C. (2003). Measuring personality and psychopathology. In J. A. Schinka, W. F. Velicer, & I. B. Weiner (Eds.), *Handbook of psychology: Vol. 2. Research methods in psychology* (pp. 377–405). New York: Wiley.

Nathan, P. E., & Langenbucher, J. W. (1999). Psychopathology: Description and classification. *Annual Review of Psychology, 50,* 79–107.

O'Boyle, M., & Self, D. (1990). A comparison of two interviews for *DSM-III-R* personality disorders. *Psychiatry Research, 32,* 85–92.

Ogles, B. M., Lambert, M. J., & Fields, S. A. (2002). *Essentials of outcome assessment.* Hoboken, NJ: Wiley.

Regier, D. A., Kaelber, C. T., Rae, D. S., Farmer, M. E., Knauper, B., Kessler, R. C., et al. (1998). Limitations of diagnostic criteria and assessment instruments for mental disorders: Implications for research and policy. *Archives of General Psychiatry, 55,* 109–115.

Robins, L. N., Helzer, J. E., Croughan, J., & Ratcliff, K. (1981). National Institute of Mental Health Diagnostic Interview Schedule: Its history, characteristics, and validity. *Archives of General Psychiatry, 38,* 381–389.

Robins, L. N., & Regier, D. A. (Eds.). (1991). *Psychiatric disorders in America: The epidemiologic catchment area study.* New York: Free Press.

Rogers, R. (2001). *Diagnostic and structured interviewing: A handbook for clinical practice.* (2nd ed.). New York: Guilford.

Rogers, R. (2003). Standardizing *DSM-IV* diagnoses: The clinical applications of structured interviews. *Journal of Personality Assessment, 81,* 220–225.

Rogers, R. (1997). *Clinical assessment of malingering and deception* (2nd ed.). New York: Guilford.

Rogers, R., Jackson, R. L., & Cashel, M. (2004). The Schedule for Affective Disorders and Schizophrenia (SADS). In M. J. Hilsenroth, D. L. Segal, & M. Hersen (Eds.), *Comprehensive handbook of psychological assessment: Vol. 2. Personality assessment* (pp. 144–152). New York: Wiley.

Rounsaville, B. J., Alarcon, R. D., Andrews, G., Jackson, J. S., Kendell, R. E., & Kendler, K. (2002). Basic nomenclature issues for *DSM-V.* In D. J. Kupfer, M. B. First, & D. E. Regier (Eds.), *A research agenda for DSM-V* (pp. 1–29). Washington, DC: American Psychiatric Association.

Rush, A. J., Pincus, H. A., First, M. B., Blacker, D., Endicott, J., Keith, S. J., et al. (Eds.). (2000). *Handbook of psychiatric measures.* Washington, DC: American Psychiatric Association.

Segal, D. L., & Coolidge, F. L. (2003). Structured interviewing and *DSM* classification. In M. Hersen & S. Turner (Eds.), *Adult psychopathology and diagnosis* (4th ed., pp. 13–26). New York: Wiley.

Shedler, J. (2002). A new language for psychoanalytic diagnosis. *Journal of the American Psychoanalytic Association, 50,* 429–456.

Skodol, A. E., Oldham, J. M., Rosnick, L., Kellman, H. D., & Hyler, S. E. (1991). Diagnosis of *DSM-III-R* personality disorders: A comparison of two structured interviews. *International Journal of Methods in Psychiatric Research, 1,* 13–26.

Spitzer, R. L., & Endicott, J. (1978). *Schedule for affective disorders and schizophrenia* (3rd ed.). New York: Biometrics Research.

Spitzer, R. L., Endicott, J., & Robins, E. (1975). Clinical criteria for psychiatric diagnosis and *DSM-III. American Journal of Psychiatry, 132,* 1187–1192.

Spitzer, R. L., Williams, J. B.W., & Skodol, A. E. (1980). DSM-III: The major achievements and an overview. *American Journal of Psychiatry, 137,* 151–164.

Summerfeldt, L. J., & Antony, M. M. (2002). Structured and semistructured diagnostic interviews. In M. M. Antony & D. H. Barlow (Eds.), *Handbook of assessment, treatment planning, and outcome for psychological disorders* (pp. 3–37). New York: Guilford.

Trull, T. J. (2001). Structural relations between borderline personality disorder features and putative etiological correlates. *Journal of Abnormal Psychology, 110,* 471–481.

Watkins, C. E., Campbell, V. L., Nieberding, R., & Hallmark, R. (1995). Contemporary practice of psychological assessment by clinical psychologists. *Professional Psychology: Research and Practice, 26,* 54–60.

Westen, D. (1997). Divergences between clinical and research methods for assessing personality disorders: Implications for research and the evolution of Axis II. *American Journal of Psychiatry, 154,* 895–903.

Westen, D., & Shedler, J. (1999). Revising and assessing Axis II, Part I: Developing a clinically and empirically valid assessment method. *American Journal of Psychiatry, 156,* 258–272.

Widiger, T. A. (2001). Structured Clinical Interview for *DSM-IV* Axis I disorders–Clinician Version. In J. Impara & B. Plake (Eds.), *The mental measurements yearbook* (pp. 1191–1193). Lincoln, NE: Buros Institute of Mental Measurements.

Widiger, T. A. (2002). Personality disorders. In M. M. Antony & D. H. Barlow (Eds.), *Handbook of assessment, treatment planning, and outcome for psychological disorders* (pp. 453–480). New York: Guilford.

Widiger, T. A., & Clark, L. A. (2000). Toward DSM-V and the classification of psychopathology. *Psychological Bulletin, 126,* 946–963.

Widiger, T. A., Mangine, S., Corbitt, E. M., Ellis, C. G., & Thomas, G. V. (1995). *Personality Disorder Interview–IV. A semistructured interview for the assessment of personality disorders. Professional manual.* Odessa, FL: Psychological Assessment Resources.

Widiger, T. A., & Samuel, D. B. (2005). Evidence-based assessment of personality disorders. *Psychological Assessment, 17,* 278–287.

Wood, J. M., Garb, H. N., Lilienfeld, S. O., & Nezworski, M. T. (2002). Clinical assessment. *Annual Review of Psychology, 53,* 519–543.

Zanarini, M. C., & Frankenburg, F. R. (2001). Attainment and maintenance of reliability of Axis I and Axis II disorders over the course of a longitudinal study. *Comprehensive Psychiatry, 42,* 369–374.

Zanarini, M. C., Frankenburg, F. R., Chauncey, D. L., & Gunderson, J. G. (1987). The Diagnostic Interview for Personality Disorders: Interrater and test-retest reliability. *Comprehensive Psychiatry, 28,* 467–480.

Zimmerman, M. (2003). What should the standard of care for psychiatric diagnostic evaluations be? *Journal of Nervous and Mental Disease, 191,* 281–286.

Zimmerman, M., & Mattia, J. I. (1999). Psychiatric diagnosis in clinical practice: Is comorbidity being missed? *Comprehensive Psychiatry, 40,* 182–191.

4. BEHAVIORAL ASSESSMENT

Stephen N. Haynes, Joseph Keawe'aimoku Kaholokula,
and Dawn T. Yoshioka

■ The Role of Assessment in Treatment Research

Treatment research is designed to estimate (a) the effectiveness of a treatment, (b) the effectiveness of a treatment relative to other treatments, (c) the treatment components that most strongly affect outcome, (d) the time course of treatment effects, (e) treatment side effects, (f) the cost-benefits of a treatment, (g) the generalizability and transportability of a treatment across treatment settings, (h) the duration of treatment effects (i.e., time to, and probability of, relapse), (i) the variables that affect posttreatment lapse and relapse, (j) the mechanisms that account for treatment effects, (k) the incremental benefits of basing treatment on case formulations, and (l) the individual differences that affect treatment outcome.

The results of treatment research are strongly affected by research designs, which are well articulated in this volume and described by Kazdin (2002) and Kendall, Butcher, and Holmbeck (1999). These sources discuss the importance of research design factors such as sampling strategies (e.g., Minke & Haynes, 2003), interrupted time series measurement (e.g., Kratochwill & Levin, 1992), and the many threats to internal and external validity.

This chapter focuses on a fundamental component of treatment research: *assessment.*[1] We discuss the best measurement strategies in treatment research and the rationale for those strategies. In treatment research, assessment is the application of the science of measurement to describe, predict, explain, and guide the process and outcome of treatment. Essentially, we measure changes in variables and how these changes are related to other variables. Measures that are valid, precise, and sensitive to change are necessary to draw valid inferences about treatment effects, the relative contributions of treatment components, the role of moderator variables, the side effects of treatment, and causal mechanisms underlying treatment effects. Invalid or imprecise measures will lead to invalid and imprecise inferences in treatment research. Ultimately, invalid assessment limits the development of effective treatments.

One system of psychological assessment with methods particularly amenable to the valid measurement of change is behavioral assessment. Behavioral assessment methods are frequently used in treatment research. Haynes and O'Brien (2000) documented the frequent use of observation methods, self-monitoring, self-report questionnaires, and interviews across a 30-year span of treatment research. For this chapter, we supplemented these data by examining the frequency with which behavioral assessment methods have been used in treatment outcome research published in two major journals: *Journal of Consulting and Clinical Psychology (JCCP)* between the years 2000 and 2006 and *Behavior Therapy* for the years 2004 and 2005. In these years (including only one issue of *JCCP* in 2006) the number of treatment outcome studies that used a behavioral assessment method was as follows: analogue observation: 27; observation in the natural environment: 13; self-monitoring: 38; focused self-report questionnaire: 229 (almost every treatment research article), psychophysiological assessment: 68; and behavior problem checklists: 61. Many studies measured important variables with multiple assessment instruments, and some used multiple assessment methods.

The main goal of this chapter is to discuss the role of behavioral assessment in treatment research. We will examine how behavioral assessment strategies are adaptable to the goals of treatment research, congruent with principles of measurement, and appropriate given the characteristics of behavior disorders and their causes. We suggest that behavioral assessment strategies can provide valid, sensitive, precise, and clinically useful data to guide judgments about treatment research. At the end of the chapter, we offer a guide for the behavioral assessment in treatment outcome research.

In our discussions of behavioral assessment in treatment research, we assume the reader has a basic background in behavioral assessment, treatment research design, and psychometry. In-depth discussions of these topics can be found in Haynes and O'Brien (2000), Haynes and Heiby (2003), Hersen (2006), Kazdin (2006), and Nunnally and Bernstein (1994).

■ What Are the Assessment Goals in Treatment Research?

Assessment strategies used in treatment research should be congruent with the goals of the research, such as evaluating the incremental benefits of case formulation, estimating the comparative effectiveness of different treatments, or identifying moderators of treatment outcome. One of the advantages of behavioral assessment is that it is composed of a set of methods that can be adapted to different assessment goals. Among these methods are observation in natural and analogue environments, self-monitoring, ambulatory psychophysiological assessment, behavior rating scales, and product-of-behavior methods. Thus, a researcher can select the method that is best suited for the specific goals of the treatment research.

Table 4.1 provides an overview of some major goals of treatment research and the behavioral assessment strategy that is congruent with each goal. Note that the measurement of "change" is a focus of all goals.

TABLE 4.1
Treatment Goals and Their Associated Assessment Strategies

Treatment goal	Description/example	Behavioral assessment strategy
Estimate *effect size, comparative effects,* and *clinical significance*	The primary goals of treatment research are to estimate the strength of effects of a treatment, the comparative effects of more than one treatment, and the degree to which treatment-related changes occur to a clinically significant degree. For between-group and single-subject research, effects are estimated by comparing pre- and posttreatment changes in the context of pretreatment variance across groups or across time and the degree to which posttreatment measures approximate those of nonclinical samples.	Assessment should include *multiple methods* that provide measures validated for the characteristics of the sample (e.g., age, ethnicity), using assessment strategies that *minimize alternative explanations,* such as regression to the mean, carryover effects, practice, or reactive effects. The *specific effects* (see next section) are also important foci and mandate the use of narrowly focused instruments.
Identify *individual differences* in response to treatment and *moderator* variables	The clinical utility of treatment research is estimated by examining individual differences in response to a treatment and the variables that affect those differences. Such data facilitate treatment decisions with individual clients and increase the probability of clinically significant effects. Moderator variables do not "explain" treatment effects but affect them. They often are treated as challenges to positive treatment outcome.	Assessment and data-analytic strategies should include measures of potential *moderator variables.* Examples of treatment moderator variables amenable to behavioral assessment include social support, comorbid behavior problems, causal attributions, and response contingencies.

continued

TABLE 4.1 (*continued*)

Treatment goal	Description/example	Behavioral assessment strategy
Describe the *time course* of treatment effects and identify treatment failures	A time course of treatment effects is treatment-outcome measures (or measures of side or collateral effects) plotted across time. Time-course plots of treatment effects are useful for estimating cost-benefits associated with additional treatment sessions (*i.e. dose-response relations*).	Measures of potential outcome variables should be collected frequently, at a rate that reflects the *dynamic nature of the behavior problems.*
Identify *treatment mechanisms* and effective *components* of effective treatment	Treatment mechanisms are the processes that account for treatment effects. They address the "why" and "how" of treatment effects: e.g., "Why do exposure treatments result in decreased anxiety responses to feared stimuli for some persons?" Such data can lead to more powerful and efficient treatments.	Assessment strategies should include measures of variables that might mediate treatment effects, such as cognitive processes, response contingencies, changes in the social environment, and neurophysiological events.
Examine the *relative cost-benefits* of a treatment and its outcome	Cost-benefits of a treatment are ratios of treatment effects as a function of costs, usually in terms of client and therapist time. Two or more treatments can be compared on their relative cost-benefits.	Assessment should include cost variables, such as time for assessment, consultation, planning, data management, report writing, and sessions, in addition to data on main and collateral effects. Benefit data can include days of work missed, medication use, and number of physician visits.

continued

TABLE 4.1 (*continued*)

Treatment goal	Description/example	Behavioral assessment strategy
Identify the effects of a treatment on the specific components of a behavior disorder	As we note in a subsequent section, most behavior problems are composed of complex arrays of response systems and symptoms, and it is important to identify the degree to which they are differentially affected by a treatment.	Because of its diverse methods and emphasis on highly specific measures, behavioral assessment is well suited to multimodal assessment and assessment of specific symptoms.

Table 4.1 is only a sample of treatment research goals, but it demonstrates the flexible set of behavioral assessment methods that are differentially useful across these goals. Although there are firm conceptual foundations of behavioral assessment (see Haynes & O'Brien, 2000; Haynes & Heiby, 2003), it is also a methodologically based assessment strategy that emphasizes the following:

- The use of multiple methods of assessment
- The selection of assessment methods on the basis of the goals of a particular assessment context
- The acquisition of data using time series measurement strategies
- The use of assessment instruments that focus on highly specific, well-defined, and minimally inferential variables
- A focus on functional relations among overt behavior, cognitive, emotional, and physiological variables, and events in the natural environment

■ What Do We Know About Principles of Measurement and Assessment?

In behavioral assessment we measure attributes of behavior and environmental events to help us understand their changes across time and the variables that influence those changes.[2] The validity of our conclusions about change depends on the degree to which the numbers assigned to them accurately reflect the attributes. If our pre- to posttreatment assessment data indicate a 25% reduction in a person's blood pressure following treatment, or in the number of a person's panic episodes, to what degree do those data accurately reflect true changes in those attributes?

There are many sources of error in measures and in the inferences derived from those measures. Examples include blood pressure measures that can be affected by movement and posture, self-reports of past moods that can reflect the current mood of the respondent, an observer who can miss critical comments in an argument between spouses, or an investigator who can overstate the clinical significance of treatment-related changes. Thus, a primary goal of treatment research is to use assessment strategies that maximize the ratio of true variance to error variance in obtained measures, and psychometry provides the guiding principles to approximate that goal.

The psychometric foundations of behavioral assessment have been discussed by Cone (1998), Haynes and O'Brien (2000), Haynes, Nelson, and Blaine (1999), Haynes (2006), Silva (1994), and Suen and Rzasa (2004). In this chapter we sample a few of the many relevant psychometric principles in behavioral assessment.

First, it is important to estimate the *accuracy* of measures within a treatment study and to then employ strategies that maximize accuracy. Behavioral assessment often involves the measurement of specific, narrowly defined events and attributes as primary targets, in contrast to other assessment paradigms that consider measures as markers of higher level constructs (e.g., personality traits). Sometimes we want to know whether a treatment changes the frequency of drug use by an adolescent, how often family members have arguments, or the rate of positive social behaviors of a psychiatric inpatient. In these examples, we are concerned with the *accuracy* of our measures, which is a form of *validity* that often requires the use of a "gold standard" criterion.

To increase confidence in the accuracy of measures, treatment studies should use *multiple measures* of important variables. One common method of estimating accuracy of measures is to use more than one observer or source of data, then examine the degree of covariance between the measures. Ultimately, accuracy estimates, based on covariances among multiple measures of the same variable, affect our confidence in the validity of our inferences in treatment research. In the absence of multiple measures of important variables within a treatment study, one cannot be confident in the degree to which measures reflect true rather than error variance. With the use of only one measure of an important variable in treatment research, confidence in the results will be attenuated. As we note elsewhere, the use of multiple measures of a precise, narrowly defined construct can also reduce the unique error variance of each measure when aggregated.

The *conditional nature of validity* is also an important consideration in designing assessment strategies in treatment research. The validity of a measure can vary across assessment contexts, such as assessment settings, states of the client at the time of assessment, age, and ethnicity. For example, the validity of measures from ambulatory heart rate monitors is inversely related to the level of physical activity at the time of measurement. Validity coefficients are high at low levels of activity but low at high levels of activity (Terbizan, Dolezal, & Albano, 2002), which is often a goal in aerobic fitness interventions. Consequently, treatment researchers should remember that *validity is not a generalizable characteristic of a measure.*

What do these guiding principles mean for behavioral assessment in treatment research? They mean that researchers should always use *multiple measures of main assessment targets and should use measures that have been previously validated in the context relevant to their study.* Researchers should be sure that the measures selected are the best available for the sex, age, ethnicity, level of severity, state of the client, and goals and other contexts of the assessment.

Another guiding principle for assessment in treatment research is to select measures that *minimize alternative explanations of change* in order to separate error and true variance and to maximize confidence in the results. A major threat to the specificity of inferences is the use of measures that are composed of multiple facets. It is important to specify what attributes and dimensions (a *dimension* refers to a quantifiable aspect, such as the frequency, duration, and intensity of an attribute) of what particular behaviors and events are important to measure in the treatment research and to then select instruments that measure them as precisely as possible. Rather than (or in addition to) using aggregated measures of treatment outcome, such as personality trait measures, measures should focus on the elements of the trait that are important—for example, specific social attributions, specific behaviors in specific social situations, specific environmental events associated with fear or self-injury. Narrowly focused measures will allow the researcher to make more confident inferences about the specific effects of treatment. With more aggregated measures, such as scale scores from many multielement questionnaires, it is difficult to attribute change to specific elements in the aggregate.

Although there is a strong focus on variables as samples rather than signs in behavioral assessment (Suen & Rzasa, 2004), measures are sometimes used as indicators of *latent variables,* which are unobservable theoretical constructs, such as depression, anxiety, coercion, neuroticism, and stress. Variance in latent variables is inferred from multiple indicators, such as summated responses on a questionnaire. For depression, as an example, indicators would include sleep efficiency, motor activity, and expectations about the future. Inferences about latent variables have additional sources of error because individual items or elements of the measure can vary in the degree to which they are relevant to the targeted latent variable. For example, a questionnaire designed to measure depression might erroneously include items that measure anxiety.

The psychometric principles that guide measures of latent variables in treatment research are the same as those that guide more specific measures of behaviors and events. To increase the validity of these measures and their contingent inferences, it is necessary to use *multiple sources and methods.* For example, in measures of post–traumatic stress disorder (PTSD), we can increase the amount of true variance by *aggregating* data from multiple informants, such as reports from family members and coworkers, assessor's observations, and psychophysiological indices. Aggregation can reduce idiosyncratic sources of error associated with individual measures when the elements of the aggregate are valid indicators without high levels of covariance or shared method variance.

It is also important in treatment outcome research to use measures with a high degree of *content validity*—the degree to which the elements of an instrument are relevant to and representative of the targeted constructs and assessment goals (Haynes, Richard, & Kubany, 1995; Haynes & O'Brien, 2000). Haynes and O'Brien (2000) outlined methods of increasing the content and other aspects of validity in assessment strategies:

- Use assessment instruments that are validated for the population, situation, and purpose for which they are being applied.
- Use assessment instruments that are congruent with the goals of the assessment; that is, they should specifically measure the behaviors and variables that are most important and provide information of greatest use for the clinical judgments that must be made.
- Measure all important dependent and independent variables.
- Measure the most important dimensions and facets of the behavior problems and causal variables.
- Use multiple methods of assessment.
- Gather data from multiple informants.
- Use instruments that are sensitive to the dynamic aspects of behavior problems and causal variables.
- Measure behavior in the most relevant settings.
- Use instruments that include elements that are relevant to and representative of the targeted constructs.

Finally, whenever possible, observe behaviors directly rather than, or in addition to, relying on subjective reports about behavior. If you are interested in changes in the dyadic communication patterns in a distressed marriage, observe how the couple tries to solve a problem in their relationship; if you are measuring changes in parenting strategies, observe parent-child interactions in a clinic or at home; and if you are interested in changes in psychophysiological reactivity of a person with an anxiety disorder, use ambulatory biosensors. While all these methods are accompanied by idiosyncratic and important sources of variance, they avoid many of the errors associated with self-reports, such as retrospective recall and selective memory biases (see the special section on self-monitoring in *Psychological Assessment* [Cone, 1999]).

■ What Do We Know About Behavior Problems?

In the previous section we provided a few examples of how psychometric principles guide behavioral assessment strategies in treatment research. Assessment strategies for treatment research are also guided by assumptions about the nature of behavior problems. For example, persons seeking help for a behavior problem often have *multiple behavior problems* with *multiple response systems* and *dimensions* that can change over time and across settings. Thus, the best assessment strategies for treatment research are those that can capture these complex characteristics of behavior problems.

In this section, we discuss several assumptions about the nature of behavior problems and how they affect behavioral assessment strategies in treatment outcome research. Table 4.2 summarizes these assumptions.

Several characteristics of behavior problems outlined in Table 4.2 are illustrated in Figure 4.1. A person can have multiple behavior problems, behavior problems can differ in their important dimensions, behavior problems are dynamic, clients with the same behavior problem can respond differently to treatment, and different behavior problems for the same client can respond differently to treatment.

Multiple Behavior Problems

People seeking help for behavior problems often have multiple or *comorbid* behavior problems (Biederman et al., 2005), as illustrated in Figure 4.1. Studies have found that 51% of adolescents and 59% of adults with anxiety-related disorders have comorbid psychiatric disorders, such as depression (Bassiony, 2005; Essau, 2003). Among people with an eating disorder, 49% also have a personality disorder (Ilkjaer et al., 2004). People seeking help can also have multiple behavior problems that do not meet criteria for formal psychiatric diagnoses, such as when interpersonal problems lead to sleep disturbances (Brissette & Cohen, 2002) or when depressed mood is associated with marital discord (Denton, Golden, & Walsh, 2003).

Haynes and O'Brien (2000) described several causal models that could account for comorbid behavior problems. Briefly, behavior problems could covary (a) because they share the same causal variable, such as when chronic pain leads to covariance between sleep disturbances and depressed mood (Davison & Jhangri, 2005); (b) when one behavior problem serves as the causal variable for another, such as when a person's social anxiety leads to alcohol abuse to ease the anxiety (Morris, Stewart, & Ham, 2005); and (c) when they are the result of different but covarying causal variables, such as when a person's recent divorce leads to a depressed mood and a change in residence leads to excessive worries about personal safety.

The presence of *comorbid* behavioral problems and their potential *functional interrelations* have several implications for assessment strategies in treatment research. Most important, assessment should focus on multiple behaviors in addition to the primary target. The measurement of multiple behavior problems within a longitudinal or time series design can help

TABLE 4.2

Characteristics of Behavior Problems That Affect Behavioral Assessment Strategies in Treatment Research

Characteristics	Description/example	Assessment strategy
People have *multiple behavior problems.*	Persons seeking treatment for substance dependence often have mood, anxiety, psychophysiological, and interpersonal problems.	Assessment should focus on multiple behavior problems and not be confined to the major treatment target.
Behavior problems have *multiple response systems* and *individual differences.*	Anxiety disorders often have cognitive, motor, and physiological modes, and the relative importance of each response system can also differ across persons with a similar behavior problem.	Assessment should be multimodal to capture the cognitive, motor, and physiological response systems of a behavior problem.
Behavior problems have *multiple dimensions.*	Manic behaviors can be characterized by rate, magnitude, duration, and latency to onset. The relative importance of these dimensions can differ across persons with a similar behavior problem.	Assessment should capture the rate, magnitude, duration, and latency of occurrence of a behavior problem and the idiosyncratic differences in response systems and their relative importance. The focus should be on specific, lower level units of behavior
Conditional nature of behavior problems.	The rate of a child's aggressive behaviors can vary across different environments (e.g., school vs. home) or states (e.g., medicated state).	Measures should be obtained on behavior problems in different environments, contexts, and states.
Dynamic nature of behavior problems.	The characteristics, probability, and conditional nature of delusional thoughts or sleep problems can change over time.	Time-sampling assessment strategies that are appropriate for the rate of change of the behavior problem should be used.

detect their functional interrelations and differences in degree or rate of change. For example, a person's alcohol use could affect mood and family interactions, or alcohol use could be a behavioral result of mood fluctuations and conflictual family interactions (see subsequent section on causal relations). These different functional relations have important implications for

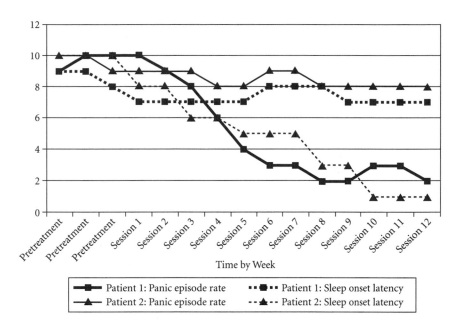

FIGURE 4.1. Time series assessment.

the focus of treatment strategies because most treatments focus on hypothesized causal variables.

Multiple Response Systems of Behavior Problems

Behavioral assessment strategies in treatment research also reflect the fact that behavior problems have *multiple response systems,* such as motor, cognitive, emotional, and physiological, which can differ in importance across time and across persons. For example, for one person, social anxiety can be most strongly manifested as disruptive thoughts and beliefs, whereas another person's anxiety can be most strongly manifested as overt avoidance behaviors or psychophysiological hyperreactivity.

Given these multiple response systems, a *multisystem assessment strategy* should be used to capture the important response systems of each behavior problem for each person. In treatment research, the assessment strategy should include measuring how participants behave, think, and respond physiologically and emotionally. Measures of behavior that are aggregates and include irrelevant response systems will be relatively insensitive to specific treatment-related changes because the apparent variance in important response systems will be attenuated by the inclusion of elements that tap less important response systems. For example, depression questionnaires that disproportionately assess for cognitive and motor symptoms may not adequately identify depression, or track the specific effects of a treatment program, among persons who have more somatic or affective symptoms of depression.

Multidimensional Nature of Behavior Problems

Our assessment strategies in treatment research are also affected by the observation, as illustrated in Figure 4.1, that behavior problems have *multiple dimensions* (quantitative attributes of behavior such as their rate, severity, and duration) that can differ in importance across time and across persons. For example, persons with a PTSD diagnosis can differ in the rate and duration at which they reexperience a traumatic event via "flashbacks," the rate at which they experience sleep disturbances, and the severity of those disturbances.

The *multidimensional* nature of behavior problems has several implications for the best assessment strategies in treatment research. First, assessment should focus on the *multiple dimensions of response systems* to capture differences in the rate, magnitude, and duration of treatment-related changes. Second, the assessment focus should be on *specific, precisely defined targets* (e.g., frequency or duration of depressive episodes) rather than on broadly defined constructs (e.g., "depression"). Measures of behavior that are aggregates across dimensions will be relatively insensitive to specific treatment-related changes because measures of variance on important dimensions will be attenuated by the inclusion of measures of variance on unimportant dimensions. It is particularly important that researchers identify the most important dimension of a behavior problem or the dimension that is most likely to be affected by a treatment.

The Conditional Nature of Behavioral Problems

Behavior problems and the effects of treatment for many persons are also *conditional.* That is, the likelihood or severity of a behavior problem and the degree of treatment-related change can vary across settings (e.g., the degree of familiarity of persons at a social gathering), states (e.g., the degree of sleep deprivation), or other contexts (e.g., the recent history of stressful life events). The onset, rate, and intensity of a child's disruptive behaviors in school can differ across teachers, subject matter being studied, the classroom setting, and time of day. Furthermore, the contexts associated with elevated conditional probabilities for a behavior problem can differ across persons. One person may be more likely to have a panic episode while driving in traffic or flying, whereas another person may be more likely to have panic episodes in response to being separated from a loved one in an unfamiliar setting (Craske & Barlow, 2001).

Given the conditional nature of behavioral problems, assessment strategies should involve measurement of behavior problems in various and well-specified situations, states, and contexts. Measures of behavior that are aggregates and include irrelevant contexts will be less sensitive to specific treatment-related changes because measures of variance in critical contexts will be attenuated by the inclusion of measures of variance in irrelevant contexts.

Dynamic and Dysynchronous Aspects of Behavior Problems

Finally, our assessment strategies are affected by the *dynamic nature* of behavior problems, as illustrated in Figure 4.1. Behavior problems can change over time in their comorbidity, importance, functional relations, most important response systems and dimensions, and conditional probabilities. Moreover, these changes may not occur in parallel. A child's aggressive behaviors could begin to escalate at school, where he hits and threatens classmates, but show no escalation at home with siblings or parents.

It is often the goal of treatment to change some dimension of a behavior problem and to measure such changes over the course of treatment. We might want to know when the maximum benefit of a treatment has occurred, catch failing therapies quickly, or note treatment effects on different dimensions of the behavior problem.

Time series assessment strategies involving frequent measurements of well-specified variables are the best approach to capturing the dynamic nature of behavior problems, particularly the changes associated with treatments. The rate of measurement should match the rate of change of a behavior problem in order to capture the time course of treatment-related changes.

■ What Do We Know About the Causes of Behavior Problems?

In addition to the principles of measurement and the nature of behavior problems, behavioral assessment strategies in treatment research are also guided by the nature of causal relations for behavior problems.[3] Causal variables and causal relations are important because they are often the targets of treatments. For example, a treatment might focus on changing parental response contingencies that are hypothesized as maintaining a child's oppositional behavior (Diamond & Josephson, 2005). We review here several aspects of causal variables and causal relations and their implications for assessment in treatment research. Haynes (1992), Haynes and O'Brien (2000), and O'Brien, Kaplar, and McGrath (2004) have discussed this topic in greater depth.

A set of causal assumptions with a strong effect on behavioral assessment strategies in treatment research consists of *dynamic, idiographic, and multivariate causality:* Behavior problems can result from different permutations of multiple causal variables, and these permutations (their strength, direction, and form of effect of causal variables) can vary across persons and across time within persons. Depressed mood, for example, can result from different combinations of biological, cognitive, social, environmental, and life event variables (Watts & Markham, 2005). The most important causal variables from this set can differ across persons with the same depressive symptoms, and their causes can change across time.

The dynamic, idiographic, and multivariate aspects of causal relations are relevant to two goals of treatment research, as outlined in Table 4.1: (a) identifying the mechanisms underlying treatment effects and (b) identifying individual difference variables that affect treatment outcome. Haynes, Kaholokula, and Nelson (1999) presented several models to illustrate that a treatment's magnitude of effect depends partly on the degree to which the treatment's mechanism of action matches the causal relations relevant to a client's behavior problem. With social anxiety, for example, a treatment's magnitude of effect in modifying self-statements would depend on the degree to which self-statements affected the probability or duration of the client's social anxiety (Scholing & Emmelkamp, 1999).

There are several implications of dynamic, idiographic, and multivariate causality for behavioral assessment strategies in treatment research. First, assessment in treatment research should focus on potential causal variables for the targeted behavior problems. This would allow researchers to estimate differential treatment outcomes as a function of causal relations. Most treatment research includes measures of behavior problem severity, but few include measures of causal relations. For example, what is the relation between the magnitude of an expectancy-oriented treatment for alcohol use and the degree to which a client's alcohol use was affected by outcome expectancies (Gilles, Turk, & Fresco, 2006)?

Second, treatment mechanisms and treatment fidelity should be measured, and individual treatment mechanisms should be introduced in a systematic manner (e.g., through interrupted time series designs or through between-group designs) that allows for the partition of outcome variance across treatment mechanisms. Given that treatments usually involve multiple components, the identification of the most powerful components can be accomplished only if mechanisms of action are measured.

Treatment research should include measures of treatment variables, such as fidelity of implementation, duration of implementation, and client adherence to treatment recommendations. For example, in a multicomponent treatment for distressed couples, in addition to outcome variables such as satisfaction and conflict, a researcher should measure the type and duration of focus on communication skills in treatment and the degree to which the couple practices recommended communication strategies outside the treatment setting. The affects of treatment mechanisms and treatment fidelity on the behavioral assessment of treatment outcome will be discussed further in a subsequent section.

Third, environmental causal variables should be measured as part of treatment outcome research. Research on posttreatment maintenance and relapse is an example of where an environmental focus would help identify important causal relations. The likelihood of relapse in alcohol abuse, for example, can be affected by work and family stressors, social environments where alcohol is present (Ramo, Anderson, Tate, & Brown, 2005), and medication use (Breese, Overstreet, & Knapp, 2005). Relapse can also be affected by outcome expectancies for alcohol use and biologically based cravings (Gilles et al., 2006). The development of effective relapse-prevention strategies depends on the measurement of these causal variables, along with the measurement of drinking behavior, in a time series format that allows for the identification of time-lagged correlations between the potential causal variables and alcohol use.

Fourth, causal relations can be conditional. The causal relations relevant to a person's behavior problems can vary across settings and contexts. Therefore, treatment research should include measures from different settings to allow for the identification of setting-specific outcomes and causal relations. For example, an intervention for aggressive behaviors by an elementary-aged child may prove effective in some but not other classrooms (Hughes, Cavell, Meehan, Zhang, & Collie, 2005), which may differ in important causal variables such as peer interactions, classroom structure or sociometry, and reinforcement systems.

Finally, causal variables can differ in their *strength of effects* across different response systems and dimensions of a behavior problem and can differ across persons with similar behavior problems. For example, a person's fearful thoughts about an anticipated social event could lead to sympathetically mediated hyperarousal, but whether or not they escalate to a panic episode could depend on how the person interprets the aroused state. For another person the social setting itself might trigger a panic episode (Craske & Waters, 2005). Therefore, measurement of causal variables should focus on their *strength of effects* on specific *dimensions* and *response systems* of a behavior problem.

We have touched on only a few of many causal assumptions that affect behavioral assessment strategies in treatment research. Other important aspects of causal relations include their additive and interactive effects, their multidimensional and multimodal nature, the modifiability of causal variables, nonlinear causal relations, and bidirectional causal relations. These are discussed in greater length in the citations previously provided. However, the causal assumptions and measurement foci that we have presented underscore our previous suggestions about the best methods and foci of assessment in treatment research. The best strategy for identifying behavior problems and their causal variables, causal relations, and treatment mechanisms is the use of specific, narrowly defined measures within a multimethod time series measurement strategy.

■ What Do We Know About Treatments?

Previously, we discussed how the nature of, and causal relations underlying, behavior problems influence behavioral assessment strategies in treatment research. We emphasized that treatment research involves the assessment of change (change in the aspects and dimensions of behavior problems) and of the variables that affect that change.

Treatments are instruments of change, and behavioral assessment strategies are influenced by their characteristics. For example, research can focus on why a treatment works (e.g., *mechanism of action*), what aspects of a treatment work best (e.g., the *components* of a treatment), how reliably and easily a treatment is applied (e.g., *treatment fidelity* and *transportability*), how fast a treatment works (e.g., the *time course* of treatment effects), or how a treatment can inadvertently affect quality of life (e.g., *treatment side effects*). Each research focus requires different assessment strategies. This section reviews some of the characteristics of treatments and their implications for behavioral assessment strategies.

Identifying Treatment Mechanism and Active Treatment Components

The *mechanism of action* for many psychosocial treatments (i.e., what accounts for change in a behavior problem) is not fully understood, even for well-studied, evidence-based treatments (EBTs), such as cognitive-behavioral therapy (CBT) for depression and anxiety (Kazdin, 2005). Most often a treatment's mechanism of action is inferred from the interpretation of treatment effects within a particular theoretical framework. For example, CBTs for depression and anxiety are believed to work, in part, by reducing a client's automatic negative thoughts and how he or she processes information. Decreases in the rate of these thoughts are presumed to be the mechanisms that account for decreases in depressed mood and anxiety symptoms during therapy.

The therapeutic effects of CBTs for depression and anxiety are well supported by many empirical studies (Butler, Chapman, Forman, & Beck, 2006; Hollon, Stewart, & Strunk, 2006). However, pharmacotherapy for depression has also been shown to affect a person's automatic negative thoughts, despite working via a presumably different treatment mechanism (i.e., biological substrate; DeRubeis et al., 1990). The identification of a treatment's mechanism of action is challenging because treatments often have *multiple components* (e.g., cognitive restructuring, social skills training, contingency management) that may differ in their relative effects across response systems and dimensions of a client's behavior problem.

To identify a treatment's mechanism of action we must measure (a) the *independent treatment variable* (e.g., time spent in, and method for, changing automatic negative thoughts in treatment); (b) the *immediate treatment mechanism variable* (e.g., client's automatic negative thoughts in the natural environment); and (c) the *ultimate outcome variable* (e.g., depressed mood). These variables must be measured within a *multivariate time series assessment strategy* in order to identify the time order and strength of functional relations. To identify (b) as a treatment mechanism underlying the effects of (a) on (c), we must show that changes in (a) precede and are significantly correlated with changes in (b) and that changes in (b) precede and are significantly correlated with changes in (c). Failure to confirm the strength or temporal direction of either of these functional relations would be inconsistent with the hypothesized treatment mechanism.[4]

The relative magnitude of effect of each component of a treatment on a behavior problem, like its mechanism of action, is also not well understood. For example, dialectical behavior therapy (DBT), a type of CBT for persons with a borderline personality disorder (BPD) diagnosis, has several distinguishable components: individual psychotherapy, group skills training, telephone consultations, and peer consultation for therapists (Palmer, 2002). Each component (except the peer consultation component) focuses on a different aspect of a client's BPD: Individual psychotherapy addresses maladaptive thoughts and behaviors, group skills training focuses on practicing more adaptive behaviors, and telephone consultations assist with problem solving of adaptive interpersonal responses and provide crisis intervention. Despite its distinguishable components and noted treatment efficacy, the relative effects of each component of DBT in treatment outcome have yet to be fully understood (Koerner & Linehan, 2000). However, this is not unique to DBT. The relative effects of a treatment's components for many psychotherapeutic approaches for various behavior problems have yet to be adequately examined (Kazdin, 2005).

A treatment's specified components are also referred to as *treatment-specific components* (or specific factors attributed to a particular treatment approach); *nonspecific treatment components* (or common factors) refer to other therapeutic aspects of a treatment commonly found across different treatment approaches (Stevens, Hynan, & Allen, 2000). Some nonspecific factors identified as having therapeutic effects across treatment approaches are warmth and empathy of a therapist, a therapist's ability to form a working alliance with clients, and a client's treatment expectations and belief in a therapist's ability to help him or her (Lambert & Barley, 2001).

Earlier treatment outcome studies found no significant difference in treatment effects across different treatment approaches (e.g., CBT vs. interpersonal), suggesting to some people that common factors were the effective components of all psychotherapies (Wampold et al., 1997). However, a more recent meta-analytical study by Stevens et al. (2000) reported larger effect sizes for treatment-specific factors ($d = .17–.19$) compared with common factors ($d = .07–.13$) across three different outcome domains: subjective well-being, symptoms, and life functioning. Further, many measures used in treatment studies are from aggregated self-report questionnaires not sufficiently sensitive to change in the main target variables.

Kazdin (2005) has commented that what actually accounts for change in a behavior problem is often overlooked in treatment outcome research and that efficacy studies need to focus on the mechanisms of psychotherapeutic change as well as treatment outcomes. In addition, he also suggested that well-designed experimental studies are needed to test common factors and their treatment effects. The examination of treatment-specific components and nonspecific treatment components can help to identify why and how a treatment works.

Research on treatment components, as with research on treatment mechanisms of action, must include well-designed assessment strategies. Not only must components be studied within appropriate interrupted time series and longitudinal between-group designs, but measures of independent and dependent variables must be precise, valid, and sensitive to change. For research on treatment components for BPD, for example, outcome measures must sensitively reflect changes in the frequency and intensity of multiple variables, such as negative emotions, physiological reactivity, interpersonal conflict, and distress in romantic relationships. As with previous treatment research foci, the use of multimethod, lower level, more specific, appropriately validated measures is necessary to achieve this goal.

Treatment Fidelity

Treatment research is also complicated by the fact that what occurs in a treatment is not always consistent with what was intended. The degree to which treatment delivered is consistent with established protocol is referred to as *treatment fidelity* (Borrelli et al., 2005). For example, research on the effects of a family-focused behavioral management program for delinquent adolescents presumes that the intervention follows a particular protocol—a sequence of foci, particular methods, and particular ways of coping with implementation challenges. When there is diversity in treatment implementation across therapists, families, or time, it is difficult to draw inferences about treatment outcome, treatment mechanisms, or the relative contribution of the treatment components. Essentially, the internal validity of all inferences about the effects of a treatment is threatened.

Research has been mixed on the effects of monitoring treatment fidelity. Some studies have found that greater treatment fidelity is associated with better treatment outcomes, whereas others have not (Henggeler, 2004; Miller & Binder, 2002). The strategies used to ensure treatment fidelity vary greatly across studies, and they are often inconsistently used (Bellg et al., 2004), which could explain the disparate findings concerning the relationship between treatment fidelity and treatment outcomes. For example, Borrelli et al. (2005) examined studies of health behavior interventions published between 1990 and 2000 in selected peer-reviewed journals. They found that only 22% of the studies examined used strategies to help maintain therapists' skills, 35% used treatment manuals, and only 12% used a combination of strategies. Interestingly, they also found that 54% of the studies examined did not use any treatment fidelity strategy, and among those that used some type of strategy, only 27% actually assessed therapists' adherence to treatment protocols using audiotapes, observations, or self-reports from therapists and participants.

Treatment fidelity can affect treatment outcome, and measures of treatment fidelity are necessary to explain treatment mechanisms or to identify effective components of treatments. Thus, treatment research should include measures of therapists' adherence to treatment protocols (see Bellg et al., 2004). This would require an assessment strategy that can measure the degree to which therapists are consistent in the delivery of treatment protocols and the degree to which treatments are delivered as intended.

Paradoxical and Unintended Effects of Treatment

A treatment can have paradoxical (i.e., contradictory) and other unintended adverse effects. In some cases, the paradoxical and unintended effects of a treatment can be more important than its main effects on the behavior problem (Bootzin & Bailey, 2005). Some treatments designed to improve problem behaviors can worsen them. For example, well-designed group interventions for youths with antisocial behaviors have had paradoxical effects on participants in which they evidenced an increase in delinquent behaviors and substance use (Rhule, 2005). Studies have found that 7% to 15% of people who undergo a psychosocial treatment for a substance use disorder show increased depression and substance use after treatment (Moos, 2005). Some psychological treatments for trauma (e.g., critical incident stress debriefing) could also inadvertently result in an escalation of emotional distress (Bootzin & Bailey, 2005). Cognitive-focused treatments that ask people to suppress anxiety-provoking thoughts could inadvertently make those thoughts more salient (Wenzlaff & Wegner, 2000).

Besides having a paradoxical effect, a treatment could improve a behavior problem but also have adverse side effects that can affect a person's quality of life, physical health, or adherence to treatment. The use of psychoactive medications to treat depression can lead to sexual dysfunctions (Fava & Rankin, 2002) and sleep disturbances (Mayers & Baldwin, 2005), whereas neuroleptics can lead to severe neurological problems, such as tardive dyskinesia (Nasrallah, 2006). Some adverse side effects of a treatment could lead to other behavior problems and premature termination of treatment, such as when sexual dysfunction from using an antidepression medication causes diminished self-esteem and sexual dissatisfaction by partners (Williams et al., 2006).

Behavioral assessment strategies in treatment research should be designed to identify potential paradoxical and other unintended effects. The assessment strategies discussed earlier in this chapter remain relevant for this focus— multivariate, multimodal, multidimensional, time series strategies, with a specific focus on a broad range of variables that could demonstrate treatment-related change. Cost-efficient but more broadly focused measures of potential unintended effects of treatment should be included. For example, behavior problem checklists collected frequently from multiple sources (e.g., client, spouse, coworkers) would allow for early identification of problems and immediate modification or termination of an ineffective or potentially harmful treatment.

■ Recommendations for Assessment Strategies in Treatment Research

We conclude this chapter with a summary of recommendations for assessment strategies in treatment research. These recommendations emphasize *a functional approach to assessment:* Assessment strategies should be based on the goals of treatment research, psychometric principles, and the characteristics of behavior disorders, causal relations, and treatments, as discussed in previous sections. Our recommendations, which are consistent with the use of behavioral assessment in treatment research, are as follows:

1. Specify the goals of the research and select strategies that are consistent with those goals.
   a. Specify the research goals of the study. Are the goals to compare two treatments? To identify moderators of treatment outcome? To identify the relative efficacy of treatment components? To identify treatment mechanisms of action? To plot the time course of treatment effects? To identify side effects of treatment? To monitor treatment fidelity?
   b. Each goal will require a different assessment strategy. Ensure that assessment instruments, the measures obtained from them, and the time-sampling strategy (the schedule of measurement) matches the goals of the treatment. Carefully consider if the data acquired will allow you to answer the questions addressed in your research.
2. Consider the psychometric properties of all measures.
   a. Although reliability and validity indices are not stable traits of a measure, you can increase the likelihood that the data will be valid by selecting measures with a history of strong validity support from multiple investigators.
   b. The validity data should be relevant to your goals. For example, if you are using the measure to evaluate treatment-related change in behavior problems over time, has the measure been shown to be sensitive to change?
   c. The validity data should be relevant to your sample. Many studies have shown that a measure can be valid when used with younger but not older persons, with one ethnic group but not another,

with persons with one level of behavior problem severity but not another.

3. Consider the characteristics of the behavior problems that you are studying and use highly focused, minimally inferential, direct measures.

   a. Which components and response systems of a behavior problem are more and less likely to be affected by the treatment? Which behaviors, thoughts, attitudes, and expectations are affected? Ensure that the measures you select provide valid and sensitive data on the specific components of interest. In most treatment research contexts, more specific, lower level measures are more helpful than less specific, higher level measures, such as general personality trait measures.

   b. Which dimensions of a behavior problem are more and less likely to be affected by the treatment? Do you expect the treatment to have greater effects on the rate, duration, or severity of a behavior problem? Ensure that the measures you select provide valid and sensitive data on the dimension of interest. Many measures (e.g., most personality trait measures) are aggregates of multiple dimensions and do not allow precise measurement of any single dimension.

4. Measure immediate, intermediate, and ultimate outcomes.

   a. To understand how treatments work (i.e., the mechanism underlying their effects), it is necessary to specify and measure immediate and intermediate outcomes, in addition to the ultimate outcomes. For example, what thoughts, behaviors, physiological reactions, and environmental events must change in order for a treatment to improve mood, reduce drinking, increase sleep efficiency, or reduce oppositional behavior? Measures that tap specified outcomes should be selected, and measures should be obtained frequently.

   b. In many cases, immediate and ultimate outcome variables will be the presumed *causal variables* that will affect the ultimate outcome. The causal variables for the targeted behavior problems that are intended for modification should be specified and measured throughout the treatment and posttreatment periods. Specification of the causal variables should include their domains or other aspects. Is it the frequency, magnitude, or duration of a causal variable that is important?

5. Measure treatment implementation.

   a. Specify the events that should occur during treatment and measure them. Often, the best method of monitoring treatment implementation and fidelity is by video recordings and subsequent ratings by trained observers.

6. Use time series assessment strategies.

   a. In order to identify failing treatments, to describe the time course of treatment effects, to understand treatment mechanisms, and to identify causal relations, measurement of all variables should occur frequently.

For example, measure mood, blood pressure, school attendance, alcohol intake, and social interactions on a daily basis or as often as possible.[5]

7. Examine the validity of measures during the research.

   a. Given that validity coefficients are not necessarily generalizable across assessment contexts, persons, and assessors, data on the performance of measures should be acquired during a study. Indices of internal consistency, temporal consistency, factor structure, interrater reliability, between-assessor agreement, and covariance among multiple methods can establish confidence in the obtained measures.

   b. In some cases, measures can be modified to provide more valid indices of a targeted construct. For example, items with low temporal consistency, behavior codes with low interrater reliability, or measures that do not correlate highly with other measures of the same construct can be omitted or refined to make them a better fit with the assessment target.[6] With refined measures, sources of error variance are reduced and estimates of functional relations are less likely to be attenuated.

8. Be cautious in the use of archival data sets in treatment research.

   a. Many studies are published in which existing treatment research data sets are reanalyzed to address new research questions. This can result in useful findings, but confidence is reduced because most archival data sets are not consistent with the functional approach to assessment in treatment research. That is, measures and measurement strategies were most likely selected with different original goals. It is likely that the archival data set does not contain the best measures to answer the new research question, and the results will be subject to alternative explanations or threats to internal validity.

9. Measure potential unintended effects of treatment.

   a. Consider potential negative and positive effects of treatment that are in addition to the main treatment foci.

10. Measure the contexts in which measures are obtained.

   a. Treatment effects can vary across environmental settings, states of the client, and other contexts. The conditions in which data are acquired should be measured so that variance in outcome can be examined.

Notes

1. We adopt definitions for several measurement terms from Haynes and O'Brien (2000):

   Assessment method: A class of procedures (e.g., self-report questionnaires, behavioral observations in the natural environment, interviews) for deriving data on the behavior of a person or on other events (e.g., life stressors, social environments).

Assessment/measurement strategy: The plan of action for deriving assessment data, which can include a set of assessment instruments, instructions to client, time-sampling parameters, and assessment context.

Measure: A number that represents the variable being measured; a score obtained from an assessment instrument (e.g., blood-pressure reading, observed rate of behavior, scale score).

Measurement: The assignment of a numerical value to a dimension of a variable.

2. Psychometric and causality terms are adapted from a behavioral assessment glossary at http://www2.hawaii.edu/~sneil/ba/.

3. A causal variable is any variable that can account for variance (e.g., changes in the magnitude, duration, frequency, or latency) in a behavior problem. Causal variables can be described in terms of strength, direction (e.g., unidirectional or bidirectional), and form (e.g., linear, quadratic, catastrophic; Haynes & O'Brien, 2000). Two variables have a causal relation when they have a functional relation, the hypothesized causal variable reliably precedes the effect, there is a logical mechanism for the hypothesized causal relation, and alternative explanations for the observed covariance can reasonably be excluded. See http://www2.hawaii.edu/~sneil/ba/ for additional definitions.

4. The identification of a treatment mechanism also requires some data analytic strategies. For example, one must show that the proportion of shared variance between (a) and (c) is significantly reduced when (b) is introduced as a mediator variable in hierarchical regression equations.

5. Many factors can affect how often data are collected in treatment research, such as the time required on the part of respondents, the cost of the assessment, the burden on the assessors, autocorrelation, and carryover effects in obtained data. But data should be collected as often as possible without jeopardizing adherence to the protocols or the validity of the data.

6. The main drawback to using modified measures is that comparisons between studies are more difficult because different measures of the same variables have been used.

■ References

Addis, M. E., Wade, W. A., & Hatgis, C. (1999). Barriers to dissemination of evidence-based practices: Addressing practitioners' concerns about manual-based psychotherapies. *Clinical Psychology: Science and Practice, 6*, 430–441.

Bassiony, M. M. (2005). Social anxiety disorder and depression in Saudi Arabia. *Depression and Anxiety, 21*, 90–94.

Beck, A. T., Steer, R. A., & Garbin, M. G. (1988). Psychometric properties of the Beck Depression Inventory: Twenty-five years of evaluation. *Clinical Psychology Review, 8*, 77–100.

Bellg, A. J., Borrelli, B., Resnick, B., Hecht, J., Minicucci, D. S., Ory, M., et al. (2004). Enhancing treatment fidelity in health behavior change studies: Best practices and recommendations from the NIH behavior change consortium. *Health Psychology, 23,* 443–451.

Biederman, J., Petty, C., Faraone, S. V., Hirshfeld-Becker, D. R., Henin, A., Pollack, M. H., et al. (2005). Patterns of comorbidity in panic disorder and major depression: Findings from a nonreferred sample. *Depression and Anxiety, 21,* 55–60.

Bootzin, R. R., & Bailey, E. T. (2005). Understanding placebo, nocebo, and iatrogenic treatment effects. *Journal of Clinical Psychology, 61,* 871–880.

Borrelli, B., Sepinwall, D., Ernst, D., Bellg, A. J., Czajkowski, S., Breger, R., et al. (2005). A new tool to assess treatment fidelity and evaluation of treatment fidelity across 10 years of health behavior research. *Journal of Consulting and Clinical Psychology, 73,* 852–860.

Breese, G. R., Overstreet, D. H., & Knapp, D. J. (2005). Conceptual framework for the etiology of alcoholism: A "kindling"/stress hypothesis. *Psychopharmacology, 178,* 367–380.

Brissette, I., & Cohen, S. (2002). The contribution of individual differences in hostility to the associations between daily interpersonal conflict, affect, and sleep. *Personality and Social Psychology Bulletin, 28,* 1265–1274.

Butler, A. C., Chapman, J. E., Forman, E. M., & Beck, A. T. (2006). The empirical status of cognitive-behavioral therapy: A review of meta-analyses. *Clinical Psychology Review, 26,* 17–31.

Cone, J. D. (1998). Psychometric considerations: Concepts, contents, and methods. In A. Bellack & M. Hersen (Eds.), *Behavioral assessment: A practical handbook* (3rd ed.; pp. 42–66). Needham Heights, MA: Allyn & Bacon.

Cone, J. D. (1999). Introduction to the special section on self-monitoring: A major assessment method in clinical psychology. *Psychological Assessment, 11,* 411–414.

Craske, M. G., & Barlow, D. H. (2001). Panic disorder and agoraphobia. In D.H. Barlow (Ed.), *Clinical handbook of psychological disorders: A step-by-step treatment manual* (3rd ed., pp. 1–59). New York: Guilford.

Craske, M., & Waters, A. M. (2005). Panic disorder, phobias, and generalized anxiety disorder. *Annual Review of Clinical Psychology, 1,* 197–225.

Davison, S. N., & Jhangri, G. S. (2005). The impact of chronic pain on depression, sleep, and the desire to withdraw from dialysis in hemodialysis patients. *Journal of Pain and Symptom Management, 30,* 465–473.

Denton, W. H., Golden, R. N., & Walsh, S. R. (2003). Depression, marital discord and couple therapy. *Current Opinion in Psychiatry, 16,* 29–34.

DeRubeis, R. J., Evans, M. D., Hollon, S. D., Garvey, M. J., Grove, W. M., & Tuason, V. B. (1990). How does cognitive therapy work? Cognitive change and symptom change in cognitive therapy and pharmacotherapy for depression. *Journal of Consulting and Clinical Psychology, 58,* 862–869.

Diamond, G., & Josephson, A. (2005). Family-based treatment research: 10-year update. *Journal of the American Academy of Child and Adolescent Psychiatry, 44,* 872–887.

Dohrenwend, B. P., Krasnoff, L., Askenasy, A. R., & Dohrenwend, B. S. (1978). Exemplification of a method for scaling life events: The PERI Life Events Scale. *Journal of Health and Social Behavior, 19,* 205–229.

Essau, C. A. (2003). Comorbidity of anxiety disorders in adolescents. *Depression and Anxiety, 18,* 1–6.

Fava, M., & Rankin, M. (2002). Sexual functioning and SSRIs. *Journal of Clinical Psychiatry, 63*(Suppl. 5), 13–16.

Gilles, D. M., Turk, C. L., & Fresco, D. M. (2006). Social anxiety, alcohol expectancies, and self-efficacy as predictors of heavy drinking in college students. *Addictive Behaviors, 31,* 388–398.

Hamilton, M. (1960). A rating scale for depression. *Journal of Neurology, Neurosurgery, and Psychiatry, 23,* 56–62.

Haynes, S. N. (1992). *Models of causality in psychopathology.* Des Moines, IA: Allyn & Bacon.

Haynes, S. N. (2006). Psychometric principles of behavioral assessment. In M Hersen (Ed.), *Clinician's handbook of adult behavioral assessment* (pp. 17–39). New York: Academic Press.

Haynes, S. N. & Heiby, E. (Eds.). (2003). *Behavioral assessment.* Vol. 3 of Michel Hersen (Series Ed.), *Comprehensive handbook on psychological assessment.* Hoboken, NJ: Wiley.

Haynes, S. N., Kaholokula, J. K., & Nelson, K. (1999). The idiographic application of nomothetic, empirically based treatments. *Clinical Psychology: Science and Practice, 6,* 456–461.

Haynes, S. N., Nelson, K., & Blaine, D. C. (1999). Psychometric issues in assessment research. In P. C. Kendall, J. N. Butcher, & G. N. Holmbeck (Eds.), *Handbook of research methods in clinical psychology* (pp. 125–154). New York: Wiley.

Haynes, S. N., & O'Brien, W. O. (2000). *Principles of behavioral assessment: A functional approach to psychological assessment.* New York: Plenum/Kluwer Press.

Haynes, S. N., Richard, D. C. S., & Kubany, E. S. (1995). Content validity in psychological assessment: A functional approach to concepts and methods. *Psychological Assessment, 7,* 238–247.

Henggeler, S. W. (2004). Decreasing effect sizes for effectiveness studies— Implications for the transport of evidence-based treatments: Comment on Curtis, Ronan, and Borduin. *Journal of Family Psychology, 18,* 420–423.

Hersen, M. (2006). *Clinician handbook of adult behavioral assessment.* New York: Academic Press.

Hollon, S. D., Stewart, M. O., & Strunk, D. (2006). Enduring effects for cognitive behavior therapy in the treatment of depression and anxiety. *Annual Review of Psychology, 57,* 285–315.

Hughes, J. N., Cavell, T. A., Meehan, B. T., Zhang, D., & Collie, C. (2005). Adverse school context moderates the outcomes of selective interventions for aggressive children. *Journal of Consulting and Clinical Psychology, 73,* 731–736.

Ilkjaer, K., Kortegaard, L., Hoerder, K., Joergensen, J., Kyvik, K., & Gillberg, C. (2004). Personality disorders in a total population twin cohort with eating disorders. *Comprehensive Psychiatry, 45,* 261–267.

Kazdin, A. E. (2002*). Research designs in clinical psychology* (4th ed.). Des Moines, IA: Allyn & Bacon.

Kazdin, A. E. (2005). Treatment outcomes, common factors, and continued neglect of mechanisms of change. *Clinical Psychology Science and Practice, 12,* 184–188.

Kazdin, A. E. (2006). Assessment and evaluation in clinical practice. In C. D. Goodheart, A. E. Kazdin, & R. J. Sternberg, (Eds.), *Evidence-based psychotherapy: Where practice and research meet* (pp. 153–177). Washington, DC: American Psychological Association.

Kendall, P. C., Butcher, J. N., & Holmbeck G. N. (Eds.). (1999). *Handbook of research methods in clinical psychology.* New York: Wiley.

Koerner, K., & Linehan, M. M. (2000). Research on dialectical behavior therapy for patients with borderline personality disorder. *Psychiatric Clinics of North America, 23,* 151–167.

Kratochwill, T. R., & Levin, J. R. (Eds.). (1992). *Single-case research design and analysis: New directions for psychology and education.* Hillsdale, NJ: Erlbaum.

Lambert, M. J., & Barley, D. E. (2001). Research summary on the therapeutic relationship and psychotherapy outcomes. *Psychotherapy, 38,* 357–361.

Mayers, A. G., & Baldwin, D. S. (2005). Antidepressants and their effects on sleep. *Human Psychopharmacology: Clinical and Experimental, 20,* 533–559.

Miller, S. J., & Binder, J. L. (2002). The effects of manual-based training on treatment fidelity and outcome: A review of the literature on adult individual psychotherapy. *Psychotherapy: Theory/Research/Practice/Training, 39,* 184–198.

Minke, K., & Haynes, S. N. (2003). Sampling issues. In J. C. Thomas & M. Hersen (Eds.), *Understanding research in clinical and counseling psychology.* Mahwah, NJ: Erlbaum.

Moos, R. H. (2005). Iatrogenic effects of psychosocial interventions for substance use disorders: Prevalence, predictors, prevention. *Addiction, 100,* 595–604.

Morris, E. P., Stewart, S. H., & Ham, L. S. (2005). The relationship between social anxiety disorder and alcohol use disorders: A critical review. *Clinical Psychology Review 25,* 734–760.

Nasrallah, H. A. (2006). Focus on lower risk of tardive dyskinesia with atypical antipsychotics. *Annals of Clinical Psychiatry, 81,* 57–62.

Nunnally, J. C., & Bernstein, I. H. (1994). *Psychometric theory* (3rd ed.). New York: McGraw-Hill.

O'Brien, W. H., Kaplar, M. E., & McGrath, J. J. (2004). Broadly-based causal models of behavior disorders. In S. N. Haynes & E. M. Heiby (Vol. Eds.), *Comprehensive handbook of psychological assessment: Vol. 3. Behavioral assessment.* Hoboken, NJ: Wiley.

Palmer, R. L. (2002). Dialectical behaviour therapy for borderline personality disorder. *Advances in Psychiatric Treatment, 8,* 10–16.

Ramo, D. E., Anderson, K. G., Tate, S. R., & Brown, S. A. (2005). Characteristics of relapse to substance use in comorbid adolescents. *Addictive Behaviors, 30,* 1811–1823.

Raskin, A., Schulterbrandt, J. G., Reatig, N., & McKeon, J. J. (1969). Replication of factors of psychopathology in interview, ward behavior and self-report ratings of hospitalized depressives. *Journal of Nervous and Mental Diseases, 148,* 87–98.

Rhule, D. M. (2005). Take care to do no harm: Harmful interventions for youth problem behavior. *Professional Psychology: Research and Practice, 36,* 618–625.

Scholing, A., & Emmelkamp, P. M. G. (1999). Prediction of treatment outcome in social phobia: A cross-validation. *Behaviour Research and Therapy, 37,* 659–670.

Silva, F. (1994). *Psychometric foundations and behavioral assessment.* Newbury Park, CA: Sage.

Stevens, S. E., Hynan, M. T., & Allen, M. (2000). A meta-analysis of common factors and specific treatment effects across the outcome domains of the phase model of psychotherapy. *Clinical Psychology: Science and Practice, 7,* 273–290.

Suen, H. K., & Rzasa, S. E. (2004). Psychometric foundations of behavioral assessment. In S. N. Haynes & E. M. Heiby (Vol. Eds.), *Comprehensive handbook of psychological assessment: Vol. 3. Behavioral assessment.* Hoboken, NJ: Wiley.

Terbizan, D. J., Dolezal, B. A., & Albano, C. (2002). Validity of seven commercially available heart rate monitors. *Measurement in Physical Education and Exercise Science, 6,* 243–247.

Wampold, B. E., Mondin, G. W., Moody, M., Stich, F., Benson, K., & Ahn, H. (1997). A meta-analysis of outcome studies comparing bona fide psychotherapies: Empirically, "all must have prizes." *Psychological Bulletin, 122,* 203–215.

Watts, S., & Markham, R. A. (2005). Etiology of depression in children. *Journal of Instructional Psychology, 32,* 266–270.

Wenzlaff, R. M., & Wegner, D. M. (2000). Thought suppression. *Annual Review of Psychology, 51,* 59–91.

Williams, V. S., Baldwin, D. S., Hogue, S. L., Fehnel, S. E., Hollis, K. A., & Edin, H. M. (2006). Estimating the prevalence and impact of antidepressant-induced sexual dysfunction in 2 European countries: A cross-sectional patient survey. *Journal of Clinical Psychiatry, 67,* 204–210.

5. Self-Report Measures

Rocío Fernández-Ballesteros and Juan Botella

A *self-report* (SR) refers to verbal information about any event reported by a given subject about him- or herself. *Self-report measures* are the most common methods for collecting data in psychology and in the social sciences in general. As an assessment method, SRs are supported not only by psychometric principles and standards but also by experimental basic research developed in the fields of cognitive psychology (language, learning, and memory), social psychology, and neuropsychology (e.g., Schwarz, 1998; Stone, Turrkan, Bachrach, Kurtzman, & Cain, 2000).

SRs are also claimed as an important method for data collection in outcome evaluation (Lambert, 1994; Maruish, 1994; Tran & Smith, 2004). Most of the instruments selected by the conference organized for identifying a core battery to be used in outcome evaluation (for different forms of psychological interventions) were SRs (Strupp, Horowitz, & Lambert, 1997). As Lambert (1994, p. 81) pointed out, in most outcome research, SRs are included as change measures. Moreover, in 25% of outcome studies, SRs are the only source of information.

Self-Report Characteristics

SRs provide information about thousands of events. Among them we provide the following categories:

1. *External and observable conditions.* These may include observation of behaviors (e.g., "How many cigarettes do you smoke?") or observation of external conditions or contexts (e.g., "Are there rehabilitation services in your neighbourhood?"). This category of SRs can be independently assessed by other sources (other informants, direct observation, etc.).
2. *Physiological responses.* This category of SR involves assessment of one's autonomic nervous system responses (e.g., "Do you have a high heart rate?"). Physiological information can also be independently assessed by physiological records, but self-report can also be used in RCT research, where self-reports can be considered as more efficient methods when physiological responses are outcomes of a given treatment.
3. *Subjective or internal events.* SRs are the most direct method for assessing subjective or internal (cognitive or emotional events; see Fernández-

Ballesteros & Staats, 1992), which cannot be observed or mechanically recorded—in other words, what subjects feel or think, their plans or wishes (e.g., "Are you feeling sad?"). Self-reports of internal events are always needed in RCTs when relevant variables (dependent variables, independent variables, intervening variables, etc.) are subjective events.

SRs should be used when subjects' evaluations, attributions, or any other subjective information about any events are relevant for outcome research. For example, training outcome expectation is a mediator variable in all intervention, and therefore it should be measured through self-report (e.g., "Do you think the treatment will improve or reduce your complaints?").

Finally, from an information-processing approach, Ericsson and Simon (1980, 1984) classify SRs in two main forms: concurrent verbal reports (those reporting information at the same time it is being processed) and retrospective verbal reports. Whereas both types of self-reports are used in RCTs, retrospective verbal reports are usually employed for assessing eligibility criteria and various dependent variables (since they usually are related to the subject's needs or complaints). However, concurrent verbal reports should always be required when cognitive variables are to be manipulated during intervention (e.g., cover conditioning).

The most well known SRs are paper-and-pencil measures that are administered in a standardized way in the clinical situation. But self-reports can also be administered in *natural* or *analogue settings.* Self-observation of verbal expressions and self-monitoring are strategies for collecting information that can be administered in natural as well as in analogue situations; both are frequently used in outcome research (Tran & Smith, 2004) as it is described in the next section.

Moreover, the assessor can take subjects' self-reports at different *levels of inference,* using different types of research *design* and different methods of *statistical analysis;* that is, they can be used *directly* as verbal data or *isomorphically* as simple measures of cognitive events (Ericsson & Simon, 1980, 1984), such as when the target behavior is "cigarette smoking" and subjects report number of cigarettes smoked. Also, a set of SRs can be used in *aggregate, indirectly,* or as a *sign* of underlying psychological structures or process using between-subjects designs and proceeding through sophisticated statistical analysis, such as if a set of self-reports are taken together as a measure of anxiety (Fernández-Ballesteros, 1991, 2004c; Fernández-Ballesteros & Staats, 1992).

Table 5.1 presents the most important sources of variations of self-reports described here. Examples of SR modalities are also included.

Type of Self-Reports

Not only can subjects report on different classes of psychological events, but as strategies for data collection, SRs have several formats (Fernández-Ballesteros,

TABLE 5.1
Self-Reports: Relevant Characteristics and Derived Modalities

Characteristics	Modalities
Type of event	Motor, physiological, cognitive responses; subjective appraisal of a given response or situation
Data verifiability	Potentially verifiable vs. not verifiable
Referred time	Past, present, future
Setting	Standard administration in clinical settings vs. self-natural and analogue situations
Assessor's level of inference	Low level of inference: molecular self-reports vs. high level of inference: aggregate self-reports taken as sign of underlined constructs

1991, 2004a). Table 5.2 shows the most important types of self-reports: referring questions, responses, item manipulations, and output. Interviews (covered extensively in Chapter 3 of this volume), questionnaires, inventories and scales, self-observation or self-monitoring in experimental situations, and think-aloud protocols are considered the most common types of self-reports.

The variations regarding the different self-reports are the following:

- Open-format versus closed-format questions (e.g., Schwarz, 1998)
- Standard or nomothetic versus idiographic statements, both questions and answers (e.g., Haynes, 1986)
- Item aggregation (i.e., the score of a combination of items) versus molecular (or single) items or simple indicators (Fernández-Ballesteros, 1994, 2004a)

Self-report starts with an oral or written question (item) given by the assessor. As is well known, self-report items range from very open *versus* very closed questions (items). Let us describe the most common SRs.

Interviews usually have an open format both in the question ("Which is your problem?" "Could you tell me something about your family?"), organized by relevant standard areas (e.g., complaints, biographical data, family history, education, profession) , and in the answer. It can be stated that interview results are processed not to quantitative but to qualitative analysis.

Questionnaires, inventories, and scales are the most well known self-report instruments (sometimes self-reports are confounded with this category). These data collection methods are constituted by a set of standard closed questions or standard (nomothetic) items. Responses have different formats: dichotomous (yes/no), multiple-choice scales (through verbal responses, iconic images, etc.),

TABLE 5.2
Type of Self-Reports

	Interview, autobiography	Questionnaires, inventories, scales	Self-observation, self-monitoring	Think-aloud protocols
Questions	Open, semiopen	Closed, nomothetic or standard questions	Open, semi-open, idiographic	Open, semi-open, idiographic
Responses	Open, semiopen	Closed, nomothetic, yes/no format Ordinal, multiple-choice scales	Closed, semiopen, idiographic	Open, idiographic
Item manipulation	No manipulation	Aggregate measures, high level of inference	Simple or molecular measures	Simple or molecular measures
Output	Qualitative data	Norms, standard scores	Qualitative data, sometimes normative data	Qualitative data

and ordinal responses (first, second, third, etc.). Perhaps the most important condition of questionnaires, inventories, and scales is, precisely, that they contain standard material in both question and answer format. Moreover, results are analyzed in aggregation, and derived scores can be converted to norms or standard scores. Questionnaires, inventories, and scales are very commonly used in outcome research (e.g., Tran & Smith, 2004); recently, Maruish (2003) has indicated the usefulness of self-report scales in treatment planning and outcome assessment.

SRs could also be the expression of the *self-observation* or *self-monitoring* in *natural* as well as in *analogue or experimental settings* (Fernández-Ballesteros, 1994, 2004a,b). It can be stated that self-observation and self-monitoring, both in natural and in analogue situations, are "idiographically" based, in the sense that the protocols developed are dependent on the relevant problematic situation or subject's complaints. In general, a self-observation protocol addresses a given situation (natural or analogue) in which the subject should observe his or her own behavior. Usually, *target* refers to an open or semiopen response to be observed; it can be collected through paper-and-pencil tests, response counters, time records, or even electronic measurement devices. Depending on the type of the target observed, results can be analyzed from a quantitative or qualitative perspective; there even are norms for some self-monitoring devices (e.g., Phillips, Jones, Rieger, & Snell, 1997).

This type of self-report is used in outcome research; as an example, consider that a measure referred to as the Personal Report of Confidence as a Speaker has been designed to assess both reported fear and confidence before, during, and after public speaking (Phillips et al., 1997) and has been presented as a typical instrument for outcome research in social phobia (e.g., see Tran & Smith, 2004). Also, the Behavioral Avoidance Test (BAT; Lang & Lazovik, 1963; see Hersen & Bellack, 2002) is a situational or analogue method for measuring anxiety that consists of the presentation of fear stimuli or situations and the assessment of the triple response system, that is, the observation of overt behavior, the SRs of both cognitive and emotional-verbal behavior, and the record of physiological responses that is commonly used in the anxiety treatment outcome. Another very common self-report instrument for assessing behavioral change in both natural and experimental situations is the Fear Thermometer, used for assessing the cognitive component of fear on a 10-point scale (Kleinknecht & Bernstein, 2002).

Finally, a *think-aloud protocol* is an open instrument for verbal-cognitive data collection (see Genest & Turk, 1981; Hollon & Kendall, 1980). In short, the subject is asked to think aloud when a task is administered, and verbal and motor responses are taped. Afterward, qualitative analyses of the verbal and motor responses are conducted (Merluzzi, Glass, & Genest, 1981; Hollon & Kendall, 1980). Although think-aloud protocols are qualitative methods for data collection and are very rare in outcome evaluation, they can be considered as a promising procedure for assessing change in pre-post design; for example, Baltes and Staudinger (2000) have tested a training program on "relativism" (one of the components of wisdom) using think-aloud protocols as their main method in a series of tasks on "life review," "dilemmas," or "life planning" (Staudinger, Marsiske, & Baltes, 1995).

All these SR methods have positive and negative characteristics. Usually, questionnaires, inventories, and scales present good numbers about the validity and reliability of their scores. Since they have norms, changes in posttreatment scores can be analyzed not only by comparison with a baseline but also by making normative comparisons. At the same time, constructs assessed have a very high level of inference and a very low level of sensitivity to change. On the contrary, molecular or simple measures coming from self-observation, self-monitoring, and think-aloud protocols in natural or analogue situations are much more reactive and obtrusive. This is because, as is well known, introspection usually interferes with monitoring of target behavior. Very few molecular or simple measures have norms, but they have a very low level of inference and can be more sensitive to treatment when the behaviors observed are carefully selected.

■ Quality of Self-Reports

In the context of RCTs, SR quality can be considered in two different ways: (a) when a self-report should be selected among the instruments already developed, and (b) when an ad hoc self-report measurement device should be developed.

An advantage of the already developed measures is that they are usually some quality indexes of their scores; by contrast, the development of a new self-report requires a long and complex process (e.g., Clark & Watson, 1995; Kogan & Edelstein, 2004). However, an advantage for the specific measures developed ad hoc is that they usually yield larger effect sizes than standardized measures (Wilson & Lipsey, 2001). This difference could be explained by assuming that specific measures probably better tap the construct under study.

Several criteria can be used for testing the psychometric quality of SRs (see the *Standards for Educational and Psychological Testing;* American Educational Research Association, American Psychological Association, & National Council on Measurement in Education, 1999). But, besides the classic dimensions of psychometric principles, such as *reliability* and *validity,* in the context of RCTs some others must be taken into account: *sensitivity* and *specificity* of the SRs to collect information for judgments related to classification and diagnoses in applying the inclusion/exclusion (I/E) criteria, and *utility,* time *efficiency*, and *sensitivity to change* in the SRs employed as outcome measures.

Reliability

Although reliability is frequently taken as a property of the measure itself, in fact it is a property of the measure's scores. A single tool, when applied to different samples in different measurement contexts, can yield scores with different levels of reliability.

Reliability is, in general terms, the degree to which the scores are free from random error. Depending on the source of the random error, the reliability can be understood as *stability,* as *internal consistency,* or as *equivalence.* Reliability as *stability* refers to the extent to which the scores from a given measure are sensitive to time. It is quantified by calculating the correlation between the scores recorded in two administrations delayed by a time interval, obtaining the so-called *retest coefficient.* Reliability as *internal consistency* refers to the degree to which the elements or components of a given measure are determined to be the same. It is tested by measuring the contribution of the covariances between the elements to the total variance of the scores. Although several indexes are available, the most frequently employed is Cronbach's (1951) alpha coefficient. Reliability as *equivalence* is the degree to which two forms of the same tool are interchangeable. It is quantified by assessing the correlation between the scores obtained with two alternative forms of the same instrument.

The degree to which a score from an SR is stable between contexts is its degree of generalizability across situations. It would represent a risk to select a tool based on the reliability reported in the manual or in a research report if the tool is to be applied in a different context than that in which the reliability was originally estimated. For example, among adolescents, females can have a higher propensity to reflect in an SR a more pervasive range of social dysfunctions (Young, Heptinstall, Sonuga-Barke, Chadwick, & Taylor, 2005). For many SRs, we lack detailed information on how reliability changes as a function of these potential sources of variation (*facets*, in terms of the theory of generalization).

Although reliability is one of the basic psychometric principles that must be present in the scores generated by any measurement tool, each type of reliability plays a different role in RCTs:

- *Temporal stability* is essential for any measure, since design in outcome research generally implies assessment at two separate times (before and after treatment). We should have information about retest reliability because treatment effects can be confounded with time effects.
- *Internal consistency* and *equivalence* are important features for aggregate measures (see Table 5.1), with high levels of inference. In aggregate measures it is necessary to check the homogeneity of the responses to the elements that are combined to tap the set of facets that jointly reflect a high-level construct.
- *Equivalence* is also required when two circumstances are simultaneously present in repeated measurements: (a) The responses can be easily remembered, and (b) the persons have a tendency to show themselves as consistent persons. To avoid the threat posited by these circumstances, it is necessary to have equivalent versions of the same test that can be administered before and after the intervention or to plan a different order of item presentation.

Validity

Validity, the most fundamental issue in psychological assessment, is considered from classical test theory as the extent to which a measurement instrument measures what it is intended to measure. However, considerations of validity have changed significantly. Modern perspectives relate validity with the adequacy of the inferences and actions based on the obtained scores and the degree to which they are empirically and theoretically supported (Messick, 1989). An important consequence of this changed perspective is that validity is no more a statistical property of the test; it is a property of the meanings of test scores that are required by their proposed uses. The focus of validation is on the relationships between the evidence and the inferences drawn from it (Messick, 1989), so that validity can be viewed as a "system of arguments" (Cronbach, 1988).

Consequently, validation of the inferences from scores for a particular purpose cannot be automatically generalized to use for other purposes. For example, perhaps scores from a measure that are valid for diagnosis are not valid to assess a treatment's outcome. Each intended inference from the scores must be validated separately.

The concept of validity today is closer to the old concept of "construct validity." It is recognized that scores are always given a meaning related to a purpose. Because the meaning is always a construct, all relevant evidence to support a given use is related to a construct. Then, validity is the degree to which a given use of a tool captures, in all its extension and the richness of appropriate subtleties, the construct that underlies the intended use. In fact, inadequate construct validity has been recognized as a threat to the putative causes and effects of an intervention (Cook & Campbell, 1979).

The last version of the *Standards for Educational and Psychological Testing* (American Educational Research Association, American Psychological Association, & National Council on Measurement in Education, 1999) assumes this view when it describes validity as "the degree to which evidence and theory support the interpretations of test scores entailed by proposed uses of tests" (p. 9).

Whereas in older versions of the standards several types of validity were described, in the last one validity is considered as a unitary concept, although evidence for validation can (and should) come from several sources. Specifically, five sources of evidence are identified.

1. Evidence based on *test content* relates to the extent to which items represent all domains covered by the concept assessed. For example, SRs for assessing marital satisfaction must cover all areas that are potentially relevant for a measure of general satisfaction and as many contexts as possible where conflict can show up.

2. Evidence based on *response processes* focuses on the detailed nature of the responses actually given. Sometimes the responses can be more influenced by specific strategies or attitudes than by the construct itself, as devised by the assessor. For example, SRs usually elicit a set of response tendencies that are independent of an item's content but can distort SRs results.

3. Evidence based on *internal structure* has to do with the degree to which the several elements of the measure show a pattern of relationships that reflects the assumed framework. For example, a tool to assess anxiety and encompass elements to tap physiological, emotional, and cognitive components must show higher correlations for the elements within each facet than for elements from different facets.

4. Evidence based on *relations to other variables* has been one of the most relevant types of validity in the classical framework.

- The predictive power of an external criterion. When selecting the criterion to be predicted, for which validity must be assessed previously, measures of different types, and not only SRs, can be chosen. In this sense, it can be said that the measurement device will measure just as the criterion predicted. Thus, different physiological indexes have shown that SRs for tobacco consumption usually have high levels of validity (e.g., Bernaards, Twisk, van Mechelen, Snel, & Kemper, 2004; Caraballo, Giovino, Pechacek, & Mowery, 2001). Logically, a high level of this type of validity when the criterion used is itself biased produces a tool with the same bias. However, when what is being assessed is phenomenological, such as well-being or self-esteem, there is no other way to assess validity than with another SR.

- The theoretical relationships with other measures. Specifically, the measure must show high correlations with measures for making inferences assumedly similar when assessing the same construct (convergent evidence) and low correlations with measures for making inferences assumedly different, as they are assessed different constructs (discriminant evidence; see Kane, 1992).

- The degree to which evidence based on a predicted criterion can be generalized to other contexts.

5. Evidence based on *consequences of testing* is the last source incorporated in the standards. It is related to the emphasis on social considerations of the intended and unintended consequences of a measurement's use (Cronbach, 1988; Messik, 1989). It captures the value implications of score interpretation as a basis for intervention, but also the consequences of test use. Especially important is the existence of any source of invalidity that impacts negatively on the test takers, yielding bias or unfairness. But the developer of a self-report cannot limit its use. Because responsibility when applying a measurement rests ultimately with the user who makes the inferences from the scores, he or she must collect and/or evaluate the evidence on whether the inferences are appropriate for the intended purpose. As indicated in the standards, this is especially important when a measure is used for a purpose that differs from that supported by the developer. The authors of an RCT who decide to use a self-report must gather and/or produce evidence that the scores obtained are valid for the specific use they are going to give them (e.g., checking the I/E criteria, assessing severity of symptoms, or measuring change). Of course, not all sources of evidence are equally important in all uses of a self-report, even within RCTs.

Recent discussions of measurement have put the focus on a new, allegedly different dimension called arbitrariness, which is strongly related to consequential validity (evidence based on consequences of testing). A reliable and valid measure can be viewed as arbitrary if it is not linked to meaningful referents of everyday life. This is especially important in clinical psychology, where sometimes reliable and valid measures are not clinically relevant (Kazdin, 2006). The improvement after treatment must be relevant and obvious to patients, but also to the people around them in everyday life. The sources of financial support for treatment often ask for this type of evidence.

Finally, although this is not the appropriate place to deal with this in detail, we wish to mention the importance of method variance in the construct measurement (whatever its level of inference). Since each method has its own source of error, a certain amount of variance is due to the method used. Therefore, method has an important influence in constructs measurement. It should be stated that no single measure can appropriately represent any construct. As has been pointed out by Cook (1985) from postpositivism, different constructs (or different objectives) should be operationalized by multiple measures and methods, but different types of self-reports cannot be considered as different methods, since they share (more than any other method) the same sources of error and explain a similar amount of variance in the construct assessment. For example, Fernández-Ballesteros (1994) reports higher correlations between self-reports assessing different constructs described by different responses than the same construct described by the same responses assessed by different methods. The most problematic issue refers to cognitive constructs that cannot be assessed by different methods; in this case the assessment of the convergence implies a homomethod (self-reports) and only different techniques of verbal data collection (questionnaire, self-observation, etc.). As a consequence, when using multiple measures and multiple operationalizations, the irrelevancies are probably different, and the measures capture better the pursued construct. A specific source of irrelevancies in RCTs is the expectations of the assessor. Of course, as with any other assessment method besides self-report, the employment of assessors without expectations is the way to circumvent this problem.

We agree with Lambert (1994) that in an ideal study of change, all parties involved who have information about change might be presented; this would include the client, the therapist, relevant (significant) others, trained judges (or observers), and societal agencies that store relevant information about the client.

Sensitivity and Specificity in Classification

SRs are often employed for classifying a person in one of several categories. Although in RCTs the selection and assessment of I/E criteria are done before the intervention, during the screening process, they could be also necessary after the intervention, when changes in classification become an outcome measure. In both cases, as I/E criteria or as an outcome measure, the self-report must fulfill the sensitivity and specificity requirements. Again, the lack of evidence for sensitivity and specificity of the scores from a given self-report should be remedied before its use.

These concepts are related to the classification rule that is applied, taking as a basis the scores in that test; they are not properties of the test itself. For a given measurement device it is possible to obtain as many values of sensitivity and specificity as rules can be defined. *Sensitivity* is the degree to which the persons pertaining to a given category (target) are classified as such. *Specificity* is the degree to which the persons not pertaining to that category are correctly excluded from it. In other words, the sensitivity reflects the probability of giving a true positive, and the specificity that of giving a true negative (Swets & Pickett, 1982). The two forms of producing wrong classifications (the complementary of the sensitivity and specificity) are called *false positive* and *false negative* (e.g., Mossman & Somoza, 1989; see Patrick et al., 1994).

The problem faced when defining classification rules is that when the rule is shifted to increase the sensitivity, then the specificity decreases, and vice versa. The setting of a rule based in a measure implies the assumption of a given compromise between both tendencies. The relationship between both values is usually represented by receiver operating characteristic (ROC) curves such as the one in Figure 5.1 (Wickens, 2002). The figure shows the probability distributions of the scores in an imaginary test by the target (T) population and another control (C) population from which it has to be discriminated. Each possible decision rule is represented by a point in the figure. Suppose that the rule "Classify in the key category whenever the person's value on X is 4 or more" is employed. Then, in the long run 90% of the target population will be correctly classified in the key category, whereas 30% of the control population will be incorrectly classified in that category.

Let us illustrate the procedure with an example. It has been claimed that self-report of smoking behavior is often inaccurate. Patrick and colleagues (1994) assessed by a meta-analysis the sensitivity and specificity of SR mea-

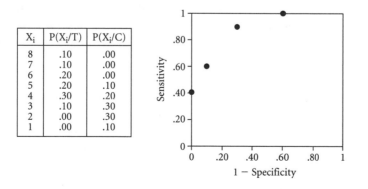

X_i	$P(X_i/T)$	$P(X_i/C)$
8	.10	.00
7	.10	.00
6	.20	.00
5	.20	.10
4	.30	.20
3	.10	.30
2	.00	.30
1	.00	.10

FIGURE 5.1. Measure X is a self-report used in the screening process to select patients with a given disease. The table shows the probability distributions of the scores for the target (T) population and for another population (C, for control) from which the target has to be discriminated. The unitary square to the right shows the sensitivity and the complementary of the specificity for four selection rules based on the test ("select those with $x \geq 6$, 5, 4, and 3," respectively). The ROC curve is plotted connecting the points that represent performance of each decision rule.

sures, taking biochemical assessments as the basis for control. That is, the biochemical assessment is employed to set the "real" category for each participant (smoker/nonsmoker). Because each participant is also self-identified as a smoker or a nonsmoker in an SR, ROC analysis can be used to assess the degree to which both measurements match. After collecting 51 statistical results, the mean sensitivity was .875, and the mean specificity was .892. More important, intervention studies for smoking cessation in student populations were identified as especially prone to low levels of accuracy. For those cases, the use of biochemical assessment instead of SR is recommended.

The costs of producing false positives and false negatives and the benefits of obtaining true positives and true negatives must be the basis for setting the rule to be employed. Furthermore, the sensitivity and specificity of a given rule can change with the type of population or context in which it is employed. For example, Zung's Self-Rating Depression Scale usually yields high levels of sensitivity and specificity, but it is especially efficient in the balance between them when applied in the elderly (Zung & Zung, 1986).

The sensitivity and specificity of SRs are important in RCTs, above all, in the process of screening. During this process, I/E criteria can be used that bias the final sample, so that although all those admitted are from the target population, some of the subtypes of that population are overrepresented, whereas others are underrepresented.

Utility

A self-report must always be reliable and valid, independently of the function for which it is used. When used for selection in the screening process, a self-report must also be sensitive and specific; when used as an outcome measure, it must have some additional properties. Utility is especially important. Thus, Tran and Smith (2004) highlight the efficiency in the time of administration and the sensitivity to change as characteristics composing clinical utility.

When the administration of a self-report takes too much time, its practical usefulness is limited. If the sessions devoted to collecting the information in the pretreatment, posttreatment, and follow-up are long and boring, the quality of the responses drops significantly. The subjects can answer to the last part in a routine, thoughtlessly way. In fact, the ideal SRs for RCTs are those that allow collecting a large amount of information in a short time, while reliability and validity remain intact. This characteristic is the so-called time efficiency in administration (Tran & Smith, 2004). Reliability and validity are necessary, but this practical characteristic should not be ignored.

The other characteristic of utility is sensitivity to change (Silva, 1993). It is related to the capacity for reflecting changes in what is intended to be changed by the intervention under study (Fernández-Ballesteros, 2002). The self-reports that assess enduring characteristics are not useful as outcome measures; an SR that is too weighted with personality characteristics will have low sensitivity to change. However, an SR that focuses on simple behaviors of the patient can have high sensitivity to change. To establish this property for an SR, it must be demonstrated that the scores change significantly as a consequence of the treatment and that the amount of change is positively related to the improvement in target behaviors.

Sensitivity to change usually covaries negatively with time efficiency. The administration of a measure that is highly sensitive to change is usually more time-consuming. The goal in selecting an SR as a measure of the outcomes of a trial is reaching a good balance between time efficiency and sensitivity to change.

In short, classical psychometric characteristics of reliability and validity are necessary but not sufficient for assessing the advantages and shortcomings of alternative measurement tools. Reliable and valid measures that take too much time or need too many resources could have low sensitivity to change, and therefore may not be useful in practical terms for an RCT.

■ Selecting Self-Report Measures for Outcome Research

In selecting a self-report method in outcome research, three conditions may be relevant: the *nature* of the event (motor, cognitive, or physiological), the *moment* in the process of experimental situation, and the *class* of variable to be assessed (dependent, independent, intervening, controlling, etc.). Self-reports are used for all these conditions.

As stated earlier, although motor and physiological responses allow direct measurement (observation and physiological records, respectively), and self-report can be considered as an "indirect" but more efficient method for assessing those responses, when assessing cognitive variables, self-report must be considered the unique measurement strategy. Nevertheless, because there are several types of self-reports (with different sources of errors), the assessor should carefully select several types of measures to test a "within-subjective" validity of the subject's cognitive verbal reports (Fernández-Ballesteros, 1994, 2004a, 2004c).

Also, outcome evaluation implies a long process (Maruish, 2004; Fernández-Ballesteros, 2004c; Nezu, Nezu, Peacock, & Girdwood, 2004) with three main steps: (a) analyzing the case, (b) planning and administering the treatment, and (c) evaluation and follow-up. Measures for testing outcomes could be collected during this process, linked to one or several steps, mainly depending on the role each variable has in the experimental design selected. Before dealing with this important issue, let us discuss the general criteria proposed by authors in this field for selecting measures in an RCT.

Criteria for Selecting Measures of Treatment Success

Although, as Lambert, Strupp, and Horowitz (1997) have pointed out, there is no consensus for selecting measures of treatment success, two main perspectives can be distinguished: *nomothetic measures* and *idiographic measures.* From the perspective of nomothetic measures, the selection of a "battery" of standard tests for a given psychopathology is emphasized. This is the case of the Outcome Measures Project and the Core Battery Conference (see Strupp et al., 1997). With idiographic measures, tailored treatments have specific measures selected individually for single cases. This distinction is important because while in our typology of SR methods, the nomothetic approach refers to standard questionnaires, inventories, and scales, the idiographic approach refers to self-observation and monitoring or to think-aloud cognitive methods.

In our opinion, the "appropriateness" of a given method depends on the extent to which the method fulfills a set of criteria. As has been mentioned earlier, from the scientific point of view of *multiplism* (Cook, 1985), authors agree that one of the most important criteria for treatment outcome is to have multiple objectives assessed through multiple methods and investigated through multiple informants.

But when consensus has to be reached in order to select a set of core measures for a given problem, political reasons usually surpass scientific ones. The most common criteria to be followed to select measures for treatment outcome (Newman & Ciarlo, 1994; Goldfried, 1997; Strupp et al., 1997; Lambert, 1994; among others) are the following:

- Relevance to the target group and independent of the treatment provided
- Simple methods and procedures
- Psychometric features: reliability, validity
- Sensitivity to change
- Standard administration and norms for replicability
- Low cost, efficiency
- Utility considerations (understandable by nonprofessional audiences, easy feedback and uncomplicated consideration, useful in clinical services, compatibility with clinical theories)

Following these criteria, most of the instruments listed for treatment outcome research of anxiety, mood, and personality disorders are self-reports (see Strupp et al., 1997).

Self-Report Measures Assessing Relevant Variables

Kerlinger (1973) said that an essential ingredient of any research is the way a given variable is operationalized with a given measure or instrument. Therefore, one of the most important decisions in outcome research has two faces:

(a) the list of target and relevant variables, and (b) the instruments or procedures used for assessing them.

The most important variables assessed through self-reports are the following: (a) subjects' characteristics and the assessment of eligibility criteria; (b) target or dependent variables; (c) instrumental, causal, independent, or mediating goals; (d) treatment intervening variables; and (d) treatment control. Let us review the use of self-reports measuring these variables.

CHECKING THE INCLUSION AND EXCLUSION CRITERIA

The setting of well-defined I/E criteria is essential for RCTs. Outcome studies without explicit criteria or with inadequate criteria, or studies whose implementation is lax, will produce biased results. Self-reports are often used for assessing I/E criteria. Frequently, the process of screening has several stages, and SRs are employed to get the relevant information in most, if not all, of them. Since other chapters in this volume deal with the process of subject selection, here we only highlight the specific sources of potential bias linked to SRs that could have an influence on this process.

All factors that threaten the quality of SRs are present when applying the I/E criteria. These include not only the more classic psychometric properties but also the vulnerability to the influence of extraneous factors (situational and response biases). But other potential sources of error are relevant here.

The first one is the desire (conscious or nonconscious) to be selected or rejected. If the candidates believe that their participation can yield a benefit for them, they can respond in the way they believe will increase the probability of being included. Faking and impression management (symptom exaggeration or reduction) are intentional distortions, but subjects also can nonconsciously deny their pathological behaviors. Although in clinical settings the use of self-report is based in the assumption of subjects' honest cooperation, this cannot be assumed in some contexts, such as when patients are hoping to receive a desired treatment (in the same vein as in personnel selection) or any other expected benefit from being selected. For example, as reported by Christensen and colleagues (2004) in some RCTs on couple therapy using self-report measures as I/E criteria, couples interested in receiving therapy (especially therapy at no cost) can exaggerate their conflicts so that their relationships look more troubled than they in fact are.

When conducting an RCT, the use of self-reports in checking the I/E criteria should be carefully taken into account. For example, to avoid intentional deception the researcher can partially and momentarily omit the final goal of the process. During the process of screening, it can be presented as a study of the problem, but without making explicit the possibility of any benefit if the person is selected and randomly assigned to the group that receives the treatment under study in the trial.

Second, whereas the self-reports that are employed as an outcome measure usually refer to the present time, many I/E criteria refer to events relatively distant in time. This is a known factor that reduces the quality of SRs because of forgetting or false remembering, but also because of the reduced precision of true old memories (Menon & Yorkston, 2000; Tourangeau, 2000). Thus, for example, the I/E criteria to enter in studies of sleep treatments (e.g., Johnson, 2003) assume relatively long histories of insomnia. If there are no records of previous events, the memories of the candidates regarding the duration and intensity of the problem must be trusted.

In summary, a self-report is useful only if honest participation is assured; outcome researchers should be sure about the characteristics of participants so that legitimate generalizations can be made from the trial. The degree of specification of the I/E criteria and their application in the process of screening are crucial. SRs are often employed in checking the I/E criteria, sometimes because of the subjective nature of what is assessed and sometimes because of the practical advantages of self-reports. When SRs are used for this function, some specific difficulties could be avoided if the goal of selection for an eventual benefit is temporarily omitted during the screening process. For other problems, it is a good idea to ask, when possible, for records that confirm specific details about the participants' reported problems.

MEASURING TARGET OR DEPENDENT VARIABLES

Target behavior or dependent variables are the ultimate goals of a given treatment. Two main conditions require the use of self-reports. *Target* refers to the patient complaints, which can be specified also as constituents of his or her psychological problem. Since patient demands usually are self-reported, in those cases, SRs are important instruments for measuring patient change. In addition, the nature of the target can be verbal-cognitive or emotional (subjective); therefore, the self-report is a fundamental method for assessing cognitive psychopathology. Nevertheless, in both cases, other overt behaviors should also be tested. In no way should SRs be the only method for evaluation of psychological interventions. Finally, let us mention that all these measures are collected in the first step of the process during the case formulation.

These two conditions are behind the fact that most of the instruments in the core battery for assessing change already described are self-reports in anxiety, mood, and personality disorders. For example, mood disorders have the following dependent variables to be assessed by self-reports: *subjective distress* (Well-being Scale of the SF-36 Health Survey) and *depressive symptoms* (measured by four very well known self-report measures; see Strupp et al., 1997).[1]

---

1. Also, rating scales and diagnostic interviews are proposed in order to assess general functioning and proceed to a diagnosis or classification.

All these measures are standard or nomothetic self-report scales or question-naires for assessing depression and distress. Nevertheless, other molecular measures of outcome target can be used. For example, in treatment outcomes of social anxiety disorders, Tran and Smith (2004) proposed the use of the Behavioural Avoidance Test to measure changes of fear—not only motor and physiological components of anxiety but also subjective (cognitive) responses—through the Subjective Units of Discomfort Scales, which are subjective discomfort ratings on a scale ranging from 0 (no anxiety) to 100 (panic or extreme anxiety). As the authors emphasized, standardized BAT results allow comparisons across studies. The idiographic variety affords researchers the most flexible procedure, as well as the lowest level of inference.

In conclusion, target variables are strongly related to subjective responses established in the first step of the assessment-treatment-evaluation process and, in pre-post experimental designs, should be reassessed after treatment and in any eventual follow-up. In sum, self-reports are indicated in outcome measures in RCT.

INSTRUMENTAL, CAUSAL, INDEPENDENT, OR MEDIATING VARIABLES

Measuring patient change should not be reduced to target or dependent variables. Outcome research should also examine to what extent other variables, with functionally related targets, have changed, or whether independent (casual) variables manipulated by treatment can be considered instrumental outcomes. As Nezu and Nezu (1993) pointed out, dependent, or ultimate, outcomes should be differentiated from "instrumental outcomes" (or independent variables; Rosen & Proctor, 1981). In cognitive and cognitive-behavioral treatments, those variables are basic behavioral repertoires that should also be measured in order to test causal hypotheses behind the treatment (Fernández-Ballesteros & Staats, 1992).

For example, following Nezu et al. (2004), theories about depression postulate the following "instrumental" outcome variables: pleasant and unpleasant variables, expectation of positive events, coping abilities, problem-solving ability, assertive behavior, management and communication skills, interpersonal skills, autonomic thoughts, negative self-evaluations, negative ruminations, unrealistically high expectations, self-punishment, flexibility and perspective taking, positive orientation to problems in living, cognitive distortions, errors in logic, irrational thinking, self-blame, negative attributions, social skills, and negative images and memories. All these postulated causal variables of depression are behavioral repertoires that could potentially be assessed by questionnaires, inventories, or scales (see Heiby & Hurtado, 1994).

Since changes in instrumental variables are expected after treatment, they should be assessed at two points in the process: before and after treatment. In summary, SRs should be employed for assessing cognitive constructs as instrumental outcomes or independent variables when treatments are manipulating those constructs.

TREATMENT-INTERVENING VARIABLES

Treatment-intervening variables are considered those relevant conditions for treatment because they could intervene in treatment outcomes. Although personality variables—of both patient and therapist—seem to have influence in therapy outcomes (see Hilsenroth, 2004), here we are dealing with two types of intervening variables: (a) those specific subjects' conditions related to the ongoing treatment, and (b) those general characteristics that could have effects in all treatments.

Regarding the former, each treatment usually has some preconditions. For example, since reinforcement implies a functional concept, when a reinforcement training by token economy is administered, the therapist should assess, before training, which are the most suitable reinforcements for clients (e.g., Hollon & Kendall, 1980). Also, all covert condition training (strategies or methods for treatment behavior) requires imagery capacities; therefore, these capacities should be assessed before proceeding to training, and there are standard methods for doing so (e.g., Cautela, 1977).

But other subjects' conditions are relevant in all training programs; for example, as has been very well established, outcome expectancy is a good predictor of treatment success (Bandura, 1969). For assessing a subject's treatment expectancy, there are both general standard self-reports (e.g., Treatment Evaluation Inventory; Kazdin, 2002) and also simple scale scores that can be standardized for a given outcome study (Fernández-Ballesteros, 2004b).

In this case, within the assessment, treatment, and evaluation process, there is only one right moment for assessing intervening variables, namely, before the treatment.

TREATMENT CONTROL

Most psychological treatments require subjects to complete homework or assignments. Therefore, self-reports on whether those assignments have been fulfilled should be administered and checked throughout treatment. For example, in bibliotherapy, subjects should read concrete texts; in thought-stopping, subjects should use this technique at home when undesirable thoughts occur. In fact, the outcome of a given treatment depends not only on the number of sessions but also on treatment compliance (see Kazdin, 1980). Self-monitoring during treatment and self-report are the main procedures for assessing the extent to which subjects are not only attending prescribed sessions but also following prescribed tasks.

In summary, SRs have extraordinary importance in RCTs not only for assessing I/E criteria and dependent or target variables but also for assessing instrumental or independent variables, for checking intervening variables in the preassessment step, and for controlling compliance during treatment.

■ Response Distortions

The response process validity of self-reports (described earlier) largely depends on the cooperation of test takers, who are generally instructed to read items carefully and provide honest responses (Baer, Rinaldo, & Berry 2003, p. 861). But a subject's answer to the question formulated by the assessor or listed in a self-report paper-and-pencil instrument (including formal conditions such as clarity, comprehensibility, etc.) not only is determined by its content (about what the participant thinks, feels, behaves, or infers) but also is influenced by several distortions coming from the participant's *tendency* to answer in a given response format and by the subject response *management.*

Response Tendencies

Questionnaires, inventories, and scales have a closed-response format; among the most common are a yes/no format and Likert scales (with 4, 5, 7, or more possible responses). As is well known in psychological assessment, the yes/no format can introduce acquiescence bias, and scales introduce the so-called range restriction, that is, the possibility of answering just in the middle or on the border of the scale. Since response distortions refer RCTs, and since we are assigning subjects at random to experimental and control conditions, it can be assumed that they are not threatened by any of these distortions.

Response Management

As Lanyon and Goodstein (1971) pointed out, "any self-report is affected or distorted by the subject's desire (conscious or not) to appear well or poorly adjusted, a need to confirm or agree with the test conditions of the examiner, a tendency to choose a particular alternative in a multiple-choice format, and a variety of recent immediate experiences such as viewing a dramatic film or failing to perform well on a task" (p. 388). These response distortions, response styles, or response set threaten not only the traditional psychological constructs (personality traits, attitudes, etc.) but also low-inference behavioral constructs and even simple reports of behavioral and contextual events (McCann, 1998; Fernández-Ballesteros, 2004a, 2004c).

Social desirability, lying, faking, malingering, and impression management (good and bad) are very closed concepts developed at the same time as the validity scales of the Minnesota Multiphasic Personality Inventory (MMPI). Recent meta-analysis of MMPI-2 faking-bad (Rogers, Sewell, Martin, & Vitacco, 2003) and faking-good (Baer & Miller, 2002) pointed out the ability of faking scales (F, Fb, F-K, Fp, and L, K, F-K, L + K, and S, respectively) to classify malingerers. In fact, MMPI validity scales for sensitivity and utility have been largely tested and found to be good strategies for controlling these distortions

(Bagby, Marshall, & Bocchiochi, 2005; Baer et al., 1995). Looking at this issue from the perspective of treatment evaluation, we agree with McCann (1998) that our concern should be the *credibility* of self-report.

Two issues should be discussed here: First, to what extent do response distortions affect self-reports in outcome research in clinical settings? Second, if we decide that such distortions should be assessed and controlled, at what stage of the process should we proceed?

All the concepts listed earlie differ along a deliberate/unaware dimension (see Fernández-Ballesteros, 1991). As Lanyon (2003) recently stated, the empirical definition of the existing assessment procedures of these concepts ignores this dimension, and they are generally viewed as deliberate behaviors for cheating (following the MMPI validity scale named "Lie"). But Lanyon proposes to recognize the presence of both type of motivations, as well as many gradations in between. He uses the term *misrepresentation* to refer to the overall field and the interchangeable terms *overstatement* and *exaggeration* as neutral concepts. Finally, he criticizes available scales for not offering a reliable way to determine whether behavior is or is not deliberate.

As has already been stated, we assume that in a clinical setting subjects are highly motivated to give honest responses. Nevertheless, it is also well known that among response distortions in the aware pole we can find *faking* (good or bad), but also, in the opposite nonaware side, *self-deception* could be a very important distortion. Following Schneider (2001), a subject's self-deception is marked by the lack of attempts to gain reality checks. It relies on an exclusively confirmatory approach to information processing and may even involve an active attempt to avoid information inconsistent with desired beliefs. Even if we assume that in clinical psychology subjects are highly motivated to be honest, and therefore it is not necessary to check aware distortions, self-deception could be a relevant variable in outcome research and could be a target for treatment.

The most problematic issue is how these response distortions (with several levels of a subject's awareness) affect outcome research. Because this book refers to RCTs, two possibilities can be distinguished across the assessment-treatment-evaluation process: (a) Our first concern refers to random assignment; it can be assumed that both experimental and control groups are affected by this distortion to the same extent. (b) The second issue refers to whether treatment can have an effect by self-deception. Most cognitive treatment acts on a subject's self-awareness, and therefore these variables should be taken into consideration. Moreover, relationships between therapist and client are increasing throughout the treatment process; it can be predicted that the subject will reduce all types of distortions because both motivation to be honest and self-awareness will increase. In both cases, nonaware response distortions should be taken into consideration and should be assessed before and after treatment.

Because very few studies have examined the impact of self-report distortions (both aware and nonaware) on outcome research, our only possibility is to call for much more investigation in this field.

■ Conclusion

Self-report is an important method for data collection in outcome evaluation. Most of the instruments selected as a core battery for psychological treatment evaluation are SRs, and in 25% of outcome studies SRs are the only source of information. The most important SRs methods for data collection in RCT are questionnaires, inventories, and scales, self-observation and self-monitoring, and think-aloud protocols in experimental or natural situations.

All these SR techniques have positive and negative characteristics. Usually, questionnaires, inventories, and scales show good reliability and validity coefficients, but at the same time, measures from these instruments have a very high level of inference and very low sensitivity to change. On the contrary, molecular or simple measures coming from self-observation, self-monitoring, and think-aloud protocols in natural and analogue situations are much more sensitive to change, but before using them, reliability and validity should be tested.

Any single measure cannot appropriately describe a construct, as has been pointed out by Cook (1985). As we know from postpositivism, different constructs (or different objectives) should be operationalized by multiple measures and methods, as well as different sources. But different types of self-reports cannot be considered as different methods, since they share (more than any other method) the same sources of error, and they explain a similar amount of variance in the construct assessment. Also, as Lambert (1994) has said, in an ideal study of change, all parties involved who have information about change might be presented; this would include the client, therapist, relevant (significant) others, trained judges (or observers), and societal agencies that store relevant information about the client.

Temporal stability, internal consistency, and equivalence are the most common criteria for testing reliability in SRs used in RCTs. After revising forms of validity, sensitivity and specificity in classification and utility are considered important criteria for evaluating SRs in RCTs. Finally, classic psychometric features of reliability and validity are necessary but not sufficient for evaluating the advantages and shortcomings of alternative measurement instruments. SRs are often employed in checking the I/E criteria because of their own subjective nature, as well as because of their practical advantages. When SRs are used for this function, some specific problems could be avoided if the goal of selection for an eventual benefit is temporarily omitted during the screening process.

SRs are also required for assessing dependent, instrumental, and treatment control variables. Target (or dependent) variables are, to some extent, subjective responses established in the first step of the assessment-treatment-evaluation process. Therefore, SRs indicated as outcome measures in RCT and in pre-post experimental designs, should be reassessed after treatment and during follow-up, should that take place. Also, changes in instrumental variables are expected after treatment and therefore should be assessed at two stages of the process: before and after treatment. Finally, during treatment follow-up, SRs are the primary methods and procedures for assessing the extent to which subjects are not only attending prescribed sessions but also following prescribed tasks.

Self-reports have two types of distortions. First, a subject's tendency to give a response elicited by the response format, independent of the actual intention of the self-report format, threatens the validity of SRs. Second, SRs can be affected by the subject's desire (conscious or nonconscious) to appear with a concrete profile. It is commonly understood that in RCTs this tendency. Nevertheless, much more research needs to be conducted in this field.

■ References

American Educational Research Association, American Psychological Association, & National Council on Measurement in Education. (1999). *Standards for educational and psychological testing.* Washington, DC: Author.

Baer, R. A., & Miller, J. (2002). Underreporting of psychopathology on the MMPI-2: A meta-analytic review. *Psychological Assessment, 14,* 16–26.

Baer, R. A., Rinaldo, J. C., & Berry, D. T. R. (2003). Self-report distortions. In R. Fernández-Ballesteros (Ed.). *Encyclopedia of psychological assessment* (pp. 851–866). London: Sage.

Bagby, R. M., Marshall, M. B., & Bocchiochi, J. R. (2005). The validity and clinical utility of MMPI-2 malingering depression scale. *Journal of Personality Assessment, 85,* 304–312.

Baltes, P. B., & Staudinger, S. (2000). Wisdom: The orchestration of mind and virtue towards human excellence. *American Psychologist, 55,* 122–136.

Caraballo, R. S., Giovino, G. A., Pechacek, T. F., & Mowery, P. D. (2001). Factors associated with discrepancies between self-reports on cigarette smoking and measured serum cotinine levels among persons aged 17 years or older: Third National Health and Nutrition Examination Survey, 1988–1994. *American Journal of Epidemiology, 153,* 807–814.

Cautela, J. R. (1977). *Behavioral analysis forms for clinical interventions.* Champaign, IL: Research Press.

Christensen, A., Atkins, D. C., Berns, S., Wheeler, J., Baucom, D. H., & Simpson, L. E. (2004). Traditional versus integrative behavioral couple therapy for significantly and chronically distressed married couples. *Journal of Consulting and Clinical Psychology, 72,* 176–191.

Clark, L. A., & Watson, D. (1995). Constructing validity: Basic issues in objective scale development. *Psychological Assessment, 7,* 309–319.

Cook, T. D., & Campbell, D. T. (1979). *Quasi-experimentation design and analysis issues for the field settings.* Boston: Houghton Mifflin.

Cronbach, L. J. (1951). Coefficient alpha and the internal structure of tests. *Psychometrika, 16,* 297–334.

Cronbach, L. J. (1988). Five perspectives on validation argument. In H. Wainer & H. Braun (Eds.), Test validity (pp. 34–35). Hillsdale, NJ: Erlbaum.

Ericsson, K. A., & Simon, H. A. (1980). Verbal reports as data. *Psychological Review, 87,* 215–251.

Ericsson, K. A., & Simon, H. A. (1984). *Protocol analysis: Verbal reports as data.* Cambridge, MA: Bradford Boos/MIT Press.

Fernández-Ballesteros, R. (1991). Anatomía de los autoinformes [Self-reports anatomy]. *Evaluación Psicológica, 7,* 263–291.

Fernández-Ballesteros, R. (2004a). Los autoinformes. In R. Fernández-Ballesteros (Ed.), *Evaluación psicológica: Conceptos, métodos y estudio de casos* (pp. 231–268). Madrid, Spain: Pirámide.

Fernández-Ballesteros, R. (2004b). Evaluación y valoración del tratamiento en un caso de depresión. In R. Fernández-Ballesteros (Ed.), *Evaluación psicológica: Conceptos, métodos y estudio de casos* (pp. 461–489). Madrid, Spain: Pirámide.

Fernández-Ballesteros, R. (2004c). Self-report questionnaires. In M. Hersen (Series Ed.) & S. N. Haynes & E. M. Heiby (Vol. Eds.), *Comprehensive handbook of psychological assessment: Vol. 3. Behavioral assessment* (pp. 194–221). Hoboken, NJ: Wiley.

Fernández-Ballesteros, R., & Staats, W. A. (1992). Paradigmatic behavioral assessment, treatment, and evaluation: Answering the crisis in behavioral assessment. *Advances in Behaviour Research and Therapy, 14,* 1–28.

Genest, M., & Turk, D. (1981). Think-aloud approaches to cognitive assessment. In T. Merluzzi, L. Glass, & M. Genest (Eds.). *Cognitive assessment* (pp. 233–269). New York: Guilford.

Goldfried, M. R. Consideration in developing a core assessment battery. (1997). In H. H. Strupp, L. M. Horowitz, & M. J. Lambert (Eds.). *Measuring patient changes in mood, anxiety, and personality disorders.* Washington, DC: American Psychological Association.

Haynes, S. N. (1986). *Models of causality in psychopathology.* Boston: Allyn & Bacon.

Heiby, E. M., & Hurtado, J. (1994). Evaluación de la depresión. In R. Fernández-Ballesteros (Ed.). *Evaluación conductual hoy* (pp. 318–348). Madrid, Spain: Pirámide.

Hersen, M., & Bellack, A. S. (2002). *Dictionary of behavioral assessment techniques.* New York: Percheron Press.

Hilsenroth, M. J. (2004). An introduction to the special issue on personality assessment and psychotherapy [Entire issue]. *Journal Personality Assessment, 83.*

Hollon, S. D., & Kendall, P. C. (1980). Cognitive self-statements in depression: Development of an automatic thoughts questionnaire. *Cognitive Therapy and Research, 4,* 383–395.

Johnson, J. E. (2003). The use of music to promote sleep in older women. *Journal of Community Health Nursing, 20,* 27–35.

Kane, M. T. (1992). An argument-based approach to validity. *Psychological Bulletin, 112,* 527–535.

Kazdin, A. E. (1980). *Research design in clinical psychology.* New York: Harper & Row.

Kazdin, A. E. (2002). Treatment Evaluation Inventory. In M. Hersen & Bellack, A. S. (Eds.), *Dictionary of behavioral assessment techniques* (pp. 485–486). Clinton Corner, NY: Percheron.

Kazdin, A. E. (2006). Arbitrary metrics. *American Psychologist, 61,* 42–49.

Kerlinger, F. N. (1973). *Foundation of behavioral research.* New York: Holt, Rinehart & Winston.

Kleinknecht, R. A., & Bernstein, D. A. (2002). Fear thermometer. In M. Hersen & A. S. Bellack (Eds.). *Dictionary of behavioral assessment techniques.* (pp. 220–221). New York: Percheron Press.

Kogan, J. N., & Edelstein, B. A. (2004). Modification and psychometric examination of a self-report measure of fear in older adults *Journal of Anxiety Disorders, 18,* 397–409.

Lambert, M. J. (1994). Use of psychological tests for outcome assessment. In M. E. Maruish, M.E. (Ed.), *The use of psychological testing for treatment planning and outcome assessment* (pp. 75–97). Hillsdale, NJ: Erlbaum.

Lambert, M. J., Strupp, H. H., & Horowitz, L. M. (1997). Introduction. In H. H. Strupp, L. M. Horowitz, & M. J. Lambert (Eds.). *Measuring patient changes in mood, anxiety, and personality disorders.* (pp. 3–10). Washington, DC: American Psychological Association.

Lang, P. J., & Lazovik, A. D. (1963). Experimental desensitization of a phobia. *Journal of Abnormal and Social Psychology, 66,* 519–525.

Lanyon, R. I. (2003). Assessing the misrepresentation of health problems. *Journal of Personality Assessment, 81,* 1–11.

Lanyon, R. I., & Goodstein, L. D. (1971). *Personality assessment.* New York: Wiley.

Maruish, M. E. (Ed.). (1994). *The use of psychological testing for treatment planning and outcome Assessment.* Hillsdale, NJ: Erlbaum.

Maruish, M. E. (2003). Outcome assessment/treatment assessment. In R. Fernández-Ballesteros (Ed.). *Encyclopedia of psychological assessment* (pp. 661–665). London: Sage.

McCann, J. T. (1998). *Malingering and deception in adolescence. Assessing credibility in clinical and forensic settings.* Washington, DC: American Psychological Association.

Menon, G., & Yorkston, E. A. (2000). The use of memory and contextual cues in the formation of behavioral frequency judgments. In A. A. Stone, J. S. Turkkan, C. A. Bachrach, J. B. Jobe, H. S. Kurtzman, & V. S. Cain (Eds.),

The science of self-report: Implications for research and practice (pp. 63–80). Mahwah, NJ: Erlbaum.

Messick, S. (1989). Validity. In R. L. Linn (Ed.), *Educational measurement* (3rd ed., pp. 13–103). New York: Macmillan.

Messick, S. (1995). Validity of psychological assessment. *American Psychologist, 50,* 741–749.

Mossman, D., & Somoza, E. (1989). Maximizing diagnostic information from the dexamethasone suppression test: An approach to criterion selection in receiver operating characteristic analysis. *Archives of General Psychiatry, 46,* 653–660.

Newman, F. L., & Ciarlo, J. A. (1994). Criteria for selecting psychological instruments for treatment outcome assessment. In M. E. Maruish (Ed.), *The use of psychological testing for treatment planning and outcome assessment.* Hillsdale, NJ: Erlbaum.

Nezu, A. M., & Nezu, C. M. (1993). Identifying and selecting target problems for clinical interventions: A problem-solving model. *Psychological Assessment, 5,* 254–263.

Nezu, A. M., Nezu, C. M., Peacock, M. A., & Girdwood, C. P. (2004). Case formulation in cognitive-behavior therapy. In M. Hersen (Series Ed.), & S. N. Haynes & E. M. Heiby (Vol. Eds.), *Comprehensive handbook of psychological assessment: Vol. 3. Behavioral assessment* (pp. 402–426). Hoboken, NJ: Wiley.

Patrick, D. L., Cheadle, A., Thompson, D. C., Diehr, P., Koepsell, T., & Kinne, S. (1994). The validity of self-reported smoking: A review and meta-analysis. *American Journal of Public Health, 84,* 1086–1093.

Phillips, G. C., Jones, G. E., Rieger, E. J., & Snell, J. B. (1997). Normative data for the Personal Report of Confidence as a Speaker. *Journal of Anxiety Disorders, 11,* 215–260.

Rogers, R., Sewell, K. W., Martin, M. A., & Vitacco, M. J. (2003). Detection of feigned mental disorders: A meta-analysis of the MMPI-2 and malingering. *Assessment, 10,* 160–177.

Rosen, A., & Proctor, E. K. (1981). Distinction between treatment outcomes and their implications for treatment evaluation. *Journal of Consulting and Clinical Psychology, 49,* 418–425.

Schwarz, N. (1998). Self-reports of behavior and opinions: Cognitive and communicative processes. In N. Schwarz, D. Park, B. Knauper, & S. Sudman (Eds.), *Cognition, aging and self-reports* (pp. 1–16). Ann Arbor, MI: Taylor & Francis Group, Psychology Press.

Schneider, S. L. (2001). In search of realistic optimism: Meaning, knowledge, and warm fuzziness. *American Psychologist, 56,* 250–263.

Schwarz, N., Park, D., Knauper, B., & Sudman, S. (Eds.). (1998). *Cognition, aging and self-reports.* Ann Arbor, MI: Taylor & Francis Group, Psychology Press.

Silva, F. (1993). *Psychometric foundations and behavioral assessment.* London: Sage.

Staudinger, U. M., Marsiske, M., & Baltes P. B. (1995). Resilience and reserve capacity in later adulthood: Potentials and limits of development across the life span. In D. Cicchetti & D Cohen (Eds.), *Developmental psychopathology* (Vol. 2, pp. 801–847). New York: Wiley.

Stone, A. A., Turkkan, J. S., Bachrach, C. A., Kurtzman, H. S., & Cain, V. S. (Eds.). (2000). *The science of self-report: Implications for research and practice.* Mahwah, NJ: Erlbaum.

Strupp, H. H., Horowitz, L. M., & Lambert, M. J. (Eds.). (1997). *Measuring patient changes in mood, anxiety, and personality disorders.* Washington, DC: American Psychological Association.

Swets, J. A., & Pickett, R. M. (1982). *Evaluation of diagnostic systems.* New York: Academic Press.

Tourangeau, R. (2000). Remembering what happened: Memory errors and survey reports. In A. A. Stone, J. S. Turkkan, C. A. Bachrach, J. B. Jobe, H. S. Kurtzman, & V. S. Cain (Eds.). *The science of self-report: Implications for research and practice* (pp. 29–48). Mahwah, NJ: Erlbaum.

Tran, G. Q., & Smith, P. S. (2004). Behavioral assessment in the measurement of treatment outcome. In M. Hersen (Series Ed.) & S. N. Haynes & E. M. Heiby (Vol. Eds.), *Comprehensive handbook of psychological assessment: Vol. 3. Behavioral assessment* (pp. 269–290). Hoboken, NJ: Wiley.

Wickens, T. D. (2002). *Elementary signal detection theory.* New York: Oxford University Press.

Wilson, D. B., & Lipsey, M. W. (2001). The role of method in treatment effectiveness research: Evidence from meta-analysis. *Psychological Methods, 6,* 413–429.

Young, S., Heptinstall, E., Sonuga-Barke, E. J. S., Chadwick, O., & Taylor, E. (2005). The adolescent outcome of hyperactive girls: Self-report of psychosocial status. *Journal of Child Psychology and Psychiatry, 46,* 255–262.

Zung, W. K. W., & Zung, E. M. (1986). Use of the Zung Self-Rating Depression Scale in the elderly. *Clinical Gerontologist, 5,* 137–148.

SECTION III

METHODOLOGICAL AND DESIGN ISSUES

6. SAMPLE SIZE AND STATISTICAL POWER

Rand R. Wilcox

From basic principles, there are two major types of errors one might commit when testing any hypothesis. The first, called a *Type I error*, is rejecting when in fact the null hypothesis is true; the second is failing to reject when the null hypothesis is false. Certainly it is undesirable to claim that groups differ when this is false. But, simultaneously, it is undesirable to fail to detect a difference that is real, particularly if the difference has important practical implications. This latter error, failing to reject when the null hypothesis is false, is called a *Type II error*, and the probability of rejecting when the null hypothesis is false is called *power*.

Another fundamental issue is determining an appropriate sample size, and again from basic principles, power and sample size are related. Roughly, a standard way of judging sample sizes is in terms of achieving some specified level of power. A related strategy is to determine sample sizes so that the resulting confidence intervals have length less than or equal to some specified value. Both approaches will be described.

There are two important cases when dealing with power and sample sizes: determining sample sizes to control power before any data are collected, and determining sample sizes to control power once pilot data are available. Methods for dealing with the first case are, perhaps, better known, but several practical issues need to be considered when they are used.

Many software packages are available for dealing with power and sample sizes. For a comparison of 29 programs, see Thomas and Krebs (1997).

■ Determining Sample Sizes Prior to Collecting Any Data

There are routinely used methods for determining sample sizes prior to collecting any data. Modern advances and insights have revealed that these techniques are based on rather restrictive assumptions. But for the moment, these issues are ignored, and attention is focused on illustrating the steps that are used. Then, practical concerns about these methods, and how they might be addressed, are discussed.

Two-Sample Case

Consider two independent groups and suppose the goal is to test

$$H_0 : \mu_2 = \mu_2,$$

the hypothesis that the means are equal. The classic solution to choosing the sample sizes is based on Student's t test, which assumes normality and that the corresponding variances, σ_1^2 and σ_2^2, are equal. For convenience, this common variance is denoted by σ^2.

To determine the sample sizes, three quantities must be specified by the investigator:

- The Type I error probability, α
- A difference between the groups that is deemed important
- The desired probability of detecting this difference

The usual way of measuring the difference between groups is with

$$\Delta = \frac{\mu_1 - \mu_2}{\sigma}$$

Cohen (1988) defines a large effect as something that is visible to the naked eye when viewing plots of the distributions to be compared. He concludes that for two normal distributions having a common variance, small, medium, and large effect sizes correspond to $\Delta = .2$, $\Delta = .5$, and $\Delta = .8$, respectively.

As a simple illustration, imagine that an investigator wants power to be .8 when $\Delta = .8$ and when testing at the $\alpha = .05$ level. Then one can simply look at Table 8.3.13 in Cohen (1988, p. 313) to determine the sample size needed to achieve the desired amount of power. Cohen's table reports power in terms of $f = .5 \Delta$. So when referring to his table, one would use $f = .4$ in the illustration considered here. In particular, power is .79 when both groups have a sample size of 6. For $\Delta = .5$, sample sizes of about 52 are needed to achieve the same level of power (also see Kraemer & Thiemann, 1987).

Solution When Using the ANOVA F

Now consider the case where two or more independent groups are to be compared with the ANOVA F. The process is the same as in the two-sample case, except that the difference among the population means is measured in a manner that takes into account the population means of all the groups. To elaborate, imagine that there are J groups having means $\mu_1, \ldots, \mu_J$; again let σ^2 represent the assumed common variance, let $\bar{\mu} = \Sigma \mu_j / J$ be the grand means, and let

$$\sigma_\mu = \sqrt{\frac{\Sigma(\mu_j - \mu)^2}{J}}$$

which measures the variation among the population mean. Cohen (1988, p. 274) takes as his measure of effect size

$$f = \frac{\sigma_\mu}{\sigma}$$

and he considers small, medium, and large effect sizes to be $f = .1, .25$, and $.4$, respectively, which is consistent with the two-sample case already discussed.

Example: Imagine that four groups are to be compared, the desired probability of a Type I error is $\alpha = .05$, and the goal is to have power $.9$ with a medium effect size. Then $f = .25$ and from Cohen (1988, p. 318), the sample size for each group needed to achieve this goal is 50.

A two-way ANOVA design is handled in a similar manner. That is, a choice for the Type I error is made, differences among the means must be specified, using a simple generalization of f, the desired amount of power must be chosen, and this yields a sample size that is appropriate when the underlying assumptions of the ANOVA F tests are true. Perhaps the easiest way of dealing with the calculations is to use one of the software packages reviewed by Thomas and Krebs (1997). One that is free, and which handles a range of experimental designs, is GPOWER, available at http://www.psycho.uni-duesseldorf.de/aap/projects/gpower/. (Alternatively, enter GPOWER into the search engine Google, and you will be taken to an appropriate link.) When dealing with a one-way design, GPOWER provides a window where one merely enters the Type I error probability, the desired power, the number of groups, and the effect size of interest. At the bottom of the window is a reminder of what are conventionally considered small, medium, and large effect sizes. When the user clicks on "calculate," the total number of observations needed is shown. GPOWER also has the ability to report the power achieved, given the sample sizes.

When dealing with a repeated measures design, or a between-by-within design, it is known that determining power with no data cannot be done in a reasonably accurate manner, even under normality. The difficulty is that the conventional F test assumes sphericity. In a one-way design, if all groups have equal variances and a common correlation, sphericity is achieved and power can be computed. But violating the sphericity assumption creates problems in terms of Type I errors, and a common method for dealing with this issue is to use something like the Huynh-Feldt corrected degrees of freedom. But because this correction is not known and must be estimated with data, it is unclear how best to determine the sample sizes to achieve a desired level of power when no data are available. However, once data are available, yielding an estimate of the Huynh-Feldt correction, power can be estimated given the sample size that was used, and GPOWER has a command to accomplish this goal.

The Huynh-Feldt correction reduces the degrees of freedom. A conservative approach when no data are available, still assuming normality, is to use the smallest possible degrees of freedom that can result due to this correction. This would result in using degrees of freedom $v_1 = 1$ and $v_2 = n - 1$. By entering these degrees of freedom into GPOWER, with values specified for the effect size, sample size, and Type I error probability desired, GPOWER will report the resulting power. By adjusting the sample size, the desired amount of power can be achieved; this provides some sense of the sample size required. A criticism is that perhaps a smaller sample size is really needed, but when using the usual F test, nonnormality complicates matters, as discussed next.

■ Some Practical Considerations

A fundamental issue is whether the methods just described and illustrated will result in sample sizes that will achieve reasonably high power when the assumptions of normality and equal variances are false. Under general conditions, if the ANOVA F is used to the exclusion of all other methods that might be used, the answer is an unequivocal no. Unequal variances, differences in skewness, and sampling from heavy-tailed distributions (roughly meaning that outliers are common) can result in power being substantially lower than what is achieved when the assumptions of normality and equal variances are true. Another fundamental concern has to do with the use of Δ and f as measures of effect size.

To elaborate, consider some population of individuals and suppose some outcome measure, X, has been chosen for study. When working with means, it is well known that the variance of a distribution, σ^2, has a direct effect on power: The larger σ^2 happens to be, the lower power will be with α and the sample sizes fixed. More generally, power is related to the squared standard error of the measure of location being used. For the sample mean, $\bar{X}$, the squared standard error is the variance of the sample mean (if a study could be repeated infinitely many times), which is

$$\text{VAR}(\bar{X}) = \frac{\sigma^2}{n}, \tag{1}$$

where n is the sample size. This connection with the variance can wreak havoc when using any method based on means. In practical terms, slight departures from normality can result in substantially less power than intended. Also, slight departures from normality can result in Δ and f being small even when from a graphical point of view, there is a large difference between two groups.

Power and Heavy-Tailed Distributions

A classic illustration of why is based on a particular mixed (or contaminated) normal distribution where with probability .9, an observation is sampled from

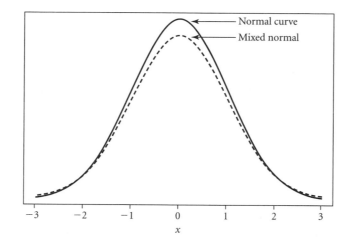

FIGURE 6.1. A mixed normal and standard normal distribution. Despite the similarity, the mixed normal has variance 10.9 versus the standard normal, which has variance 1.

a standard normal distribution; otherwise sampling is from a normal distribution having standard deviation 10. Figure 6.1 shows the standard and mixed normal distributions. The mixed normal is said to have thick or heavy tails because its tails lie above the normal curve, which implies that unusually small or large values, called outliers, are more common when sampling from the mixed normal versus the normal. As is evident, the two distributions are very similar in a certain sense, but there is a crucial difference: The standard normal has variance 1, but the mixed normal has variance 10.9. This illustrates the well-known result that an arbitrarily small change in any distribution, including normal distributions as a special case, can cause the variance to become arbitrarily large. That is, σ^2 is extremely sensitive to the tails of a distribution. One implication is that arbitrarily small departures from normality can result in low power (relative to other methods we might use) when comparing means.

To provide an explicit illustration regarding the effect of nonnormality on power when using means, suppose 25 observations are randomly sampled from each of two normal distributions both having variance 1, the first having mean zero, and the second having mean 1. Applying Student's t test with $\alpha = .05$, the probability of rejecting (power) is .96. But if sampling is from mixed normals instead, with the difference between means again 1, power is only .28.

For the situation just described, if instead medians are compared with the method in Wilcox (2003, section 8.7.1), power is approximately .8 when sampling from the normal distributions. So a practical issue is whether a method can be found that improves upon medians when sampling from normal distributions and continues to have relatively high power when sampling from a heavy-tailed distribution such as the mixed normal. Such methods are available and are described later in this chapter.

Cohen argues that under normality and equal variances, from a graphical perspective, $\Delta = 1$ would be considered a very large effect size. With the mixed normal distributions considered in the illustration, again from a graphical perspective, the effect size is large, but the variances are large as well, $\Delta = .3$, which ordinarily would be judged to be somewhere between a small and a medium effect size. One possibility is simply to use the difference between the means as a measure of effect size. But if we do this, it is no longer possible to control power, as a function of the sample sizes, without data (Dantzig, 1940).

Student's t Can Be Biased

To illustrate the effects of skewness on power when using Student's t, suppose 20 observations are sampled from the (lognormal) distribution shown in Figure 6.2, which has a mean of .4658. From basic principles, inferences about the mean assume T has a Student's t distribution with $n - 1$ degrees of freedom. In particular, the distribution of T is assumed to be symmetrical about zero, but when sampling from an asymmetrical distribution, this is not the case. For the situation at hand, the distribution of T is given, approximately, by the asymmetrical curve shown in Figure 6.3, which is based on values for T generated on a computer. The symmetrical curve is the distribution of T under normality. The main point here is that the mean (or expected value) of T is not zero—it is approximately $-.5$. This might appear to be impossible because under random sampling the expected value of the numerator of T, $\bar{X} - \mu$, is zero, which might seem to suggest that T must have a mean of zero as well. However, for nonnormal distributions, $\bar{X}$ and s are dependent, and this dependence makes it possible for the mean of T to differ from zero. (Gosset, who derived Student's t distribution, was aware of this issue.) This property is important be-

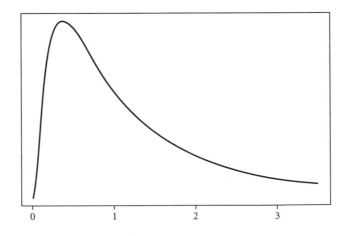

FIGURE 6.2. A lognormal distribution.

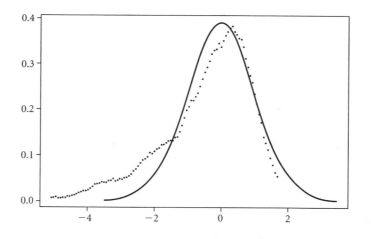

FIGURE 6.3. The ragged line is the plot of T values based on data generated from a lognormal distribution. The smooth, symmetrical curve is the distribution of T under normality.

cause it has practical implications about power—power can actually decrease as we move away from the null hypothesis. That is, situations arise where there is a higher probability of rejecting when the null hypothesis is true versus situations where the the null hypothesis is false. In technical terms, Student's t test is *biased*.

To provide perspective, Figure 6.4 shows the power curve of Student's t with $n = 20$ and when δ is added to every observation. That is, when $\delta = 0$, the null hypothesis is true; otherwise the null hypothesis is false, and the difference between the true mean and the hypothesized value is δ. In this case, power initially decreases as we move away from the null hypothesis, but eventually it

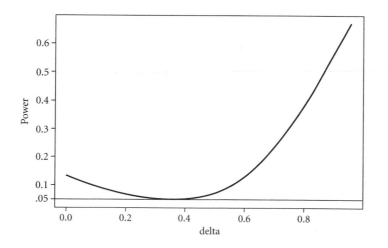

FIGURE 6.4. Power curve of T when sampling from a lognormal distribution.

goes up (cf. Sawilowsky, Kelley, Blair & Markham, 1994). The value $\delta = .6$ represents a departure from the null value of slightly more than one fourth of a standard deviation. That is, moving a quarter standard deviation from the null, power is approximately the same as when the null hypothesis is true.

The central limit theorem implies that (under random sampling) with a sufficiently large sample size, the distribution of T will converge to a normal distribution. It is known that for a lognormal distribution (which is a skewed, relatively light-tailed distribution among the class of g-and-h distribution derived by Hoaglin, 1985), even with 160 observations, there are practical problems with obtaining accurate probability coverage and control over the probability of a Type I error. (Westfall and Young, 1993, note that for a one-sided test, the actual probability of a Type I error is .11 when testing at the .05 level.) With about 200 observations, these problems become negligible. But when sampling from a skewed, heavy-tailed distribution, a sample size greater than 300 might be required. It remains unclear how quickly practical problems with bias disappear as the sample size increases.

The properties of the one-sample t test, when sampling from a skewed distribution, have implications about comparing two independent groups. To get a rough indication as to why, consider the sample mean from two independent groups: $\bar{X}_1$ and $\bar{X}_2$. If the two groups have identical distributions, and equal sample sizes are used, then the difference between the means has a symmetrical distribution, and problems with bias and Type I errors substantially higher than the nominal level are minimal. But when distributions differ in skewness, practical problems arise because the distribution of $\bar{X}_1 - \bar{X}_2$ will be skewed as well. This is not to suggest, however, that bias is not an issue when sampling from symmetrical distributions. For example, even when sampling from normal distributions, if groups have unequal variances, the ANOVA F test can be biased (e.g., Wilcox, Charlin, & Thompson, 1986).

A possible criticism of the problems with Student's t illustrated by Figures 6.3 and 6.4 is that, in theory, the actual distribution of T can be substantially asymmetrical. But can this problem occur in practice? Using data from various studies, Wilcox (2001, 2003) illustrates that the answer is yes. Consider, for example, data from a study conducted by Pedersen, Miller, Putcha, and Yang (2002), where $n = 104$. Figure 6.5 shows an approximation of the distribution of T based on resampling with replacement 104 values from the original data, computing T, and repeating this process 1,000 times (i.e., a bootstrap-t method was used). In fact, all indications are that problems with T are underestimated here for at least two reasons. First, an extreme outlier was removed. If this outlier is included, the approximation of the distribution of T departs in an even more dramatic manner from the assumption that it is symmetrical about zero. Second, studies of the small-sample properties of the bootstrap-t suggest that Figure 6.7 underestimates the degree to which the actual distribution of T is skewed.

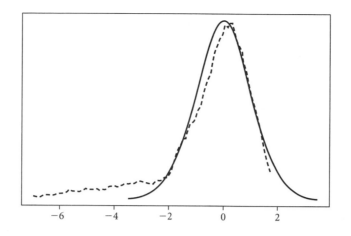

FIGURE 6.5. An approximation of the distribution of T based on data with $n = 104$.

■ Some Possible Solutions

Given the problems just described, how might they be addressed? In particular, do the methods assuming normality have any practical value?

One possibility is to perform a standard power analysis as previously indicated, but rather than compare means, use some alternative measure of location. In particular, one might consider a measure of location that achieves about the same amount of power under normality as methods based on means, but which continues to perform well when sampling from heavy-tailed distributions such as the mixed normal. The median guards against low power when distributions have heavy tails, but it does not perform that well under normality.

Recall that the median is computed by putting the observations in ascending order and, if the sample size is odd, trimming all but the middle value. If the sample size is even, all but the two middle values are trimmed, and the remaining two observations are averaged. So, under normality, the median does not perform well, roughly because it trims too much of the data. Nevertheless, as the number of outliers increases, eventually the median can have a relatively low standard error, which might translate into relatively high power. Many strategies have been proposed for comparing medians, but the better known methods are known to be unsatisfactory (Wilcox, in press). Currently, the only method that seems to perform well in simulations, particularly when tied values occur, is based in part on a percentile bootstrap method.

Another approach is simply to trim less data. A 20% trimmed mean, for example, trims the smallest 20%, trims the largest 20%, and averages the values that remain. With 20% trimming, very little power is lost under normality, and substantially higher power is achieved when sampling from the mixed normal previously described. Another advantage of using a 20% trimmed mean is that it reduces the bias problem, due to skewness, which was previously described.

It is stressed that when testing hypotheses, however, simply applying methods for means to the data not trimmed is highly unsatisfactory from a technical point of view, but effective methods are available that also allow heteroscedasticity Wilcox (2003, 2005).

Two other possibilities are to use what is called a robust M-estimator (based on Huber's psi) or a modern generalization of the Wilcoxon-Mann-Whitney test. Details about both of these approaches can be found in Wilcox (2003, 2005). Both methods perform reasonably well under normality and they provide protection against the deleterious effects of heavy-tailed distributions. Extensions of these techniques to more complicated designs are summarized in Wilcox (2003).

An important point is that in terms of power, no single method dominates. One reason is that when distributions are skewed, comparing means is not the same as comparing medians, trimmed means, or M-estimators or using some rank-based method. Wu (2002) compared the power of several methods using data from 24 dissertations. In some cases, methods based on means performed well, but on average they had the worst power. Using 20% trimmed means was not always optimal, but typically this approach had the most power. (Yet another approach worth considering is called the *shift function*, which is described in Wilcox, 2003.)

■ Strategies When Pilot Data Are Available

Stein-Type Methods for Means

When some hypothesis is rejected, power is not an issue—the probability of a Type II error is zero. But when we fail to reject, the issue becomes why. One possibility is that the null hypothesis is true, but another possibility is that the null hypothesis is false and we failed to detect this. How might we decide which of these two possibilities is more reasonable? When working with means, one possibility is to employ what is called a Stein-type two-stage procedure. Given some data, these methods are aimed at determining how large the sample sizes should have been to achieve power equal to some specified value. If few or no additional observations are required to achieve high power, of course this provides some assurance that power is reasonably high based on the number of observations available. Otherwise the indication is that power is relatively low due to using a sample size that is too small. Moreover, if the additional observations needed to achieve high power are acquired, methods for testing hypotheses have been derived that are typically different from the standard methods covered in an introductory statistics course.

Stein's original method was limited to making inferences about the mean associated with a single group, but extensions to two or more groups have been derived. Included are both ANOVA and multiple comparison procedures that do not require equal variances. The extension to ANOVA, when comparing the means of J independent groups, was derived by Bishop and Dudewicz (1978). Stein-type multiple comparisons procedures were derived by Hochberg (1975) and Tamhane (1977). One crucial difference from the Bishop-Dudewicz ANOVA is that direct control over power is no longer possible. Rather, these methods control the length of the confidence intervals, which of course is related to power. When sample sizes are small, both methods require critical values based on the quantiles of a Studentized range statistic. For software, see Wilcox (2003).

A practical concern about Stein-type methods for means is that when sampling from heavy-tailed distributions, this can result in relatively large sample variances, which can mean that relatively large sample sizes are needed to achieve the desired amount of power. A possible way of avoiding this problem is to use extensions of Stein-type methods aimed at comparing trimmed means. For computational details and easy-to-use software, see Wilcox (2005).

■ Concluding Remarks

The main message is that ensuring high power is a complex and difficult problem. Major advances have been made regarding how to achieve this goal, but it seems prudent to keep in mind the issues outlined in this chapter. Another major point is that, although no single method is optimal, the choice of statistical method is far from academic. A general rule is that methods based on means perform well under normality, but other methods have nearly the same amount of power for this special case yet maintain relatively high power in situations where methods based on means perform poorly. At a minimum, use a heteroscedastic rather than a homoscedastic method. Robust measures of location and rank-based methods represent the two main alternatives to means, with each giving a different and useful perspective on how groups differ. There is empirical evidence that, on average, 20% trimmed means are a good choice for general use, but the only certainty is that exceptions will occur.

■ References

Bishop, T., & Dudewicz, E. J. (1978). Exact analysis of variance with unequal variances: Test procedures and tables. *Technometrics, 20,* 419–430.

Cohen, J. (1988). *Statistical power analysis for the behavioral sciences* (2nd Ed.). Hillsdale, NJ: Erlbaum.

Dantzig, G. (1940). On the non-existence of tests of "Student's" hypothesis having power functions independent of σ. *Annals of Mathematical Statistics, 11,* 186.

Hoaglin, D. C. (1985). Summarizing shape numerically: The g-and-h distributions. In D. Hoaglin, F. Mosteller, and J. Tukey (Eds.), *Exploring data tables, trends, and shapes* (pp. 461–515). New York: Wiley.

Hochberg, Y. (1975). Simultaneous inference under Behrens-Fisher conditions: A two-sample approach. *Communications in Statistics, 4,* 1109–1119.

Kraemer, H. C., & Thiemann, S. (1987). *How many subjects?* Newbury Park, CA: Sage.

Pedersen, W. C., Miller, L. C., Putcha, A. D., & Yang, Y. (2002). Evolved sex differences in sexual strategies: The long and the short of it. *Psychological Science, 13,* 157–161.

Sawilowsky, S., Kelley, D. L., Blair, R. C., & Markman, B. S. (1994). Meta-analysis and the Solomon four-group design. *Journal of Experimental Education, 62,* 361–376.

Tamhane, A. (1977). Multiple comparisons in model I one-way ANOVA with unequal variances. *Communications in statistics: Theory and methods, A6,* 15–32.

Thomas, L., and Krebs, C. J. (1997). Technological tools. *Bulletin of the Ecological Society of America, 78,* 126–139.

Westfall, P. H., & Young, S. S. (1993). *Resampling based multiple testing.* New York: Wiley.

Wilcox, R. R. (2001). *Fundamentals of modern statistical methods.* New York: Springer.

Wilcox, R. R. (2003). *Applying contemporary statistical methods.* San Diego, CA: Academic Press.

Wilcox, R. R. (2005). *Introduction to robust estimation and Hypothesis testing* (2nd ed.). San Diego, CA: Academic Press.

Wilcox, R. R. (in press). Comparing medians. *Computational Statistics and Data Analysis.*

Wilcox, R. R., Charlin, V. L., & Thompson, K. (1986). New Monte Carlo results on the robustness of the ANOVA *F, W,* and *F** statistics. *Communications in Statistics—Simulation and Computation, 15,* 933–944.

Wu, P.-C. (2002). *Central limit theorem and comparing means, trimmed means one-step M-estimators and modified one-step M-estimators under non-normality.* Unpublished doctoral dissertation, University of Southern California.

7. SUBJECT SELECTION

David S. Festinger and David DeMatteo

One of the foremost aims when conducting a clinical trial is being able to draw valid inferences about a larger population based on the results obtained with a specific study sample. To maximize the validity of these inferences, it is generally accepted that the study sample must be representative of the larger population from which it was selected (see Kazdin, 2003). Although findings obtained with nonrepresentative samples may provide some preliminary data on the feasibility of an intervention, or perhaps even initial support of a concept, these findings may in fact be no more valuable than a case study in terms of their generalizability to the population from which the sample was drawn (Clarke, 1995; Copas & Li, 1997; Shadish, Cook, & Campbell, 2002; Weisz & Weiss, 1989; see Stirman, DeRubeis, Crits-Christoph, & Brody, 2003). Therefore, for studies that seek to extend their findings beyond their immediate cohort of study participants, an important consideration is ensuring that the target sample is reasonably representative of the target population from which the sample was drawn.

Despite the inherent limitations of using nonrepresentative, overly homogeneous samples of study participants, researchers often make use of such samples—for example, volunteer samples and samples of convenience—when conducting psychotherapy outcome research. Importantly, the use of such samples can have serious implications for the usefulness of a study's findings. In this chapter, we will examine the importance and process of selecting study participants in the context of psychotherapy outcome research. Among other things, this chapter will focus on defining a sampling frame, choosing between random and nonrandom sampling techniques, and determining appropriate and study-specific inclusion and exclusion criteria. Although *selecting* a representative study sample has long been recognized as being an effective way to enhance the internal and external validity of a study's findings, a related and equally important consideration is making sure that a representative study sample *remains* representative throughout the participant selection process and the duration of the study. Therefore, this chapter will also discuss the importance of monitoring the research study for evidence of selection biases.

Throughout this chapter, we will repeatedly refer to a hypothetical psychotherapy outcome research study as a means of illustrating the key concepts related to participant selection and demonstrating how the process of subject selection actually works in real-world research. As will be shown, researchers are often forced to strike a difficult balance between scientific ideals and the practical constraints of real-world research. For the purpose of providing an ongoing example, we have chosen a hypothetical research study that is a randomized controlled trial comparing two psychosocial interventions for the treatment of major depressive disorder. As new concepts are introduced, we will build upon this example and demonstrate the application of the principles we discuss throughout this chapter.

Awareness of the methodological issues surrounding the process of participant selection in psychotherapy outcome research is important for a variety of reasons. First, systematic biases in participant selection can dramatically affect the way that study findings are interpreted, because the factors responsible for the biased inclusion or exclusion of participants may be systematically related to demographic, diagnostic, or clinical factors that may influence the study's outcome. Second, participant selection biases may affect the generalizability of a study's findings because findings obtained in controlled laboratory research settings with homogeneous samples of participants may have limited relevance and generalizability to real-world clinical settings and heterogeneous groups of patients. Finally, from an ethical perspective, selection biases may lead to the underrepresentation of certain demographic groups in psychotherapy outcome research. The exclusion of certain demographic groups has the unfortunate effect of preventing researchers from examining the efficacy of certain treatments among members of these groups (American Psychological Association, 2003; Quintana, Troyano, & Taylor, 2001). According to the *NIH Guidelines on the Inclusion of Women and Minorities as Subjects in Clinical Research,* because research is designed to provide scientific evidence that could lead to a change in health policy or a standard of care, it is imperative to determine whether the intervention being studied affects both genders and diverse racial and ethnic groups differently (see Chapter 20 of this volume). Given these important considerations, it is clear that sampling and participant selection are among the most important elements of psychotherapy outcome research. No matter how well a study is ultimately conducted, if the sample is not properly selected or is biased in some manner, confidence in the study's findings as they relate to the larger population will be dramatically reduced.

Sample Versus Population

Before turning our attention to the important process of participant selection, we must first make a distinction between a population and a sample. This distinction may seem rather elementary, but having a proper understanding of this basic but important distinction is necessary if one is to truly grasp the fundamental importance of participant selection and its potential effects on the internal and external validity of a study's findings. As such, we believe that a brief refresher on the distinction between a population and a sample would be helpful, even for the more advanced readers.

In broad strokes, a population can be conceptualized as all individuals who are of interest to a researcher (see Marczyk, DeMatteo, & Festinger, 2005). More specifically, a population is the set of people (or entities) to which a study's findings are ultimately to be generalized. In practice, this usually means all individuals who occupy a certain geographic area or setting (e.g., all patients at an outpatient treatment clinic) or all individuals involved in a common pursuit (e.g., all patients seeking treatment for a particular disorder or a set of symptoms or problems). As a general rule of thumb, if the unit can be expressed using the word *all*, then it is a population. However, given time, financial, and other practical real-world constraints, researchers typically must set certain limits on the population of individuals about which they are seeking to make inferences. In most contexts, the parameters of the population of interest will involve some combination of geographic, individual, and diagnostic characteristics (e.g., all adults aged 21 and over in a specific treatment clinic who have been diagnosed with a mood disorder in the past 2 weeks). As will be discussed, these population parameters are further and more clearly defined through the articulation of study-specific inclusion and exclusion criteria.

As is evident from the preceding discussion, the population of interest is usually defined by the purpose of the research and the research question itself. For example, the purpose of our hypothetical research study is to examine the differential efficacy of two different psychosocial interventions for individuals diagnosed with major depressive disorder (MDD). As such, our target population will be individuals diagnosed with MDD. This target population will be further defined by specifying our research question, which may be the following: "Does Therapy A or Therapy B have better efficacy in reducing the symptoms of MDD?" In addition to serving as a source of hypotheses, the articulation of a research question often serves the important role of clarifying the population of interest, in this case, individuals who have been diagnosed with MDD. The target population would likely be further defined by geographic limitations (e.g., individuals diagnosed with MDD who live within a particular catchment area or reside in a specific treatment clinic) and the articulation of study-specific inclusion and exclusion criteria, which will be discussed later in this chapter.

In the majority of research contexts, studying the entire population of interest, although theoretically desirable from a methodological viewpoint, is simply not practical. Accordingly, researchers must typically study a smaller subset of the population of interest, or a sample. In broad terms, a study sample can be conceptualized as a chosen cohort drawn from the larger population of interest. Depending on the specific goals of the research, there are various ways of choosing a sample, which will be discussed in the next section of this chapter. However, in most types of research, it is particularly important—if not essential—that the study sample be *representative* of the population from which it was selected. As noted previously, using a representative sample of participants is perhaps the most effective method of enhancing the validity and generalizability of a study's findings.

In the following sections, we present a discussion of several ways of selecting participants for a research study, with a particular focus on the process of participant selection in the context of psychotherapy outcome research. Broadly speaking, the process of sampling participants can be divided into random selection and nonrandom selection, and these different sampling techniques have important implications regarding the internal and external validity of a study. Because random selection typically yields the most representative sample of participants, it is among the most widely used methods of selecting participants. As such, most texts focus almost exclusively on random selection and its effects on the generalizability of a study's findings. It is important to note, however, that a variety of other sampling techniques are available to researchers when random selection is either impractical or impossible. As will be discussed, researchers conducting psychotherapy outcome research often must make use of these alternative sampling techniques. Therefore, we will discuss several of these participant sampling techniques in the sections that follow.

Random Selection

Random selection of participants refers to the equal probability that individuals from the population of interest can be selected to participate in a particular research study (Christensen, 2004; Cochran, 1977; Kazdin, 2003). In other words, every member of the population of interest has an equal likelihood of being selected for the sample because participants are chosen at random and there is no bias in terms of who is ultimately selected for inclusion in the research study. Employing random selection, which is alternatively referred to as *probability sampling,* is the best way of selecting a cohort that is representative of the population from which it was drawn. Importantly, as will be discussed later in this chapter, random selection helps control for extraneous influences because it minimizes the impact of selection biases. If random selection can be accomplished and the sample is sufficiently large (typically more than 100 participants), then one can be reasonably confident that the sample is indeed representative of the population from which it was drawn.

As such, random selection enhances the external validity (i.e., generalizability) of a study's findings. More specifically, for researchers to make valid inferences about the population based on the study results obtained with their sample of participants, it is essential that the sample be representative of the population. Put simply, representativeness is most effectively achieved by randomly selecting a sample of participants from the population of interest. More technically, the generalizability of a research study's results depends on the representativeness of the participants in the sample to those individuals who were *not* chosen for inclusion in the particular study. In other words, if the individuals chosen for inclusion in a study differ in important respects from those individuals who were not chosen for inclusion in the study, the sample is not representative and the researchers cannot be confident that the study findings will generalize to the population from which the sample was drawn. In this regard, it is noteworthy that random selection is the only sampling technique that enables a researcher to accurately estimate how different the sample is from the population from which it was drawn.

It is important to note that random selection is rather difficult to accomplish unless the population of interest is specifically defined. For example, in our hypothetical research study, it would be unrealistic to define the population as "all individuals diagnosed with MDD." If taken literally, this would mean that we were proposing to randomly select participants from all the individuals who have ever been diagnosed with MDD in the entire world. Alternatively, we could more specifically define the population as "all adults who respond to an advertisement in XYZ Newspaper for a study on depression and who are subsequently found to meet *DSM-IV* diagnostic criteria for MDD." By randomly selecting participants from this more circumscribed group of people, we would more clearly know the population of individuals to whom our study results (obtained from a representative sample) would apply.

Therefore, when selecting a random sample of participants, an important first step is identifying the sampling frame, which is simply a list of the population from which the sample will be drawn. The sampling frame may consist of a list of individuals, households, organizations, or any other units of analysis, depending on the type and purpose of the research. In the context of psychotherapy outcome research, the sampling frame is typically a list of individuals. Using this list, individuals may then be numbered and selected for inclusion in the research study according to some predetermined random selection procedure. If our hypothetical research study were taking place in an inpatient treatment clinic, for example, we could decide to include every third person who is diagnosed with MDD and satisfies other inclusion and exclusion criteria. The important point to keep in mind is that researchers must first narrowly define the population of interest and then randomly select the required number of participants from the population. Following this procedure greatly enhances the generalizability of a study's findings to other, similar populations.

A notable consequence, however, of narrowly defining the population of interest is that it ultimately reduces the representativeness of the sample vis-à-vis the larger population (e.g., all individuals diagnosed with MDD). To counter this unfortunate result, researchers often conduct large multisite trials to increase the representativeness of a sample. These trials are often conducted in specifically targeted catchment areas around the United States in an attempt to achieve more geographically and sociodemographically representative cohorts of participants. Given the huge expense associated with large multisite trials, it may not be practical to conduct such studies. Therefore, another approach is to conduct a series of smaller research studies to examine the generalizability of a study's findings among different populations. In other words, replicating a study's findings is an effective method of demonstrating the generalizability of the study's results.

Nonrandom Selection

Several sampling techniques are available to researchers who are unable, or choose not, to use random sampling in their studies. Although many nonrandom sampling techniques exist, some of them (e.g., expert sampling, critical case sampling) have little relevance in the context of psychotherapy outcome research. We will therefore limit our discussion to nonrandom sampling techniques that could potentially be used in psychotherapy outcome research. Despite the obvious appeal of these alternative techniques in situations where randomization is impractical or impossible, they all share the same disadvantage to one degree or another. Specifically, all nonrandom sampling techniques have a negative impact on the generalizability of a study's findings.

AVAILABILITY SAMPLING

Because of the often impractical nature of random selection in many research contexts, researchers must often make use of availability sampling by selecting a sample of convenience. A *sample of convenience* is simply a potential source of research participants that is easily accessible to the researcher. This sampling technique is alternatively referred to as *haphazard sampling*. For example, individuals are often chosen to participate in a research study because they are present in a convenient location, such as a hospital waiting room or inpatient psychiatric clinic. Another example of a commonly used sample of convenience is undergraduate psychology students, who often serve as research participants in a study to satisfy a course requirement or earn extra credit. Importantly, however, as noted by Kazdin (2003), researchers often use samples of convenience without having a clear rationale as to why a particular sample is important, useful, or relevant to their study. Many times, researchers make use of these "captive" samples of participants simply because they are available and easy to access, yet the rationale for using a particular sample of participants is not well developed. As a result, the relationship between the particular sample of participants and the research question may not always be apparent.

Samples of convenience are frequently used in psychotherapy outcome research to examine the therapeutic effects of specific psychosocial interventions. The primary advantage of using a sample of convenience is that it provides the researcher with a ready-made, easily accessible, and oftentimes large sample of participants who share some important (in terms of the research question) characteristic. In some contexts, for example, researchers may have relatively easy access to a large group of psychiatric patients, and using such a sample of convenience may seem methodologically logical and logistically attractive. In our hypothetical research study, for example, we could make use of a sample of convenience by conducting our study using a sample of patients diagnosed with MDD in a specific inpatient treatment facility. Among other things, this would certainly make it easier for us to ensure that the participants were actually getting the different interventions being compared (i.e., client adherence) and that the interventionists were actually delivering the interventions according to protocol (i.e., therapist fidelity), both of which are important considerations in controlled psychotherapy outcome research.

Importantly, however, the use of samples of convenience, which are often highly specialized and circumscribed, raises some rather serious concerns. In particular, the primary disadvantage of using a sample of convenience is the negative impact that it can have on the generalizability of a research study's findings, in that samples of convenience are rarely representative of the larger population. Many times, the features that contribute to the convenience of a particular sample of convenience—such as geographic location and psychiatric diagnosis—may end up restricting the generalizability of the research study's findings. Therefore, when using a sample of convenience (or any sample, for that matter), researchers bear the burden of demonstrating why the particular sample they chose to use in their study is well suited to the specific question being addressed by the research. Moreover, the researcher must examine whether the unique features of the sample are in some way contributing to the study's results and perhaps limiting the generalizability of the results. For example, in our hypothetical research study, if our sample consisted entirely of inpatients diagnosed with MDD from one psychiatric facility, it is possible, and perhaps likely, that the participants are not representative of inpatients diagnosed with MDD from other psychiatric facilities, and they are most certainly not representative of all individuals diagnosed with MDD. As such, the findings obtained in our research study may not generalize beyond our immediate sample of participants.

QUOTA SAMPLING

Quota sampling is a variant of availability sampling, with the added constraint that proportionality by strata be preserved (King, 1986). For example, as a way of improving the representativeness of a sample of participants, researchers may decide to include a certain number of participants of a particular gender, race, ethnicity, or socioeconomic status in the sample. The goal is to choose a sample that is maximally representative—in terms of proportions of participants who exhibit key variables of interest—of the target population of interest. In some circumstances, researchers may intentionally seek participants who exhibit maximal differences on the variables of interest; this variant of quota sampling is referred to as *maximum variation sampling*. The principle behind maximum variation sampling is that if you intentionally include participants who exhibit large differences on the variables of interest, their aggregate answers are likely to be a good reflection of the population from which the sample was chosen. For example, in our hypothetical MDD study, we may decide to intentionally obtain a diverse sample in terms of demographic characteristics and levels of depression to increase the likelihood that our sample is an accurate reflection of the population from which it was drawn.

CHAIN REFERRAL SAMPLING

This sampling technique, which is alternatively referred to as *snowball sampling* or *network sampling*, involves selecting a few participants who display a characteristic of interest, such as inclusion in a particular group (e.g., member of a private club), and then asking the participants for referrals for additional research participants (Penrod, Preston, Cain, & Starks, 2003; see also Biernacki & Waldorf, 1981). For researchers working with highly specific or exclusive groups, this may be an effective way of obtaining a sample of participants.

Subject-Selection Biases

As discussed previously, one of the most important questions facing psychotherapy outcome researchers is whether and to what degree their study samples are representative of the population of interest. As noted, using a representative sample of participants is an effective way of enhancing the generalizability of a research study's findings. Conversely, using a sample of participants that is somehow biased reduces the likelihood that the study's results will be generalizable to the population from which the sample was drawn. In this section, we will discuss the effects of subject-selection biases on the generalizability of a research study's findings. Broadly defined, *subject-selection biases* are influences that are attributable to the types of participants who enter research studies (Kazdin, 2003), and different selection biases can operate at different points in a research study. We will discuss two significant sources of participant-selection biases that are commonly encountered in psychotherapy outcome research: the use of special samples and participant attrition. The first source of bias operates during the participant recruitment phase of the study, and the second source of bias can occur at any time during the study.

USE OF SPECIAL SAMPLES

A common criticism of psychotherapy outcome research is the restricted range of populations that are sampled. As noted previously, psychotherapy outcome researchers often make use of samples of convenience, which has important implications in terms of the generalizability of a research study's findings. Besides using a sample of college students (which should raise obvious concerns about the generalizability of a study's findings), psychotherapy outcome researchers often use other samples of convenience. For example, it is not uncommon for researchers to test hypotheses on a sample of participants that was originally recruited for another, entirely separate purpose. In these situations, the sample may be well suited for the original question but not for the new question. In this circumstance, the researcher bears the burden of demonstrating why a particular sample is appropriate vis-à-vis the research question being addressed.

The use of volunteers is another potential source of selection biases, and one that is encountered frequently in psychotherapy outcome research. In most types of social science research, and probably all types of psychotherapy outcome research, all participants are technically volunteers in the sense that they must agree to participate in the research study (Kazdin, 2003). Ethical guidelines governing researchers make it clear that potential research participants must be adequately informed of important aspects of the research study, such as study purposes, duration of participation, potential risks and benefits of participation, and the volunteer nature of participation, before agreeing to participate in a study. In a more narrow sense, however, we can think of volunteers as being individuals who respond to newspaper or radio advertisements for a study, or other types of solicitations designed to attract potential participants. In this situation, some people agree to be in a study and others do not, and the important question for our purposes is whether the volunteers differ significantly in any important respects from the nonvolunteers. This would be a relevant and important question if the sample for our hypothetical research study consisted of individuals recruited through a newspaper or radio advertisement for a depression study. Among other things, it would be important to know whether our sample differs in important respects from those individuals with MDD who responded to the advertisement yet ultimately chose not to participate (or were ineligible to participate) in the study.

A great deal of research has compared individuals who volunteer to participate in research studies to those who do not volunteer to participate in studies. Although the findings are dated and somewhat equivocal, there appears to be sufficient evidence to conclude that individuals who volunteer to participate in psychological studies differ on a number of demographic and personality variables from nonvolunteers. For example, volunteers are more likely to be female, better educated, less authoritarian, younger, and more intelligent (e.g., Rosenthal & Rosnow, 1975). Researchers have also looked at the association between specific psychiatric diagnosis and likelihood of participating in a research study. For example, some studies suggest that patients with schizophrenia are less likely to participate in research studies than patients with other psychiatric disorders (e.g., Carr & Whittenbaugh, 1968; Schubert, Patterson, Miller, &

Brocco, 1984; *cf* Jaskiw et al., 2003; Thomas et al., 1997). Differences between those who agree to be in a study and those who do not have also been found in studies of patients diagnosed with substance abuse and dependence (e.g., Edlund, Craig, & Richardson, 1985).

The role of motivation in terms of an individual's likelihood of volunteering to participate in a research study also warrants some comment. It is likely that individuals who volunteer to participate in a research study may be more motivated (to change) than those individuals who choose not to participate in a study. This differential motivation may ultimately mean that the study findings are generalizable only to highly motivated individuals, and the results may indeed have little relevance for individuals who have no desire to change. The potential for this bias is virtually ubiquitous in clinical psychotherapy outcome research, and it ultimately limits the confidence that can be placed in the external validity of virtually all treatment effects. Unfortunately, there is no agreed-upon solution for this bias, and it is something that researchers must be aware of when interpreting and reporting their findings.

In the context of psychotherapy outcome research, it is particularly important to examine the influences of volunteer samples of participants on a research study's outcomes and generalizability (see Larzelere, Kuhn, & Johnson, 2004). As with other areas of research, the key question is whether volunteers and nonvolunteers differ in ways that can have a negative impact on the generalizability of the study's findings. It is possible, for example, that findings obtained with a volunteer sample of participants—for example, correlations among variables, interaction effects—may differ considerably from what would be found in the larger population of interest. Although this is a concern in any research context, it may be particularly important when researchers are seeking to establish the efficacy of an intervention for treating a specific psychiatric disorder. Positive findings obtained with a volunteer sample of participants may not always translate into positive findings among the population from which the sample of participants was drawn.

For example, in our hypothetical research study, it is possible that the volunteers who were ultimately included in the research study had less severe depression than those individuals who either did not respond to the study advertisement or responded to the advertisement but did not end up in the final sample. As a result, our study sample is limited in terms of severity of illness, and we would be unable to conclude that our treatments, if shown to be efficacious in our study, would also be efficacious among a more severely depressed group of individuals. It is also possible that the volunteers differ from nonvolunteers (or volunteers who ultimately did not end up in the sample) in terms of other important variables, such as cultural characteristics, intelligence, socioeconomic status, and age, which could interact with the treatment conditions. These interaction effects may make it difficult to reach broad conclusions regarding the efficacy of the interventions we examined in the study.

To identify differences between volunteers and nonvolunteers, researchers often conduct representativeness analyses. These between-group analyses compare individuals who chose to participate in a study with those who refused to participate (or were ineligible to participate) on any number of available demographic or other participant characteristics. Because individuals who either refused to participate or were ineligible to participate do not provide informed consent, these analyses are generally conducted using aggregate (i.e., nonidentifying) clinic or public records on the nonparticipants. Identifying specific differences between participants and nonparticipants allows researchers to more clearly define the population to which their study findings may be generalizable.

Despite the concerns associated with volunteer samples, it is important to recognize that using a volunteer sample does not sound the death knell in terms of a research study's generalizability. In some contexts, findings simply may not be significantly influenced by whether participants were volunteers. Moreover, as noted by Kazdin (2003), it is possible that conclusions drawn from studies that use volunteer samples may vary merely in terms of the magnitude of performance on the dependent variables. For example, the reduction in symptoms related to a particular treatment for MDD may simply be less evident, although still present, among the population from which the volunteer participants were recruited. In other words, the effect size of the intervention would likely be smaller if the intervention were tested in the larger, more heterogeneous population. This in turn could substantially affect the power estimates employed in the study (see Chapter 6 of this volume). The bottom line is that researchers must be careful not to draw overly broad conclusions about the effects of an intervention without simultaneously acknowledging the role that participant selection may play in terms of limiting the generalizability of the study's findings.

ATTRITION

According to Kazdin (2003), attrition is a threat to several types of validity. For example, attrition is a threat to that has obvious implications in terms of the generalizability of a study's findings. First, it affects the study's internal validity because it can alter group equivalence, which may result in comparing groups that differ on variables other than the variable being investigated. Second, attrition is a threat to external validity because it limits the applicability of findings to a specific group; the more limited a group is in terms of representativeness, the less likely it is that the results will generalize beyond the cohort being examined. Third, attrition is also a threat to external and construct validity because it raises the prospect that the intervention, combined with special participant characteristics, accounts for the conclusions that the researcher would like to attribute exclusively to the intervention being examined. Finally, attrition affects statistical conclusion validity by reducing the sample size, which in turn reduces the statistical power to detect between-group differences that truly exist. As such, attrition deserves special attention from researchers, particularly, as will be shown, in the context of psychotherapy outcome research.

There are several ways in which attrition can be troublesome in the context of psychotherapy outcome research. First, and perhaps most obviously, if too many participants drop out of a study, it may no longer be possible (from a statistical perspective) to reach valid conclusions about the effects of the interventions being examined. Small sample sizes may not yield sufficient statistical power to detect between-group differences. Second, there may be significant differences between those participants who drop out of the study and those participants who remain in the study on demographic, personality, and/or diagnostic variables, and it is possible that any observed between-group differences are attributable to these differences (i.e., these variables may be interacting with the intervention) rather than the intervention itself. Third, group equivalence may be affected if a disproportionate number of participants drop out of one condition. For example, in studies comparing a psychotropic medication with talk therapy, it is possible that more participants in the medication condition may drop out of the study due to the development of unpleasant side effects. Alternatively, it is possible that more participants in the talk therapy condition may drop out of the study due to the delayed therapeutic effects of talk therapy. In either situation, between-group comparisons may become suspect in the face of such differential group attrition. Finally, dropouts may differ systematically across conditions. In other words, participants who drop out of one condition may differ systematically from those participants who drop out of another condition, and the remaining participants in each condition may then differ considerably. Without having group equivalence, it would be difficult to attribute changes in an outcome measure to the intervention being examined in the study.

One strategy related to participant selection that can potentially minimize attrition is identifying variables shown to be correlated with attrition, and then using this information when deciding on a sample of participants. For example, if prior psychotherapy outcome research suggests that younger participants drop out at a significantly higher rate than older participants, researchers may decide to limit participation in the study to older participants. It is important to note, however, that restricting the study sample in such a way has an obvious downside in that the resulting sample will likely be less representative than a sample that has no restrictions, which could further limit the generalizability of the research study's findings. As with many methodological issues, researchers are often forced to strike a difficult balance between sound methodology and practical realities. In our hypothetical MDD study, for example, we may decide to exclude participants from a certain geographic area if prior research experience suggests that individuals from that area tend to drop out of research studies at a higher rate than individuals from other areas (perhaps due to transportation difficulties). Although this could limit the generalizability of the findings if the end result is a more homogeneous sample, the practical realities of conducting real-world research (i.e., obtaining a sufficiently large cohort of participants and minimizing attrition) may dictate this course of action.

Inclusion/Exclusion Criteria

The issue of participant selection is centrally concerned with the important question of who will participate in a particular research study. However, the composition of a particular study sample does not begin with random selection or any other sampling technique; rather, it is usually a conceptual issue that is addressed by developing well-defined, study-specific inclusion and exclusion criteria. Inclusion and exclusion criteria are often the first step in defining and narrowing down a population of interest. As such, it is important that these criteria be well conceived, properly defined, and accurately measured. Perhaps most important, inclusion and exclusion criteria should relate back to the question that will be addressed in the research study.

According to the National Institutes of Health (2006), inclusion/exclusion criteria are defined as the standards that determine whether individuals should be permitted to enter a clinical trial. These criteria may include variables such as age, gender, the type and stage of an illness, previous treatment history, and other medical conditions. Perhaps the best way to discuss inclusion and exclusion criteria is through our ongoing hypothetical research study. As noted previously, it is essential to specifically define the study sample so that we know to which population the study results will ultimately generalize. Therefore, the first step is to define the participants we want to include in the study (i.e., inclusion criteria). Importantly, inclusion criteria typically flow logically and directly from the research question and hypothesis. Because the primary aim of our hypothetical study is to examine the efficacy of two psychosocial interventions for adults suffering from MDD, we may decide to include only individuals who (a) have a current diagnosis of MDD, and (b) are between the ages of 18 and 65.

After articulating the inclusion criteria, the next step is defining the characteristics of individuals who should be excluded from the study (i.e., exclusion criteria). These criteria serve to maintain the homogeneity of the sample and ensure that the study is truly measuring the efficacy of the treatments for individuals with MDD. For our hypothetical study, for example, we may decide to exclude individuals who (a) meet *DSM-IV* diagnostic criteria for another Axis I mood or anxiety disorder, (b) are currently taking antidepressant or other psychotropic medications, (c) report current suicidal ideation, and (d) are currently incapable of providing informed consent.

These inclusion and exclusion criteria were selected for a number of reasons. As mentioned previously, the inclusion criteria of MDD diagnosis and being between age 18 and 65 were chosen because we wish to test a treatment for adults with MDD. The exclusion criteria, however, may seem a bit more idiosyncratic, and indeed they are. In our hypothetical study, we chose to exclude individuals with other mood or anxiety disorders because those disorders may interfere with the treatment and not allow for a clean test of the two interventions for MDD. Essentially, they would add "noise" to the study. The reason for excluding individuals currently taking antidepressants or other psychotropic medications should be obvious. To accurately test the effects of psychotherapy, we would not want individuals to be receiving another form of treatment because this could confound the findings. We chose to exclude individuals with current suicidal ideation as a protective measure for the potential participants. Because the hypothetical treatments we are examining are experimental, we have decided that it is far too risky to test the interventions on individuals who are at heightened risk of suicide. Finally, we decided to exclude individuals who are incapable of providing informed consent, which was designed to protect potential participants who are incapable of making informed, intelligent, and voluntary decisions about whether to participate in the research project.

Although there are no universally agreed-upon guidelines for establishing inclusion and exclusion criteria, there are at least four important questions that should be considered when defining a research study's inclusion and exclusion criteria: (a) How do the criteria affect the internal and external validity of the study, (b) are the criteria necessary for the safety of the participants, (c) are the criteria ethical, and (d) how will the criteria be measured?

VALIDITY

As discussed previously, there is s sort of catch-22 when it comes to defining a study's inclusion and exclusion criteria. If the criteria are too broad and inclusive, they may add error variance to the study and reduce confidence in the study's findings. Alternatively, if the criteria are too narrow or circumscribed, they may limit the generalizability of the findings to the population of interest. In recent years, findings from laboratory research and other efficacy trials have been increasingly criticized for their limited generalizability to real-world settings. For example, one might question how well the findings from our hypothetical study will generalize to patients in community clinics who may have comorbid disorders or suicidal ideation, which are common occurrences among those with MDD. Regrettably, there is no hard-and-fast solution for this problem. Ultimately, the researcher must decide how narrow or broad the criteria should be based on the specific objectives of the study. During the early stages of research, which are often aimed at determining preliminary efficacy of interventions rather than effectiveness, it may be more time and cost efficient to use small, narrowly defined samples. Once an intervention's efficacy has been established, researchers may want to extend the research to more representative samples of participants.

SAFETY

As illustrated by the hypothetical study, it is sometimes necessary to consider safety issues when developing inclusion and exclusion criteria. Typically addressed through the study's exclusion criteria, these safety-related criteria are aimed at preventing undue harm or adverse effects that could potentially be caused by participating in the experimental intervention. In human subjects research, initial efficacy studies for novel interventions are typically conducted with low-risk samples. Once efficacy for the novel intervention gains some degree of empirical support, researchers may then use more high-risk samples. Moreover, it is also possible that some interventions may actually be harmful for certain individuals. For example, although antidepressant therapy may be highly effective for those with MDD, it can potentially have iatrogenic effects for individuals with bipolar disorder, due to the possibility that it could precipitate a manic or hypomanic episode. Similarly, prescribing a psychotropic medication that has a high abuse potential, such as a fast-acting benzodiazepine, could be contraindicated among participants with histories of substance abuse. The message here is fairly straightforward; that is, it is imperative that researchers consider the characteristics of the participants that may alter the risk-benefit ratio of participating in the study.

ETHICS

The debate regarding the appropriate composition of study samples is no longer exclusively in the domain of researchers. In addition to protecting vulnerable populations from wrongful inclusion in research, the principal of justice, provided by the Belmont Report (National Commission for the Protection of Human Subjects of Biomedical and Behavioral Research, 1979), also protects persons from systematic exclusion from research. In 1993, President Bill Clinton signed into law the NIH Revitalization Act of 1993 (PL 103–43), which directed the National Institutes of Health (NIH) to establish guidelines for the inclusion of women and minorities in clinical research. On March 9, 1994, in response to the mandate contained in the NIH Revitalization Act, the NIH issued *NIH Guidelines on the Inclusion of Women and Minorities as Subjects in Clinical Research* ("*NIH Guidelines*"). As noted previously, because research is designed to provide scientific evidence that could lead to a change in health policy or a standard of care, the *NIH Guidelines* state that it is imperative to determine whether the intervention being studied affects both genders and diverse racial and ethnic groups differently. As such, all NIH-supported biomedical and behavioral research involving human participants is required to be carried out in a manner that elicits information about individuals of both genders and from diverse racial and ethnic backgrounds. According to the Office for Protection From Research Risks, which is part of the U.S. Department of

Health and Human Services, the inclusion of women and minorities in research will, among other things, help to increase the generalizability of the study's findings and ensure that women and minorities benefit from the research. Although the *NIH Guidelines* apply only to studies conducted or supported by the NIH, all researchers and research institutions are encouraged to include women and minorities in research studies and to avoid the systematic exclusion of any particular group of individuals.

MEASUREMENT

As with any other study variables, the integrity of a study's inclusion and exclusion criteria is only as good as the instrument or means used to measure them. Unfortunately, although most studies carefully consider the reliability and validity of dependent measures, they often pay less attention to the integrity of the measures used to measure the inclusion and exclusion criteria. The most obvious explanation for this is that these measures are used to screen for participation and therefore must be administered to a much larger number of individuals. Depending on the specific criteria and their base rate in the population, this may mean conducting dozens of screenings for every one eligible participant, which could substantially increase the time and costs of the study. Nevertheless, unless valid and reliable measures are used to determine eligibility, equally substantial resources (e.g., assessments, treatment hours) could be expended for individuals who do not actually meet study criteria. In this case, the even larger cost may be the invalidity of the study itself. For example, what is the value of a study of treatments for depression if a large proportion of the study sample did not actually meet diagnostic criteria for depression?

In our hypothetical study, for example, we could use the mood disorders section of the Structured Clinical Interview for DSM-IV Axis I Disorders (First, Spitzer, Gibbon, & Williams, 1994) to screen for MDD, as well as to rule out the presence of comorbid psychiatric disorders. We could also choose to administer a brief mini–mental status exam to determine an individual's capacity to consent, and a brief assessment of current suicidal ideation. Depending on size of the study and the available funding, it may be necessary to truncate the screening battery. However, this should be done judiciously to maintain the integrity of the study.

■ Summary

This chapter provided an overview of the principal considerations involved in planning subject selection for a randomized clinical trial in the context of psychotherapy outcome research. In particular, it provided a review of the major considerations related to defining a sampling frame, selecting study participants,

TABLE 7.1
Considerations Relevant to Participant Selection

- Determine the target population (to whom do you want your results to generalize?).
- Determine the sampling methodology (e.g., random selection, convenience, volunteer).
- Determine specific inclusion criteria (what characteristics must participants possess to adequately test your hypothesis?).
- Determine specific exclusion criteria (what chacteristics might confound the implications of the study or the ability to accurately generalize to the target population?).
- Determine the presence of any ethical issues regarding inclusion/exclusion criteria (are specific groups being intentionally or unintentionally excluded from participation?).
- Consider the possibility of differential attrition across conditions, and how to identify methods for addressing these concerns if they arise.
- Determine whether certain exclusion criteria may be necessary to ensure the safety of study participants (will certain participants be harmed or have adverse reactions to the experimental intervention?).
- Select appropriate measures for assessing inclusion/exclusion criteria (e.g., self-report, collateral interviews, record checks, standardized tests, physical examinations).
- Specify procedures for monitoring sample demographics and oversampling as necessary.
- Specify procedures for identifying potential selection biases (e.g., attrition analysis, randomization check).

monitoring and addressing potential selection biases, and determining appropriate and study-specific inclusion and exclusion criteria. To assist researchers in applying the lessons learning in this chapter, Table 7.1 provides a checklist that may help to facilitate the incorporation of these considerations into future clinical trials.

■ References

American Psychological Association. (2003). Guidelines on multicultural education, training, research, practice, and organizational change for psychologists. *American Psychologist, 58,* 377–402.

Biernacki, P., & Waldorf, D. (1981). Snowball sampling: Problems and techniques of chain referral sampling. *Sociological Methods and Research, 10,* 141–163.

Carr, J. E., & Whittenbaugh, J. A. (1968). Volunteer and nonvolunteer characteristics in an outpatient population. *Journal of Abnormal Psychology, 73,* 16–17.

Christensen, L. B. (2004). *Experimental methodology* (9th ed.). Boston: Allyn & Bacon.

Clarke, G. N. (1995). Improving the transition from basic efficacy research to effectiveness studies: Methodological issues and procedures. *Journal of Consulting and Clinical Psychology, 63,* 718–725.

Cochran, W. G. (1977). *Sampling techniques.* New York: Wiley.

Copas, J. B., & Li, H. G. (1997). Inference for non-random samples. *Journal of the Royal Statistical Society, Series B, 59,* 55–95.

Edlund, M. J., Craig, T. J., & Richardson, M. A. (1985). Informed consent as a form of volunteer bias. *American Journal of Psychiatry, 142,* 624–627.

First, M. B., Spitzer, R. L., Gibbon, M., & Williams, J. B. W. (1994). *Structured Clinical Interview for DSM-IV Axis I Disorders (SCID-I).* Arlington, VA: American Psychiatric Press.

Jaskiw, G. E., Blumer, T. E., Gutierrez-Esteinou, R., Meltzer, H. Y., Steele, V., & Strauss, M. E. (2003). Comparison of inpatients with major mental illness who do and do not consent to low-risk research. *Psychiatry Research, 119,* 183–188.

Kazdin, A. E. (2003). *Research design in clinical psychology* (4th ed.). Boston: Allyn & Bacon.

King, B. F. (1986). Surveys combining probability and quota methods of sampling. *Journal of the American Statistical Association, 80,* 890–896.

Larzelere, R. E., Kuhn, B. R., & Johnson, B. (2004). The intervention selection bias: An underrecognized confound in intervention research. *Psychological Bulletin, 130,* 289–303.

Marczyk, G., DeMatteo, D., & Festinger, D. (2005). *Essentials of research design and methodology.* New York: Wiley.

National Commission for the Protection of Human Subjects of Biomedical and Behavioral Research. (1979). *The Belmont Report: Ethical principles and guidelines for the protection of human subjects of research.* Washington, DC: U.S. Government Printing Office.

National Institutes of Health. (2006). *Glossary of clinical trials terms.* Retrieved April 27, 2006, from http://www.clinicaltrials.gov/ct/info/glossary

Penrod, J., Preston, D. B., Cain, R. E., & Starks, M. T. (2003). A discussion of chain referral as a method of sampling hard-to-reach populations. *Journal of Transcultural Nursing, 14,* 100–107.

Quintana, S. M., Troyano, N., & Taylor, G. (2001). Cultural validity and inherent challenges in quantitative methods for multicultural research. In J. G. Ponterotto, J. M. Casas, L. A. Suzuki, & C. M. Alexander (Eds.), *Handbook of multicultural counseling* (2nd ed., pp. 604–630). Thousand Oaks, CA: Sage.

Rosenthal, R., & Rosnow, R. L. (1975). *The volunteer subject.* New York: Wiley.

Schubert, D. S., Patterson, M. B., Miller, F. T., & Brocco, K. J. (1984). Informed consent as a source of bias in clinical research. *Psychiatry Research, 12,* 313–320.

Shadish, W. R., Cook, T. D., & Campbell, D. T. (2002). *Experimental and quasi-experimental designs for generalized causal inference.* Boston: Houghton Mifflin.

Stirman, S. W., DeRubeis, R. J., Crits-Christoph, P., & Brody, P. E. (2003). Are samples in randomized controlled trials of psychotherapy representative of community outpatients? A new methodology and initial findings. *Journal of Consulting and Clinical Psychology, 71,* 963–972.

Thomas, M. R., Stoyva, J., Rosenberg, S. A., Kassner, C., Fryer, G. E., Giese, A. A., et al. (1997). Selection bias in an inpatient outcomes monitoring project. *General Hospital Psychiatry, 19,* 56–61.

Weisz, J. R., & Weiss, B. (1989). Assessing the effects of clinic-based psychotherapy with children. *Journal of Consulting and Clinical Psychology, 57,* 741–746.

8. Research Participant Recruitment and Retention

Joan S. Grant, James L. Raper, Duck-Hee Kang, and Michael T. Weaver

Randomized controlled trials (RCTs) often extend beyond the funding period because of problems in obtaining required sample sizes (Gross, Mallory, Heiat, & Krumholz, 2002; McDaid, Hodges, Fayter, Stirk, & Eastwood, 2006; Puffer & Torgerson, 2003). The typical number of screened and subsequently enrolled participants is a ratio of at least two to one in behavioral and psychosocial trials (Gross et al., 2002; Motzer, Moseley, & Lewis, 1997; Sears et al., 2003). Potential participants who fail to meet eligibility criteria often are large (McMillan & Weitzner, 2003), and enrollment and attrition rates range from 16 to 60% (Cooley et al., 2003; McMillian & Weitzner, 2003). Funding agencies also may suspend, terminate, or phase out awards if recruitment and retention efforts fall significantly below cumulative targets (National Institutes of Mental Health, 2005), emphasizing the need for investigators to continually examine the effectiveness of their recruitment and retention plans.

This chapter discusses strategies investigators can use to recruit and retain research participants in conducting RCTs for psychosocial interventions. A trial with family caregivers of stroke survivors who participated in a social problem-solving telephone program (SPTP; i.e., problem solving that occurs in a natural environment, such as the home) program is used to illustrate issues and strategies concerning recruitment and retention (Grant, Elliott, Weaver, Bartolucci, & Giger, 2002).

■ Preliminary Steps

Initial empirical efforts should examine the effectiveness of specific psychosocial interventions in achieving desired study outcomes. Subsequent trials often vary patient characteristics, such as ethnicity, socioeconomic and educational levels, and severity and types of illnesses. Investigators also examine the effectiveness of these interventions by setting (e.g., inpatient vs. home setting), intervenor characteristics (e.g., ethnicity, age, gender, discipline, educational background/preparation, relationship/role [health care professional vs. family member]), and strength (e.g., intensity and duration of contacts) of the intervention. Further, these trials examine the differential effectiveness of individual intervention components when investigators do not know whether all or only specific elements are important in achieving specific outcomes (Sidani & Braden, 1998). Important preliminary steps in recruiting and retaining participants for these RCTs are examining potential participants' personal, physical, and psychosocial characteristics and their available resources; considering theoretical propositions relevant for specific intervention components and processes for achieving outcomes; evaluating characteristics of sources for obtaining research participants; and establishing quality relationships with key people in selected study sites.

Examining Participants' Characteristics and Resources

Examining potential participants' personal, physical, and psychosocial characteristics and their available resources are important in selecting appropriate research participants to examine research hypotheses and questions. Personal (e.g., sociodemographic characteristics, learning style preference, cognitive functioning), physical (e.g., severity and stage of illness, signs and symptoms, functional ability), and psychosocial characteristics and available resources (e.g., coping strategies, social support) are relevant factors in selecting participants. For example, specific technical skills (e.g., using computers) and language skills (e.g., ability to read English at a specific grade level), access to certain equipment (e.g., Internet access, telephone), and cognitive and functional (e.g., physical activity and self-care) abilities may be eligibility criteria in testing psychosocial interventions. Certain medical conditions and associated distress levels also may be criteria for participation. Further, pragmatic and financial considerations, such as participants' ability to travel and attend face-to-face individual or group counseling sessions, also are important.

Linking Theory, Processes, and Outcomes

Considering theoretical propositions relevant for specific intervention components and processes for achieving outcomes also is important in conducting these trials and in selecting appropriate participants who will benefit by interventions (Nezu, Nezu, Felgoise, McClure, & Houts, 2003). Preliminary studies and familiarity with the target population assist in identifying the intensity, duration, and acceptable methods of delivering the intervention (e.g., face-to-face individual or group counseling sessions; by telephone); necessary abilities (e.g., memory) or skills to receive the intervention; and acceptable adaptations for target populations. Consideration of these linkages enables investigators to evaluate the availability of potential participants regarding eligibility criteria that limit the effect of extraneous variables on the interaction between independent and dependent variables.

For example, theoretical guidance for providing the SPTP intervention was derived from work on social problem-solving theory (Chang, D'Zurilla, Sanna, 2004; D'Zurilla, Nezu, & Maydeu-Olivares, 2004; Nezu & Nezu, 1991) and family caregiver social problem solving (Grant, 1999; Grant, Elliott, Giger, & Bartolucci, 2001; Houts, Nezu, Nezu, & Bucher, 1996). In the SPTP intervention, a registered nurse trained family caregivers over 8 months to use social problem-solving skills to manage caregiving problems and cope with stresses of caregiving. These caregivers had initial primary nonremunerative responsibility for stroke survivors an average of at least 6 hours per day postdischarge. Further, they had no severe visual impairment or debilitating diseases that limited or prevented them from engaging in caregiving or significantly influenced study outcomes (e.g., a history of *DSM-IV* schizophrenia, alcoholism, dementia, Alzheimer's disease, head injury, or other neuromuscular diseases; Grant et al., 2002). Empirical data and theoretical propositions suggested eight contacts were sufficient for these caregivers to learn effective problem-solving skills (Nezu et al., 2003; Toseland, Labrecque, Goebel, & Whitney, 1992).

Preliminary studies indicated stroke survivor functional deficits influenced caregiver outcomes. Delimiting the study to caregivers who cared for stroke survivors with moderate functional abilities assisted in controlling for this confounding variable. The sampling criterion related to functional abilities also enrolled caregivers who would find the intensity and duration of the intervention acceptable and beneficial because of the level of care and severity of problems they experienced. Except for the first home visit, delivery of the SPTP program was by telephone, a useful strategy for caregivers who previously indicated they were unwilling to leave the stroke survivor alone postdischarge (Grant, 1996; Grant & Davis, 1997; Grant, 1999).

Evaluating Characteristics of Sources for Recruitment

Investigators often use more than one source to obtain participants, such as acute, transitional, long-term (e.g., skilled, intermediate, or residential), and ambulatory (e.g., clinics, schools) care facilities; hospice; professional, civic, advocacy, and faith-based organizations; community centers; occupational and work sites; churches; and other community events or groups (NIMH, 2005). Evaluating characteristics of these sources concerning their role in trials (i.e., recruitment vs. testing of intervention programs); institutional support for testing interventions; access and convenience to participants who are representative of target populations (Mitchell & Abernethy, 2005); and the adequacy of physical layouts (e.g., obtaining baseline data collection), equipment (e.g., computers, telephone), and materials to administer interventions is essential. Other relevant characteristics include their organizational, political, and social norms and culture; standards and protocols of care (in determining their similarity if using more than one source); composition and skill mix of health care providers; and type of facility (private, public, community, rural, etc.; Sidani & Braden, 1998).

For example, the SPTP program used two rehabilitation facilities, representing both private and public facilities, that served stroke survivors and their family caregivers with a wide range of sociodemographic characteristics, offered similar discharge programs, and had similar composition and skill mix of health care providers and lengths of stay. The physical layout, equipment, and space allocation for both facilities were adequate to recruit research participants and collect baseline data, but delivery of the intervention was in the home for both pragmatic reasons and to avoid cross-contamination of study groups. Health care professionals at both study sites supported and facilitated research efforts.

Establishing Effective Relationships With Key People at Study Sites

Establishing effective relationships with key people at study sites who are knowledgeable of the availability of potential participants and methods to gain access to them is essential in facilitating successful recruitment. Key study site personnel may include managers, directors, health care providers (e.g., physicians, nurse practitioners, physiatrists, nurses, and therapists), and data resource and other significant personnel. These individuals commonly understand local procedures for potentially gaining facility/institutional approval, know about current trials, and serve as valuable resources essential to implementing successful recruitment strategies. Investigators should inquire about (a) the ability to obtain participants who meet eligibility criteria, (b) strategies for contacting potential participants, and (c) facilitators and barriers to recruitment.

In establishing liaisons, investigators and research personnel should understand study sites' culture along with their experience with previous successful and unsuccessful recruitment routines and operational activities. This understanding provides insight concerning how and when to communicate best with designated study site liaisons, personnel (e.g., health care professionals, teachers in school settings), and potential research participants in the least disruptive and most efficient manner. Whereas potential participants such as patients and students often seek opinions of their health care providers or teachers and tend to trust their opinions about whether or not to consider participating in RCTs, eliciting their goodwill and advice is essential. Further, seeking their input and expertise early is critical. Some study site personnel may function as coinvestigators because of their expertise (e.g., specific diseases, study populations) and role.

If possible, target groups with which the research team already has ongoing relationships and maintain visibility with them. If recruiting participants from clinical sites, a variety of health care professionals play a pivotal role by introducing trials to patients, showing their support, and raising their initial interest. By supporting their potential value, health care providers are more likely to raise interest in potential participants about RCTs. Research personnel subsequently provide further information about specific psychosocial intervention programs.

In negotiating access to their facilities, investigators can use short letters and offer to meet with key individuals and groups to discuss the potential usefulness of psychosocial interventions in improving participants' health and well-being. These busy professionals appreciate clarity, conciseness, and short overviews about proposed trials. Few health care providers are interested in facilitating recruitment efforts if they fail to understand potential benefits to their patients. Similarly, nonclinical sources (e.g., schools) of potential participants value their role and responsibility to individuals they represent. Facility managers and providers typically are interested in trials' purpose and duration; risks and potential benefits; sample and inclusion/exclusion criteria; methodology; space requirements; effect on operations; and degree of involvement by their personnel. Minimizing interruptions of personnel responsibilities and meetings to discuss recruitment strategies while adhering to Health Insurance Portability and Accountability Act (HIPAA) privacy regulations are essential in assuring the success of recruitment efforts.

Also, discuss steps for keeping personnel informed about recruitment, enrollment, and dissemination of research findings. Nothing deters managers and providers more than to refer participants or facilitate recruitment efforts and never get feedback. Feedback (e.g., success of recruitment and enrollment efforts) also should be timely. Therefore, provide enrollment reports (e.g., monthly) and schedule frequent (e.g., weekly) contacts by research personnel at these study sites (McNees, Dow, & Loerzel, 2005). Strategically posted charts, tables, and graphs (e.g., work areas, lounges) can be efficient, informative means of communication to motivate personnel, especially when recruitment efforts are below targeted enrollment. Contact these key individuals to obtain their renewed commitment at least on an annual basis. These individuals also appreciate public acknowledgment and rewards for their participation. Therefore, study-related plaques, local newspaper stories, and recognition and appreciation for their participation and cooperation in staff meetings and on special occasions are useful.

Customize formats for disseminating findings to assure they are most useful for different communities, such as participants and their families, consumers, and health care professionals (NIMH, 2005). For example, participants and other community members appreciate short handouts or other media to share how findings potentially may improve their health. Abstracts or short handouts summarize findings for health professionals.

For example, in the SPTP program, the investigator initially contacted a high-level manager in each rehabilitation facility, emphasizing the potential importance of the program to family caregivers of stroke survivors discharged home. This manager identified names of individual managers of clinical units who commonly admitted stroke survivors and other personnel who could provide demographic data concerning specific eligibility criteria. In these discussions, individual managers identified names of various health providers (e.g., physicians) to contact for permission to recruit family caregivers of stroke survivors and refine recruitment procedures. These contacts and subsequent discussions occurred over several months, involving both individual and group meetings with various health care professionals, such as physicians; nurses; unit personnel; psychologists; physical, occupational, and speech therapists; and social workers to answer questions, obtain information, and gain their support for the trial.

Key personnel (e.g., data resources personnel) in the two facilities provided information regarding stroke type, functional recovery, discharge status, and demographic data concerning age, gender, race, and other variables. Nursing personnel were useful in providing information about the percentage of survivors who had family members to assist with their care. Other personnel, such as social workers, accurately estimated those who had access to a telephone, an inclusion criterion for the study (Grant & DePew, 1999). These data assisted in evaluating dyads' representativeness and the feasibility of enrolling an adequate number who met study eligibility criteria.

■ Ethical Considerations Regarding Recruitment and Retention Issues

Obtaining institutional review board (IRB) approval may occur either before or after obtaining funding. Some funding agencies require IRB approval as a criterion for their review. However, investigators often obtain this approval after they are relatively confident of receiving moneys because successful funding efforts often require multiple submissions. Universities, hospitals, and other health care agencies that apply for federal grants or contracts involving biomedical or behavioral research substantiate in grant applications that they have established IRBs to review studies (U.S. Department of Health and Human Services, 2005).

Whereas entities receiving federal funds (e.g., large universities) commonly have IRBs, those with no federal grants or contracts frequently have their own research advisory boards. These boards confirm proposed trials' congruence with institutional policies, procedures, and mission. They also compare proposed trials with competing ones and their impact on personnel and potential participants.

HIPAA privacy regulations require health care professionals to protect patient health information regulating disclosure of information for research beyond those currently monitored by IRBs (U.S. Department of Health and Human Services, 2003). Therefore, HIPAA privacy regulations influence investigators' recruitment efforts, requiring either potential participants' authorization or a full or partial IRB waiver of HIPAA authorization for recruitment. Depending on recruitment methods, signed authorizations may be either part of informed consents or separate documents (Olsen, 2003; U.S. Department of Health and Human Services, 2004a, 2004b, 2005).

Personnel at covered entities can make participants aware of studies and obtain signed authorizations to give their names to investigators. IRBs may grant investigators' requests for partial waivers of patients' authorization for recruitment and screening (e.g., to prepare a research protocol; Olsen, 2003; U.S. Department of Health and Human Services, 2004a, 2004b, 2005). Partial waiver requests commonly relate to (a) advertising; (b) telephone screening; and (c) reviewing select data (e.g., medical records, schedules, patient lists) of potential participants and subsequently contacting those who potentially meet eligibility criteria, after meeting specific guidelines (e.g., with concurrence of the primary treating health care provider). After obtaining a partial waiver, investigators may cosign recruitment letters with primary health care providers from recruitment sites (Olsen, 2003; U.S. Department of Health and Human Services, 2004a, 2004b, 2005). Alternately, mailing separate letters by investigators without personal salutations, accompanied by health care providers' personal letters, assures potential participants of their protection.

Often, potential participants are unaware that studies are approved by sponsoring institutions' review board. Therefore, affixing recruitment materials with the IRB approval stamp or specifying that a board reviewed the study to assure protection of human rights is useful. To increase potential participants' confidence, investigators may indicate they shared study information with key individuals (e.g., medical review boards, administrators) who approved use of their institution or facility. Investigators may also need to explain the role of these boards to potential participants.

■ Issues Regarding the Recruitment and Retention of Minority Populations

Adequate representation of women and members of minority groups is essential to assure findings are applicable to these diverse populations (National Institutes of Health, 2000a). Further, health care professionals need to be confident that psychosocial behavioral interventions are useful with these groups. With less diversity, limited variability and subsequent ceiling effects occur if study participants are more advantaged and less likely to benefit from interventions (Yancey, Ortega, & Kumanyika, 2006). Therefore, selecting essential eligibility criteria and appropriate sources for recruitment to assure adequate participant representation is an important element in the success of RCTs.

Primary impediments to the recruitment and retention of certain minority populations are distrust of medical and scientific communities, ineffective recruitment and retention strategies, cultural and language barriers, and concerns about the research process and use of results (Shavers-Hornaday, Lynch, Burmeister, & Torner, 1997). Financial constraints also are a major obstacle to research participation for many people, especially the elderly and racial/ethnic minorities (Wilbur et al., 2006). These groups may have limited moneys available for child care, transportation, and other trial participation costs. Inadequate flexibility in screening these participants also limits their enrollment (Morss et al., 2004; Swanson & Ward, 1995). African Americans and middle-income individuals are less likely to participate in clinical trials than White Americans and low-income individuals. Those who receive information about clinical trials from their health care providers are knowledgeable about such research, and have time available are more likely to participate in RCTs (Baquet, Commiskey, Mullins, & Mishra, 2006).

To address these barriers, network with existing community-based organizations and research advisory boards with diverse members to plan and address problems (NIMH, 2005). Interact with community leaders and members of the targeted population to develop culturally sensitive studies and incorporate traditions, beliefs, and lifestyles into recruitment materials, creating participant ownership and enthusiasm. Often, board members know about upcoming community events to recruit potential participants. Using familiar community sites with easy access promotes trust (Swanson & Ward, 1995). Further, reimburse participants for study-related expenses. Although it is valuable for both, community involvement appears more important in retaining rather than in recruiting African American and Latino participants (Northouse et al., 2006; Yancey et al., 2006). Unsurprisingly, potential African American participants who had to contact investigators to participate had lower attrition rates prior to randomization than those contacted directly by investigators (Ahluwalia et al., 2002).

The importance of ethnic/racial matching of research personnel and participants varies with accessible populations. Some studies support using research personnel of the same ethnic group as research participants to facilitate trust (Herring, Montgomery, Yancy, Williams, & Fraser, 2004; Swanson & Ward, 1995), but other reports are inconsistent regarding the importance of matching to assure enrollment and retention (Ashing-Giwa, Padilla, Tejero, & Kim, 2004; Frye, Baxter, Thompson, & Guinn, 2002; Unson et al., 2004; Warren-Findlow, Prohaska, & Freedman, 2003). Therefore, familiarity with the targeted population, characteristics of psychosocial interventions, and input from community members guide investigators in deciding whether matching is necessary in RCTs.

■ Recruitment of Research Participants

Effective recruitment and retention of research participants, especially from clinical populations, is a challenging task. Patients and their families are frequently under considerable stress with psychologically, physically, and financially demanding illnesses and treatments. Often, they are overwhelmed with unfamiliar information, uncertainty of their illness trajectory, and other family- and work-related issues. Mental and physical fatigue, pain, and illness-specific symptoms add to their burden. During this stressful period, patients may have little reserve to participate in psychosocial interventions unless they perceive direct and indirect benefits. Therefore, core elements in facilitating the success of trials are adequate research personnel and recruitment funds; using media, other written information, and telephone and personal contacts to recruit participants; and providing participants' personal and monetary incentives.

Assuring Adequate Research Personnel and Recruitment Funds

Adequate research personnel and recruitment funds avoid adding additional workload responsibilities for physicians and other health care providers and personnel. Often, using a sampling frame, such as a list of potential participants to approach about enrolling, is much more effective than relying on busy personnel and health care professionals to remember to refer potential participants (Ruffin & Baron, 2000). Systematic evaluation of the effectiveness of these strategies regarding costs and success in recruiting participants is essential. Strategies that are more successful should replace those that are less successful.

Using Media, Written Information, and Telephone and Personal Contacts

Television, radio and newspaper ads, newsletter articles, Web sites, public service announcements, press releases, and interviews on radio or television are examples of media successfully used to recruit participants (NIMH, 2005; Nystuen & Hagen, 2004). In optimally using media, investigators may share information about various RCTs from the same institution using collaborative advertising. Collaborative newspaper advertising offers several advantages. For example, local advertising agencies use eye-catching and professional ad templates. Significant contributions and positive images of institutions also increase credibility of advertisements. Finally, this approach maximizes recruitment moneys by dividing costs among those utilizing the collaborative advertising. Often, two or three exposures cost the same as one advertisement.

In advertising, human-interest angles concerning psychosocial interventions that appeal to and gain potential participants' awareness and are consistent with selected media are important in obtaining potential participants' responses.

Linking recruitment to special events (e.g., National Stroke Awareness Month or National Breast Cancer Awareness Month), holidays, and optimal recruitment seasons (i.e., spring and fall) potentially increases response rates. Investigators must be prepared to handle responses promptly and plan to rerun media messages after a few weeks. Use of answering machines is essential to avoid missing calls from potential participants (NIH, 2004).

Flyers, FAQ sheets, posters, pamphlets, and letters are examples of written information (NIMH, 2005; Nystuen & Hagen, 2004). Table 8.1 depicts important guidelines in developing recruitment materials regarding content, visual design/format, writing style, printing, and mailing. Regarding content, avoid providing too much detail and using terms with which participants are unfamiliar. These materials, usually culturally appropriate and written at no higher than a fifth- or sixth-grade reading level, contain short, concise information about a trial. Keep in mind the purpose—to give essential information— and value of a study, primary eligibility criteria, study requirements, and names of persons to contact for further questions. This information facilitates potential participants deciding if they wish to know more about a trial (NIH, 2004).

Reporting enrollment rates and time remaining to enroll participants on written recruitment materials (e.g., recruitment brochures, letters) is useful for individuals who are thinking about enrolling. For example, "Thus far, we have enrolled *20* people. About *10* months remain to enroll *40* more caregivers in our telephone partnership program to evaluate its usefulness to family caregivers of stroke survivors after they are discharged home."

To use visual design/formatting and writing style optimally, create study logos and catchphrases for recruitment materials. Use illustrations and bulleted lists along with short, simple words, phrases, and sentences to emphasize two or three important points. Pictures, diagrams, or symbols representing key concepts (e.g., a picture of health care providers and family members of both genders and varied races/ethnicity in the SPTP program) also are useful. In these materials, use the active voice, be direct and positive, and do not be afraid to use the word *you* (NIH, 2004).

With written materials, develop several versions of formats, styles, colors, and content and select the version with the most desirable features. Ask colleagues who are familiar with people typical of the target population to give feedback concerning the content, visual message, clarity, and readability (font size, reading level). Always ask for suggestions to improve the materials. Perhaps most important, assess whether these materials achieve their primary purpose—people who meet study eligibility criteria call for further information about a trial.

Focus groups also are useful in developing and customizing these materials. For example, Wilbur and colleagues (2006) used a small focus group of five community women who gave input concerning colors, logos, photographs, content, and testimonials in developing recruitment materials for a home-based walking

TABLE 8.1
Guidelines for Developing Recruitment Materials

Content
- Put most important points first and last.
- Be brief and only include information for potential participants to decide if they wish to contact you and find out more about the trial.
- Use about a fifth- or sixth-grade reading level.
- Pilot test materials with people similar to the target population and ask what they (1) notice, (2) remember, and (3) should do? Further, ask for ways to improve these materials.
- Acknowledge the funding agency on materials.

Visual design
- Put study logos and catchphrases on all recruitment materials.
- Allow lots of white space in margins and between blocks of text.
- Use visuals and illustrations that draw the eye to two or three key points.
- Consider using institutional seals for credibility.
- Use a 12-point or larger ($\geq$13 for older adults) serif font (NIH, 2004). Serif fonts have small appendages at the top and bottom (The Internet Digest, 2003).
- Do not use all capital letters, even in titles or headings. Instead, use upper and lower case letters, larger and bolder print, and underlining.

Writing style
- Use short and simple words, phrases, and sentences.
- Limit each sentence to one idea.
- A sentence structure of subject, verb, and object is best.
- Use the active voice; be positive, direct and personal and not afraid to use the word *you*.
- Bulleted lists make it easier to scan and identify important points.
- Avoid large blocks of text.
- Minimize medical terminology and technical words (e.g., *about* rather than *approximately*).

Printing
- Use camera-ready copy rather than photocopies.
- Black print on white or yellow paper is easiest to read.
- Put letters on institutional or referring agencies' letterheads with official signatures and recent dates.
- Print on 60-pound paper, or heavier, if double-sided. If using self-mailers, 65-pound paper is good.

Mailing
- Type (if time and cost are prohibitive) or handwrite addresses on envelopes.
- Avoid mailing to the same individual more than three times.

program. These materials provided a brief description of the program; screening expectations; primary eligibility criteria (e.g., race, age, and physical activity level); location of screening and data collection sites; and a toll free telephone number at each data collection site to call for further information.

Both telephone and personal contacts are effective techniques to recruit participants. Often, the telephone is effective when used to screen participants, convey general information, and answer questions concerning a trial. In testing psychosocial intervention programs, however, personal contacts often are essential because involvement required by participants is significant (Grant & DePew, 1999; Grant et al., 2002). Indicating pleasant, positive, professional, caring, and competent behaviors by research personnel is essential in these contacts (Caldwell et al., 2005; Mann, Hoke, & Williams, 2005; Ruff, Alexander, & McKie, 2005). Further, investigators and research personnel provide personal incentives in conveying a trial's value while giving accurate information about the role, time, and commitment required of participants. Often, time and aggravation are the most significant influence on recruitment. Because perceived barriers may not really exist, explaining study realities to participants is important (Ruffin & Barron, 2000). Further, graceful verbal (i.e., both telephone and personal contacts) and nonverbal (i.e., personal contacts) acceptance (e.g., body language) of potential participants' agreements and refusals are inherent in discussing psychosocial trials.

Providing Personal and Monetary Incentives

People often wish to contribute to society and assist those who are experiencing the same problem that they have faced. Others participate because they have or are at risk for a disease or problem, and they feel RCTs provide access to interventions that will improve or treat their problem. Therefore, personal incentives for many participants concern how a trial is important for refining and developing future programs and helping people similar to them. Often, participation relates to support and agreement by other significant family members, and allocating time for either research personnel or potential participants to discuss a trial with them is important. For example, in the SPTP program, African American primary caregivers often discussed the study with their spouses, brothers, sisters, or other relatives before agreeing to participate in the study.

Travel time and related expenses are disincentives for participation (Ruffin & Barron, 2000). Making decisions about offering incentives includes remuneration. Although some investigators indicate money is an important incentive to encourage participation (Martinson et al., 2000; Ulrich & Grady, 2004), others have found it of little value (Laken & Ager, 1995). However, Mapstone, Elbourne, and Roberts (2002) found monetary incentives to be beneficial in retaining research participants in 15 RCTs ($n = 33,719$ participants). Ethical concerns for research participants are whether monies will (a) unduly influence them to take part in research, (b) lessen concerns about study risks, (c) motivate them to either conceal relevant information or change their responses on study measures, and (d) preferentially attract vulnerable populations. Threats to internal validity are an issue if incentives cause participants to alter their responses (Mapstone et al., 2002).

A number of remuneration models are available. "Market," "wage-payment," "reimbursement," and "fair-share" models are examples, each with its own strengths and weaknesses (Dickert & Grady, 1999). Expenses and compensation commonly include transportation (e.g., mass-transit passes, cab vouchers), meals, lodging, mileage, and parking. Reimbursement for short-term day care or respite care for family members (e.g., children, care recipients) also is appropriate in psychosocial intervention trials. Table 8.2 summarizes NIH (2000b) guidelines for remuneration of research participants as a valuable tool for investigators. Investigators may reimburse participants for expenses, to reduce financial sacrifices, to compensate for their time and effort, and as incentives to facilitate recruitment and retention and lessen attrition. Although deviations from these guidelines are permissible, justification is necessary.

For example, in the telephone partnership, research participants received $25 ($10 at 5 weeks, and $15 at the end of 13 weeks). Some participants accepted the money for themselves; others gave it either to charitable organizations or to

---

TABLE 8.2
NIH Guidelines for Remuneration of Research Participants

Remuneration for participating in research

- Includes travel and related expenses, such as meals, lodging, and parking
- Avoids being so excessive as to be the only or primary reason for being in a study
- Is prompt and appropriate to offer for the inconvenience, time, and effort it takes to participate in research
- Is given to participants who have multiple, lengthy, and repeated contacts before they withdraw, are discharged early by the investigator (including those who are disqualified through no fault of their own), or otherwise fail to complete a study; partial payments relate to study time, effort, and discomfort
- Uses either a per-day, per-visit, or per-procedure schedule, or some combination thereof
- Can be contingent upon study completion if involving only one visit/contact
- Is offered to both healthy and patient participants
- While common, is not restricted to people in protocols offering little or no prospect of direct benefit to themselves
- Is fair, offering similar amounts of reimbursement to all persons who participate in similar research procedures in protocols
- Generally, completion bonuses should not exceed 50% of total remuneration. Do not offer large bonuses in studies with higher risks and discomforts or long-term commitments (NIH, 2000b).

---

their grandchildren. Although research participants accepted the $25 as a token for their efforts, they also iterated how team members' caring behaviors were critical in retaining them in the trial (Grant & DePew, 1999; Grant et al., 2002).

■ Retention of Research Participants

Because of the relationship between participant recruitment and retention rates, adequate attention to both is essential. Higher dropout rates are present in either intervention or control groups in which disincentives clearly outweigh benefits from the time and commitment required of study participants. Common reasons for attrition are mortality, changes in eligibility status, and lack of time or interest in continuing participation because of additional stress and study protocols that fail to meet participants' needs (e.g., assignment to attention control or control group). Personal and family attitudes toward protocols and research personnel, lengthy data collection, and relocation to another area or loss of contact influence recruitment and retention of participants (Cooley et al., 2003; Given, Keilman, Collins, & Given, 1990; Grant & DePew, 1999; Motzer et al., 1997; Northouse et al., 2006; Ruffin & Barron, 2000; Swanson and Ward, 1995). Therefore, strategies for retaining participants are developing positive and trusting relationships between research personnel and participants; selecting and training suitable personnel; balancing rigidity and flexibility in implementing study protocols; designing protocols relevant for participants' lives and situations; and systematically obtaining pertinent information from participants to facilitate locating them.

Developing Relationships Between Research Personnel and Participants

Acknowledging research participants as individuals first and as participants second is essential in building positive and trusting relationships. Research personnel who inquire about participants and their family members and communicate their commitment to them and their community demonstrate supportive approaches. Postcards, newsletters, e-mail messages, and telephone calls can be effective tools to convey caring, appreciation, information, and commitment of research team members (Ruffin & Barron, 2000). The principal investigator, project manager, or site coordinator may send greeting cards and thank-you letters regularly, taking care to assure participants do not become dependent on specific project personnel (Hellard, Sinclair, Forbes, & Fairley, 2001; Robinson & Marsland, 1994). For example, project personnel may send handwritten or formal thank-you letters after enrollment, after completing significant phases of a trial, and at the end of a trial.

Creating a project identity reinforces participants' bond with research personnel and the study and lessens concerns regarding its credibility (Motzer et al., 1997; Ribisl et al., 1996). As mentioned previously, using study logos and catchphrases in personal contacts and on business cards, correspondence, certificates (e.g., for students in schools), advertisements, and study materials creates a positive project identity (Ruffin & Barron, 2000). Quarterly newsletters also keep participants informed about the progress of RCTs, although selected content must avoid contaminating control group participants (Kelly & Cordell, 1996; Ribisl et al., 1996). Pertinent information about research personnel, such as their names, specific role (e.g., the person who will collect information from you), and personal information they are willing to share about themselves and their family, builds these relationships.

Selecting and Training Research Personnel

Selecting and training research personnel is essential to assure adequate knowledge, experience, and interpersonal skills related to study objectives, protocols, their role, the study population, and associated problems and issues. Research personnel who display professional, competent, and caring behaviors are essential (Caldwell et al., 2005; Mann et al., 2005; Ruff et al., 2005). Further, personnel who indicate their commitment to and enthusiasm about a trial and show concern for others create motivated study participants. Although using consistent personnel is important in developing relationships, personnel turnover requires balancing more inexperienced and experienced personnel. Ongoing and refresher training for replacement and all personnel, respectively, is essential (NIMH, 2005).

Training research personnel regarding study protocols and how to respond to questions or issues is important to avoid attrition. In facilitating and refining these skills and behaviors, taping and critiquing training sessions are important (Pletsch, Howe, & Tenney, 1995). Further, regularly scheduled meetings among research personnel to promptly address protocol problems and other issues help to retain research participants (Given et al., 1990).

For example, a research nurse with experience in adult neuroscience nursing implemented the SPTP intervention program. Graduate nursing students collected data from stroke survivors and their family caregivers, providing trained research personnel with interpersonal skills. Research personnel practiced personal and telephone recruitment contacts and protocols based on their role with people from different cultural backgrounds, responding to various questions or statements. These sessions also focused on telephone etiquette, how to ask and respond to questions concerning sensitive exclusion criteria (e.g., history of mental illness), and other issues (e.g., family conflicts). Assessment of treatment adherence and competence of research personnel routinely occurred (e.g., through treatment manuals, training protocols, audiotaping; Grant & DePew, 1999; Grant et al., 2001; Grant et al., 2002).

Balancing Rigidity and Flexibility in Implementing Study Protocols

Balancing flexibility and rigidity in executing protocols avoids high attrition because participants find study requirements too bothersome to incorporate into their current lifestyles. Protocols that specify acceptable time frames for making contacts and collecting data create a welcoming environment and promote participants' value by allowing them some flexibility to incorporate study contacts into their busy schedules. Depending on the situation, telephone calls, personal letters, and e-mail messages serve to confirm dates, times, and the nature of contacts, allowing participants to call if they need to change their appointment. User-friendly recruitment plans, such as using familiar locations and convenient study sites for targeted populations, also are important.

Recognizing the importance of participants' personal lives and their busy schedules is critical in arranging contact times. In coordinating appointments, calling participants before scheduled visits is useful. Providing contact numbers with an answering machine and e-mail addresses where participants can leave messages also is important. Organization concerning contacts minimizes waiting time, paperwork, and inconvenience for participants. Protocols that assure accurate data collection minimize unnecessary follow-up and frustration by both participants and research personnel in later obtaining missed but valuable information (Grant & DePew, 1999; Kelly & Cordell, 1996; Motzer et al., 1997).

In balancing flexibility and rigidity in executing protocols, investigators make decisions regarding the type and method of data collection. Using quantitative instruments, higher retention rates are associated with shorter, easy-to-complete questionnaires (Hellard et al., 2001). In selecting methods for collecting quantitative data, investigators must balance the time required to collect data; essential data concerning process, outcome, and other variables; and characteristics of the target population. Further, evaluating whether obtaining data from all measures is necessary at each data collection time is useful. If instrument psychometric properties are adequate for the target population and study purpose, mailing out questionnaires and then contacting participants by telephone approximately 1 week later for the answers is an alternative. Returning questionnaire answers, such as by facsimile and e-mail, also has have been effective (Aitken, Gallagher, & Madronio, 2003).

For example, in the SPTP program, initial data collection occurred 1 to 2 days prior to rather than on the day of discharge for several reasons. The day of discharge often is hectic for both family members and stroke survivors attending therapy and discussing plans with various hospital personnel. Subsequent data collection was at caregivers' convenience and occurred in their homes because of their strong commitment to assuring the physical and psychosocial well-being of the stroke survivor. Early in the trial, caregivers indicated the best times to make personal and telephone contacts, allowing them to consider employment, household, and caregiving activities in conjunction with stroke survivor appointments and therapy sessions in scheduling contacts. Reminder phone calls by project personnel occurred about 1 week before a planned visit and again on the morning of each scheduled contact, lessening the number of missed appointments. As arranged, family caregivers called and left a message on an answering machine if they were unable to keep appointments. Research personnel promptly called caregivers to reschedule missed appointments (Grant & DePew, 1999; Grant et al., 2002).

Designing Relevant Protocols

Participants sometimes also withdraw from psychosocial intervention trials because study protocols fail to meet their needs (e.g., assignment to attention control or control group). Study goals, theoretical frameworks, the quality of existing and proposed interventions, the target population and related problems/issues, and study site factors influence protocols (Barkauskas, Lusk, & Eakin, 2005). Therefore, a very practical and critical issue in retaining research participants is to design protocols relevant to participants' needs, lives, and situations. Although this criterion sounds simple, these protocols often are difficult to design, especially for those assigned to attention control/control groups. In developing these protocols, a key question concerns hypothesized differences expected by control versus intervention protocols.

For example, all groups received usual discharge planning services in the SPTP program. Caregivers randomly assigned to the sham intervention (i.e., attention control) group received the same number of contacts as those in the intervention group. Participants randomly assigned to the sham intervention group answered questions concerning health care services either they or the stroke survivor had received since the last contact. The protocol for this group was relevant for dyads of stroke survivors who received rehabilitative services (e.g., physical, occupational, and speech therapy) and their family caregivers. Further, work on social problem-solving theory (D'Zurilla et al., 2004) and family caregiver social problem solving (Houts et al., 1996; Nezu & Nezu, 1991) indicated that this protocol should not significantly improve study caregiver outcomes (e.g., depressive behavior).

In support of this premise, compared with the sham intervention and control groups (who received only data collection), caregivers who participated in the SPTP program had better problem-solving skills, preparedness, and general health (i.e., concerning vitality, social functioning, mental health, and role limitations related to emotional problems) and less depression. Satisfaction with health care services decreased over time in the control group while remaining comparable in the intervention and sham intervention groups (Grant et al., 2002).

Obtaining Participant Information to Facilitate Retention

Investigators also must systematically obtain pertinent information from participants to facilitate locating them when they move to other locations and change their addresses and telephone contact numbers, especially in longitudinal designs. A practical suggestion for locating participants is to ask them for current addresses and telephone numbers at each measurement time (or more frequently for longer time intervals between measurement) and for names and telephone numbers of people who will always know how to contact them (relatives, friends, etc.). Ask their full birth dates (this helps to confirm identities when using search engines) and first names (rather than initials or nicknames), and ask about first names and initials of significant others (e.g., spouses). First names and initials of significant others are useful when participants are only listed in telephone books under those names (Lyons et al., 2004). A good question to ask is, "Would you mind sharing the names of persons (and how to contact them) who typically know how to reach you in case you change either your address or your contact numbers?"

Web-based telephone directories also are useful for locating participants. These search engines commonly provide full names, ages, addresses, length of time at residence, and telephone numbers; others are useful for locating people by their name and state (e.g., full name and middle initial, their age, last known city, and state of residence; Lyons et al., 2004). Of course, HIPAA regulations and protection of human rights require approval for obtaining this type of information and procedures for protecting participants.

Frequently remind participants to notify project personnel if their residential address or telephone number changes. This request can be included on newsletters/materials mailed to participants, along with tokens (magnets, pens, calendars, or mugs) that show appreciation for their time and effort while making it easy to contact research personnel. Providing participants with a toll-free number facilitates their contacting the research team freely (Lyons et al., 2004).

In summary, this chapter describes strategies investigators can use to recruit and retain research participants in RCTs. Anticipating challenges and utilizing effective strategies increases chances of obtaining sufficient sample sizes for adequate statistical power and participants who are representative of target populations.

■ References

Ahluwalia, J. S., Richter, K., Mayo, M. S., Ahluwalia, H. K., Choi, W. S., Schmelzle, K. H., et al., (2002). African American smokers interested and eligible for a smoking cessation clinical trial: Predictors of not returning for randomization. *Annals of Epidemiology, 12,* 206–212.

Aitken, L., Gallagher, R., & Madronio, C. (2003). Principles of recruitment and retention in clinical trials. *International Journal of Nursing Practice, 9,* 338–346.

Ashing-Giwa, K. T., Padilla, G. V., Tejero, J. S., & Kim, J. (2004). Breast cancer survivorship in a multiethnic sample: Challenges in recruitment and measurement. *Cancer, 101,* 450–465.

Baquet, C. R., Commiskey, P., Mullins, C. D., & Mishra, S. I. (2006). Recruitment and participation in clinical trials: Socio-demographic, rural/urban, and health care access predictors. *Cancer Detection and Prevention, 30,* 24–33.

Barkauskas, V. H., Lusk, S. L., & Eakin, B. L. (2005). Selecting control interventions for clinical outcome studies. *Western Journal of Nursing Research, 27,* 346–363.

Caldwell, J. Y., Davis, J. D., Du Bois, B., Echo-Hawk, H., Erickson, J. S., Goins, R. T., et al. (2005). Culturally competent research with American Indians and Alaska natives: Findings and recommendations of the first symposium of the work group on American Indian research and program evaluation methodology. *American Indian and Alaska Native Mental Health Research, 12*(1), 1–21.

Chang, E. C., D'Zurilla, T. J., & and Sanna, L. J. (Eds.). (2004). *Social problem solving: Theory, research, and training.* Washington, DC: American Psychological Association.

Cooley, M. E., Sarna, L., Brown, J. K., Williams, R. D., Chernecky, C., Padilla, G., et al. (2003). Challenges of recruitment and retention in multisite clinical research. *Cancer Nursing, 26,* 376–384.

Dickert, N., & Grady, C. (1999). What's the price of a research subject? Approaches to payment for research participation. *New England Journal of Medicine, 341,* 198–203.

D'Zurilla, T. J., Nezu, A. M., & Maydeu-Olivares, A. (2004). Social problem solving: Theory and assessment. In E. C. Chang, T. J. D'Zurilla, & L. J. Sanna (Eds.), *Social problem solving: Theory, research, and training* (pp. 11–27). Washington, DC: American Psycological Association.

Frye, F. H., Baxter, S. D., Thompson, W. O., & Guinn, C. H. (2002). Influence of school, class, ethnicity, and gender on agreement of fourth graders to participate in a nutrition study. *Journal of School Health, 72,* 115–120.

Given, B. A., Keilman, L. J., Collins, C., & Given, C. W. (1990). Strategies to minimize attrition in longitudinal studies. *Nursing Research, 39,* 184–186.

Grant, J. S. (1996). Home care problems experienced by stroke survivors and their family caregivers. *Home Healthcare Nurse, 14,* 892–902.

Grant, J. S. (1999). Social problem-solving partnerships with family caregivers. *Rehabilitation Nursing, 24,* 254–260.

Grant, J. S., & Davis, L. (1997). Living with loss: The stroke family caregiver. *Journal of Family Nursing, 3,* 36–56.

Grant, J. S., & De Pew, D. D. (1999). Recruiting and retaining research participants for a clinical intervention study. *Journal of Neuroscience Nursing, 31,* 357–362.

Grant, J. S., Elliott, T., Giger, J. N., & Bartolucci, A. (2001). Social problem-solving telephone partnerships with family caregivers of persons with stroke. *International Journal of Rehabilitation Research, 24,* 181–189.

Grant, J. S., Elliott, T. R., Weaver, M., Bartolucci, A. A., & Giger, J. N., (2002). A telephone intervention with family caregivers of stroke survivors after rehabilitation. *Stroke, 33,* 2060–2065.

Gross, C. P., Mallory, R., Heiat, A., & Krumholz, H. M. (2002). Reporting the recruitment process in clinical trials: Who are these patients and how did they get there? *Annals of Internal Medicine, 137,* 10–16.

Hellard, M. E., Sinclair, M. I., Forbes, A. B., & Fairley, C. K. (2001). Methods used to maintain a high level of participant involvement in a clinical trial. *Journal of Epidemiology and Community Health, 55,* 348–351.

Herring, P., Montgomery, S., Yancy, A. K., Williams, C., & Fraser, G. (2004). Understanding the challenges in recruiting Blacks to a longitudinal cohort study: The Adventist Health Study. *Ethnicity and Disease, 14,* 423–430.

Houts, P. S., Nezu, A. M., Nezu, C. M., & Bucher, J. A. (1996). The prepared family caregiver: A problem-solving approach to family caregiver education. *Patient Education and Counseling, 27,* 63–73.

Kelly, P. J., & Cordell, J. R. (1996). Recruitment of women into research studies: A nursing perspective. *Clinical Nurse Specialist, 10,* 25–28.

Laken, M., & Ager, J. (1995). Using incentives to increase participation in prenatal care. *Obstetrics and Gynecology, 85,* 326–329.

Lyons, K. S., Carter, J. H., Carter, E. H., Rush, K. N., Stewart, B. J., & Archbold, P. G. (2004). Locating and retaining research participants for follow-up studies. *Research in Nursing and Health, 27,* 63–68.

Mann, A., Hoke, M. M., & Williams, J. C. (2005). Lessons learned: Research with rural Mexican-American women. *Nursing Outlook, 53,* 141–146.

Mapstone, J., Elbourne, D., & Roberts, I. (2002). Strategies to improve recruitment to research studies. *The Cochrane Database of Methodology Reviews, 3,* Art. No. MR000013.pub2. DOI: 10.1002/14651858.MR000013.pub2.

Martinson, B. C., Lazovich, D., Lando, H. A., Perry, C. L., McGovern, P. G., & Boyle, R. G. (2000). Effectiveness of monetary incentives for recruiting adolescents to an intervention trial to reduce smoking. *Preventive Medicine, 31,* 706–713.

McDaid, C., Hodges, Z., Fayter, D., Stirk, L., & Eastwood, A. (2006). Increasing participation of cancer patients in randomised controlled trials: A systematic review. *Trials, 7,* 16.

McMillan, S. C., & Weitzner, M. A. (2003). Methodological issues in collecting data from debilitated patients with cancer near the end of life. *Oncology Nursing Forum, 30,* 123–129.

McNees, P., Dow, K., & Loerzel, V. (2005). Application of the CuSum Technique to evaluate changes in recruitment strategies. *Nursing Research, 54,* 399–405.

Mitchell, G. K., & Abernethy, A. P. (2005). Investigators of the Queensland Case Conferences Trial; Palliative Care Trial. A comparison of methodologies from two longitudinal community-based randomized controlled trials of similar interventions in palliative care: What worked and what did not? *Journal of Palliative Medicine, 8,* 1226–1237.

Morss, G. M., Jordan, A. N., Kinner, J. S., Dunn, A. L., Church, T. S., Earnest, C. P., et al. (2004). Dose-response to exercise in woman aged 45–75 (DREW): Design and rationale. *Medicine and Science in Sports and Exercise, 36,* 336–344.

Motzer, S. A., Moseley, J. R., & Lewis, F. M. (1997). Recruitment and retention of families in clinical trials with longitudinal designs. *Western Journal of Nursing Research, 19,* 314–333.

National Institutes of Health. National Heart Lung and Blood Institute. (2004). Women's Health Initiative. *Recruitment.* Vol. 2, Section 3, 1–24. Retrieved July 23, 2006, from http://www.nhlbi.nih.gov/resources/deca/whios/studydoc/procedur/3.pdf

National Institutes of Health. Office of Human Subjects Research. (2000a). OHSR Information Sheets/Forms. *Inclusion of women and minorities in study populations: Guidance for IRBs and principal investigators.* Retrieved October 4, 2006, from http://ohsr.od.nih.gov/info/sheet11.html

National Institutes of Health. Office of Human Subjects Research. (2000b). OHSR Information Sheets/Forms. *Remuneration of Research Subjects in the Intramural Research Program.* Retrieved October 4, 2006, from http://ohsr.od.nih.gov/info/sheet20.html

National Institutes of Mental Health. (2005). Policy for the recruitment of participants in clinical research. Retrieved July 24, 2006, from http://www.nimh.nih.gov/researchfunding/nimhrecruitmentpolicy.cfm

Nezu, A. M., & Nezu, C. M. (1991). Problem-solving skills training. In V. E. Cabello (Ed.), *Handbook of behavior modification and therapy techniques* (pp. 527–553). Madrid, Spain: Siglo Veintiuno de Espana Editores.

Nezu, A. M., Nezu, C. M., Felgoise, S. H., McClure, K. S., & Houts, P. S. (2003). Project Genesis: Assessing the efficacy of problem-solving therapy for distressed adult cancer patients. *Journal of Consulting and Clinical Psychology, 71,* 1036–1048.

Northouse, L. L., Rosset, T., Phillips, L., Mood, D., Schafenacker, A., & Kershaw, T. (2006). Research with families facing cancer: The challenges of accrual and retention. *Research in Nursing and Health, 29,* 199–211.

Nystuen, P., & Hagen, K. B. (2004). Telephone reminders are effective in recruiting nonresponding patients to randomized controlled trials. *Journal of Clinical Epidemiology, 57,* 773–776.

Olsen, D. P. (2003). HIPAA privacy regulations and nursing research. *Nursing Research, 52,* 344–348.

Pletsch, P. K., Howe, C., & Tenney, M: (1995). Recruitment of minority subjects for intervention research. *Image: Journal of Nursing Scholarship, 27,* 211–215.

Puffer, S., & Torgerson, D. (2003). Recruitment difficulties in randomised controlled trials. *Controlled Clinical Trials, 24*(3S), S214–S215.

Ribisl, K. M., Walton, M. A., Mowbray, C. T., Luke, D. A., Davidson, W. S., & Bootsmiller, B. J. (1996). Minimizing participant attrition in panel studies through the use of effective retention and tracking strategies. *Review and Recommendations, Evaluation and Program Planning, 19,* 1–25.

Robinson, S., & Marsland, L. (1994). Approaches to the problem of respondent attrition in a longitudinal panel study of nurses' careers. *Journal of Advanced Nursing, 20,* 729–741.

Ruff, C. C., Alexander, I. M., & McKie, C. (2005). The use of focus group methodology in health disparities research. *Nursing Outlook, 53,* 134–140.

Ruffin, M. T., IV, & Baron, J. (2000). Recruiting subjects in cancer prevention and control studies. *Journal of Cellular Biochemistry, 77*(S34), 80–83.

Sears, S. R., Stanton, A. L., Kwan, L., Krupnick, J. L., Rowland, J. H., Meyerowitz, B. E., et al. (2003). Recruitment and retention challenges in breast cancer survivorship research: Results from a multisite, randomized intervention trial in women with early stage breast cancer. *Cancer Epidemiology Biomarkers and Prevention, 12,* 1087–1090.

Shavers-Hornaday, V., Lynch, C., Burmeister, L., & Torner, J. (1997). Why are African Americans under-represented in medical research studies? Impediments to participation. *Ethnicity and Health, 2,* 31–45.

Sidani, S., & Braden, C. J. (1998). *Evaluating nursing interventions: A theory-driven approach.* Thousand Oaks, CA: Sage.

Swanson, G. M., & Ward, A. J. (1995). Recruiting minorities into clinical trials: Toward a participant friendly system. *Journal of the National Cancer Institute, 87,* 1747–1759.

The Internet Digest. (2003). Web-safe fonts for your site. Retrieved September 16, 2006, from http://www.theinternetdigest.net/archive/websafefonts.html

Toseland, R. W., Labrecque, M. S., Goebel, S. T., & Whitney, M. H. (1992). An evaluation of a group program for spouses of frail elderly veterans. *Gerontologist, 32,* 382–390.

Ulrich, C. M., & Grady, C. (2004). Financial incentives and response rates in nursing research. *Nursing Research, 53,* 73–74.

Unson, C. G., Ohannessian, C., Kenyon, L., Case, A., Reisine, S., & Prestwood, K. (2004). Barriers to eligibility and enrollment among older women in a clinical trial on osteoporosis: Effects of ethnicity and SES. *Journal of Aging and Health, 16,* 426–443.

U.S. Department of Health and Human Services. Office for Human Research Protections. (2005). *Code of Federal Regulations. Title 45, Part 46. Protection of human subjects.* Retrieved September 2, 2005, from http://www.hhs.gov/ohrp/humansubjects/guidance/45cfr46.htm

U.S. Department of Health and Human Services. Office of Civil Rights (2003). *Standards for privacy of individually identifiable health information. HHS Code of Federal Regulations, Title 45, Parts 160 & 164.* Retrieved July 23, 2006, from http://www.hhs.gov/grantsnet/adminis/fedreg45.htm

U.S. Department of Health and Human Services. National Institutes of Research. (2004a). *Clinical research and the HIPAA privacy rule.* Retrieved August 12, 2006, from http://privacyruleandresearch.nih.gov/clin_research.asp

U.S. Department of Health and Human Services. National Institutes of Research. (2004b). *Protecting personal health information in research: Understanding the*

HIPAA Privacy rule. Retrieved August 12, 2006, from http://privacyrulean-dresearch.nih.gov/pr_02.asp

Warren-Findlow, J., Prohaska, T. R., & Freedman, D. (2003). Challenges and opportunities in recruiting and retaining underrepresented populations into health promotion research. *Gerontologist, 43*(Spec. No. 1), 37–46.

Wilbur, J., McDevitt, J., Wang, E., Dancy, B., Briller, J., Ingram, D., et al. (2006). Recruitment of African American women to a walking program: Eligibility, ineligibility, and attrition during screening. *Research in Nursing and Health, 29,* 176–189.

Yancey, A. K., Ortega, A. N., & Kumanyika, S. K. (2006). Effective recruitment and retention of minority research participants. *Annual Review of Public Health, 27,* 1–28.

9. Random Assignment Procedures

Louis M. Hsu

Detailed and generally excellent descriptions and evaluations of more than two dozen random assignment (also called random allocation) methods that are used in randomized clinical trials (RCTs) are available in Kalish and Begg (1985), Pocock (1979, 1983), Lachin, Matts, and Wei (1988), Lee (1980), Fleiss (1986), and Shadish, Cook, and Campbell (2002). Kalish and Begg (1985), Pocock (1979, 1983), and Lachin et al. (1988) focus primarily on medical applications of these methods; Lee (1980) discusses applications that involve time-related outcome measures (e.g., length of remission); Fleiss (1986) discusses random assignment in a wide variety of health-related disciplines; and Shadish et al. (2002) describe the methods mainly in relation to behavioral science objectives.

The random assignment methods presented in this chapter are motivated primarily by two problems that are frequently encountered in treatment efficacy studies: (a) heterogeneity of patients on prognostic factors (covariates), and (b) sequential rather than simultaneous entry of patients into the trial. The methods in Sections 1 and 2 illustrate two ways of handling the first problem. Section 1 methods rely on random assignment to control effects of prognostic factors (especially the biasing effects caused by nonequivalence of contrasted groups on these factors) and to justify statistical significance tests; identification, observation, or measurement of these factors is not necessary for use of these methods, or for the validity of tests of hypotheses used in the data analyses. In contrast, Section 2 methods require identification, observation, and measurement of prognostic factors. This information is used to construct "strata" of patients that are homogeneous (within strata) with respect to the prognostic factor(s), prior to random assignment. Both methods in Section 1 and those in Section 2 may use order of entry of patients into the trial to construct "blocks" of patients that are (relatively) homogeneous (within blocks) in terms of times of entry into the trial, prior to (or after) random assignment. Data analysis and interpretation implications of whether random assignment methods (discussed in Sections 1 and 2) are (or are not) preceded by random sampling are presented in Section 3.

■ Section 1. Randomization Methods That Ignore Prognostic Factors

As noted earlier, methods discussed in Section 1 do not require observation or measurement of prognostic factors, or awareness of their relative importance, and in fact do not even require knowledge of the identity of these factors. Nevertheless, they are useful (when the number of patients is sufficiently large) in controlling for bias-causing nonequivalence of treatment groups on prognostic factors and in providing the justification for hypotheses tests and confidence intervals relevant to the relative efficacy of alternative treatments. As noted by Meier (1975), "Randomization [distributes] the effects of baseline variables, both the measured ones and those not observed, in such a way that the statistical analysis makes due allowance for them" (p. 519). Methods in Section 1.1. differ from those in Section 1.2. in terms of whether the random assignments methods result in expected or targeted balance (or imbalance) over the many replications of the study, or in actual intended balance (or imbalance) in individual studies.

1.1. Random Assignments That Yield Expected Desired Distributions

1.1.1. SIMPLE RANDOM ASSIGNMENT (SIMPLE RANDOMIZATION) FOR EXPECTED EQUAL ALLOCATION OF PATIENTS TO TREATMENTS

The expression *simple random assignment*[1] or *simple randomization* will be used in this chapter in a manner that is consistent with that in Shadish et al. (2002) and Hodges and Lehmann (1970): Consider that (a) the decision concerning what treatment to administer to a patient is made immediately *after* it has been determined that this patient is eligible for the trial, and (b) the decision is made by a process that ensures a probability of $(1/K)$ of administration of any one of the K treatments to this patient, irrespective of treatments received by the other patients. This method prevents the investigator from knowing ahead of time a patient's treatment assignment, and therefore prevents bias that might occur because of "conscious or unconscious selection of patients to receive a preferred treatment. For example, when the next allocation is [known to be] to a 'treatment' group (rather than to a 'control' group), the investigator may give preferential consideration to a patient with poorer prognosis for entry into the trial" (Kalish & Begg, 1985, p. 134; see also Section 1.2.3).

To illustrate this type of simple random assignment method, suppose that the object of a study is to determine the relative efficacy of K = 6 treatments and that patients become available for participation in the study at various points in time. (Note: availability of patients at different time points rather than availability of all patients at the same time point appears to be the rule rather than the exception in treatment efficacy studies; see, e.g., Pocock, 1979, p. 183). Simple random assignment of patients to treatments can be carried out using a (six-sided) die; as each eligible patient becomes available for treatment, the die is tossed, and the outcome of the toss determines this patient's treatment ($1 \rightarrow$ Treatment A, $2 \rightarrow$ B, ..., $6 \rightarrow$ F). Given a symmetrical six-sided die, this method of assignment ensures that the probability of assignment of each treatment to each patient is 1/6. Furthermore, given our knowledge of the behavior of dice, it is reasonable to expect that this probability (of 1/6) would not be affected by outcomes of die tosses for patients who entered treatment at other time points.

Other physical devices than dice (e.g., roulette wheels, spinners) can be used to ensure that the probability of assignment of each of the K treatments to each patient is $(1/K)$, and to ensure that the treatment assignment for a patient who enters treatment at time T is independent of assignments of other patients who enter treatment at other times. However, for a variety of reasons (see Shadish et al., 2002, for some real-world examples of limitations of physical randomization devices), alternatives to the use of physical devices for simple random assignment are generally preferable (except, perhaps, in the determination of a starting point in a table of random numbers—see below).

The principal alternatives include the use of (a) tables of random digits and tables of random permutations (available in experimental design and statistics textbooks, e.g., Fleiss, 1986; Lee, 1980; Pocock, 1983), and (b) random number and random permutation generating software (now available with virtually all popular statistical software packages, such as SYSTAT, SAS, and SPSS; see Shadish et al., 2002). In contrast with the use of physical devices, both of these alternatives easily allow permanent records of the randomization actually used by researchers; for example, in the case of tables of random numbers, researchers can photocopy pages of random numbers used in the execution of their trials.

Using Tables of Random Numbers for Simple Random Assignments
Tables of random numbers list the digits 0, 1, 2, ..., 9, so that all 10 digits occur, on the average, the same number of times, and so that "there is no discernible pattern of digit values" (Pocock, 1984, p. 73). The first 43 digits in a table of random numbers provided in Pocock (1983, p. 74) are listed in row 1 of Table 9.1.

Choosing a starting point. In order to use a table of random numbers for simple random assignment of 6 treatments (A, B, C, D, E, F) to patients, a researcher would first select a starting point at random: Shadish et al. (2002) suggest that numbers should be picked "haphazardly" to identify "the page, column and row for the random start" (p. 296). Interpreting *haphazardly* to mean "randomly," suppose that the tables were located on 2 pages, with 6 rows and 6 columns per page; 1 toss of a coin (head = Page 1, tail = Page 2) and 2 tosses of a die could be used to determine the page, row, and column that would determine the random starting point. Symmetrical dice with fewer or

TABLE 9.1
Using Tabled Random Numbers to Determine Assignment of Patients to Treatments

Table entries	0	5	2	7	8	4	3	7	4	1	6	8	3	8	5	1	5	6	9	6	8	1	8	0	4	7	8	8	7	4	5	9	7	2	4	0	2	3	6	3	1	8	5
Relevant digits		5	2			4	3		4	1	6		3		5	1	5	6		6		1			4					4	5			2	4		2	3		3	1		5
Treatment		E	B			D	C		D	A	F		C		E	A	E	F		F		A			D					D	E			B	D		B	C		C	A		E

more than 6 sides are available (e.g., 4, 8, 10, 12, 20) and could also be used as needed to determine the random starting point.

Suppose that the starting point that is picked is the "0" on the left of Row 1 in Table 9.1. In order to randomly assign the treatments (in the earlier example) to incoming patients using Table 9.1, so that the probability of assignment of each treatment to each patient would be 1/6, the digits 1, 2, 3, 4, 5, and 6 might be matched with Treatments A, B, C, D, E, F, respectively, as shown in Table 9.1. Treatments would then be assigned as listed in Row 3. Thus, the 1st patient (Patient 1) would receive Treatment E, the 2nd Treatment B, . . . , and the 24th Treatment E. Assuming that only 24 patients took part in the study, the number of patients receiving each treatment would be as listed below (see Row 3 of Table 9.1):

Treatments	A	B	C	D	E	F
Number of Patients	4	3	4	5	5	3

Perfect balancing (defined as equality of ns across all treatments) would have occurred if 4 patients had been assigned to each treatment, so that in this illustration treatment groups are not exactly balanced. In general, tables of random numbers could be used to ensure that each treatment has a probability of $1/K$ of assignment to each patient, regardless of the value of K, by matching treatments with digits as illustrated earlier. With up to 10 treatments, designated 0, 1, 2, . . . , 9, single digits would be matched with treatment numbers (for $K<10$ treatments, irrelevant digits in the table would be ignored, as in the illustration); with 11 to 99 treatments, consecutive *pairs* of digits could be matched with treatment names (and irrelevant digit pairs in the table ignored), and so forth. The table of random numbers could be used, reading rows from left to right, and lines from top to bottom (as in the reading of ordinary text) until all N patients had been assigned.

Unplanned Imbalance: A Limitation of Simple Random Assignment
Unintended but large imbalance is generally considered one of the most serious limitations of simple random assignment. The predictability of serious imbalance is in fact calculable, as illustrated by Pocock (1979), who provides a table showing, for $K=2$ and $N=10, 20, 50, 100, 200, 500$, and 1000, the sizes of imbalances that would be expected to occur about 5% of the time. For example, for $N=20$ and $K=2$, imbalances at least as extreme as 6 or 14 (i.e., 6 or fewer patients, or 14 or more patients assigned to Treatment A) would be expected 11.54% of the time. Thus, it would not be very unlikely (i.e., probability = .1154) to have more than twice as many patients in one treatment as in the other.

Imbalance often results in (a) non-orthogonality and therefore collinearity of effects in factorial designs (see, e.g., Myers & Well, 1995), (b) lack of robustness of hypotheses tests (see, e.g., Maxwell & Delaney, 2004), and, most important, (c) loss of efficiency and statistical power (given that the total number of patients included in the trial is fixed) of tests of relative efficacies of the treatments (see, e.g.,

Hsu, 1993; Cohen, 1988). For example, for the preceding illustration ($N = 20$ and $K = 2$) the F test statistic ordinarily used to test the hypothesis that two treatments are equally effective is expected (with $N = 20$, $K = 2$, and a 6/14 degree of imbalance) to be only 84% the size of the corresponding F based on balanced (10/10) allocation of the 20 patients to the two treatments. When psychosocial interventions actually differ in efficacy, the loss of power associated with imbalance implies an unnecessarily large number of incorrect "dodo bird verdicts"—that is, decisions or conclusions that alternative treatments do not differ in efficacy.

1.1.2. RANDOM ASSIGNMENT FOR EXPECTED OPTIMAL IMBALANCE

The loss of statistical power caused by imbalance (unequal ns), noted earlier, refers to the relative powers of unbalanced versus balanced designs, when the total sample size N is constant across (balanced vs. unbalanced) designs. This would be relevant to a study in which a research grant allowed treatment of a fixed number of patients, irrespective of how these patients were assigned to treatments. However, when it is the total *cost* (measured in terms of dollars, researcher time, researcher effort, etc.) that is constant regardless of how patients are allocated to treatments (e.g., when a researcher has received a fixed-sized grant for a comparative efficacy study) and when the cost per patient is not constant across treatments, optimally *unbalanced* designs are generally more powerful than balanced designs (see Cochran, 1963; Nam, 1973; Hsu, 1994; McClelland, 1997). When this is the case, a random assignment method may be adopted that targets some optimal imbalance rather than perfect balance. For example, suppose that in a study concerned with the relative efficacy of two treatments, the per-patient cost of Treatment A is six times that of Treatment B. Then (assuming random sampling) the optimal imbalance (i.e., the imbalance that maximizes the probability of rejecting the dodo bird verdict if the treatments differ in efficacy) would be 71/29, that is, about three times as many patients assigned to the less expensive treatment as to the more expensive treatment (see Hsu, 1994, p. 101). A researcher might then choose to randomly assign treatments to patients (using physical devices, tables of random numbers, or software that generates random numbers—as discussed previously) so that the probability of assignment of each patient to Treatment A was 0.29 and the probability of assignment of each patient to Treatment B was 0.71. Table 9.2 (adapted from Hsu, 1994) shows the relative statistical powers of balanced versus optimally unbalanced plans for four Cohen effect sizes given that the total cost of the study allowed using 24 patients in the optimally unbalanced design. Thus, given a large difference in efficacy of two treatments ($d = .93$), the probability of correctly rejecting the dodo bird verdict (i.e., the null hypothesis) would be .776 with optimal unbalanced allocation of patients to treatments but only .706 with perfectly balanced allocation. In general, optimal randomized unbalanced allocation of patients to treatments can be expected to result in

TABLE 9.2

Statistical Powers Associated With Balanced and Optimally Unbalanced Randomized Designs When the Cost Ratio Is 6/1, and When the Total Cost of the Trial Allows Using 24 Patients in the Optimally Balanced Design

	Cohen Effect Sizes (d)			
	.68	.85	.93	1.03
Balanced design power	.480	.638	.706	.782
Optimally unbalanced design	.544	.710	.776	.846

modest increases in statistical power at no extra cost to the researcher. However, it should be noted that even optimally unbalanced randomized designs may fail to yield conventionally acceptable levels of statistical power unless the smaller of the two samples is itself quite large (see Hsu, 1993). For example, even if a very large difference in efficacy of two competing treatments is present (say, Cohen $d = 1.00$), the maximum attainable power of a t test of the dodo bird verdict (null hypothesis), assuming the researcher works at the conventional $\alpha = .01$ level, would be approximately 0.67 if the smaller treatment group was of size 10 (regardless of the size of the larger group; Hsu, 1993). A power of .67 is well below the conventionally recommended level of 0.80.

1.2. Randomly Permuted Blocks: Desired Balance or Imbalance in Actual Trials

A major limitation of random assignment methods in Section 1.2.—regardless of whether balance or optimal imbalance is targeted—is that, in any given trial, the proportions of patients actually assigned to the treatments can differ considerably from the targeted proportions. Although this problem is likely to be present only in the case of small trials, it should be noted that the typical sample sizes in studies of relative efficacies of psychosocial interventions are small (i.e., about 12 per treatment group; see Hsu, 1989, 2000; Shapiro & Shapiro, 1983). Furthermore, even with large trials, researchers may want to compare treatments in the trial's early stages, when only a small fraction of patients have completed treatment: An early answer concerning the relative efficacy of treatments could lead to an ethically desirable and cost-saving decision to terminate the trial and to administer only one treatment to all patients (see Meier, 1975). Imbalance in early stages of a large trial could prevent such a decision. Finally, certain time-related factors may affect the patients so that those who enter the trial early may be affected differently than those who enter late. Randomly permuted blocks (RPBs) were proposed specifically for the purpose of addressing problems such as these (see, e.g., Fleiss, 1990; Zelen, 1974). When all blocks are complete (i.e., no missing patients in any blocks), RPBs can be used to attain either (a) balance or (b) optimal imbalance, in *actual* studies (as opposed to balance or optimal imbalance in the long run), not just at the completion of the trial but also at various time points after the start of the trial (viz., end of each block). RPBs can also be used to parcel out possible effects of the time-related factors and to examine possible interactions of these factors with treatments.

Given that patients become available at different points in time to participate in a study of the relative efficacy of K treatments, and given that a total of nK patients are to be treated, one RPB option is to assign patients to n consecutive blocks of K. Thus the first group of K patients who seek treatment would constitute the first block, the second group of K patients would constitute the second block, and so forth. Balance is attained with this RPB by assigning one patient to each treatment within each block. Within each block patients can be assigned to treatments in K! ways (defined as $K! = (K)(K-1)(K-2) \ldots (3)(2)(1)$) assuming that one patient is to be assigned to each treatment. RPBs require selecting at random 1 from the $K!$ ways of matching patients with treatments, for each of the n blocks. For example, if $K = 3$, there would be $3! = 3.2.1 = 6$ different ways of assigning the 3 patients in the first block to the $K = 3$ treatments. Suppose the patients in each block are tagged "1," "2," and "3," to indicate their order of entry into the trial.[2] These patients could be assigned to the 3 treatments in 6 different ways, as shown in Table 9.3.

Each of the ways of assigning patients to treatments is a permutation (ordering) of patients (relative to the treatments). When there are 6 possible permutations, the decision of which permutation to use for each block could be determined by the toss of a die (matching each face of the die with one of the permutations). A table of random permutations of 3 numbers could be generated by randomly sampling (with replacement) from the "population" of permutations listed in Table 9.3.

1.2.1. USING TABLES OF RANDOM PERMUTATIONS TO CREATE RANDOMLY PERMUTED BLOCKS

Tables of random permutations of sets of numbers are available (e.g., Fleiss, 1986; Moses & Oakford, 1963; Pocock, 1983) and are generally considered

TABLE 9.3

Different Ways of Assigning 3 Patients (1, 2, 3) in Each Block to 3 Treatments (A, B, C)

Treatments	Allocations of patients					
A	1	1	2	2	3	3
B	2	3	1	3	1	2
C	3	2	3	1	2	1

preferable to physical devices (e.g., dice) for the determination of treatment assignments. Moses and Oakford (1963) provide an extensive set of random permutation tables; Fleiss (1986) includes 26 pages of random permutations of the first 100 integers. Pocock (1983) has a table of random permutations of 20 numbers $(00, 01, 02, \ldots, 19)$ in which each row represents one permutation of these numbers. The first two rows of Pocock's table are reproduced in Table 9.4.

It should be noted that there are $20! = 20 \times 19 \times 18 \times \ldots 3 \times 2 \times 1 = 2.4329 \times 10^{18}$ different permutations of 20 numbers. Thus, given a block of 20 patients to be assigned to 20 treatments (with one per treatment), there would be 2.4329×10^{18} different ways of permuting these patients relative to the treatments—that is, of matching patients with treatments. For this block to be labeled a "randomly permuted block," the permutation, used to determine treatment assignment for the 20 patients in this block, would have to be randomly drawn from this population of 2.4329×10^{18}. In practice researchers often rely on tables that list (in random order) randomly drawn permutations of 20 numbers. It might be noted that any book listing permutations of 20 numbers can, at best, include only a tiny fraction of the population of all the possible 2.4329×10^{18} permutations.

The two permutations listed in Table 9.4 (from Pocock, 1983) can be used to illustrate a wide variety of plans for randomly assigning $c \le 20$ patients (per block) to $K \le 20$ treatments so as to obtain exactly the desired numbers of patients in each treatment, for each block. Tables of random permutations of 100 numbers (available in Fleiss, 1986, and Moses and Oakford, 1963) could similarly be used for a wide variety of larger designs $(c \le 100, K \le 100)$. For even larger designs, random permutations can be obtained from interactive Internet sites (e.g., calculators.stat.ucla.edu/perm.php). Each plan can be defined in terms of a combination of ,

> K, the number of treatments,
> c, the block size,
> n, the number of blocks, and
> $n_A, n_B, \ldots$, the numbers of patients to be assigned to each treatment within each block (except for Plan 7, below), and $c = n_A + n_B + \ldots$

(Note that K, c, n, and $n_A, n_B, \ldots$ are italicized to distinguish the above from similar treatment names, (designated K, C, N). For all plans, it will be assumed that the two permutations in Table 9.4 have been drawn at random from the population of 2.4329×10^{18} possible permutations of the 20 numbers $(00, 01, \ldots, 19)$. Thus, if the table had (say) 1,000 lines, each corresponding to one random permutation of the 20 numbers, random digit software (included in SPSS, SYSTAT, SAS, etc.) could be used to generate 3 consecutive digits that would identify the first permutation (e.g., 367 would result in selection of the 367th permutation from the table).

Plan 1: Number of Treatments = Block Size = Size of Tabled Permutation (viz., 20)
Number of Blocks = 2 (i.e., $K = 20$, $c = 20$, $n = 2$, $n_A = n_B = \cdots = n_T = 1$)

TABLE 9.4
Using Two Random Permutations of the Numbers 00, 01, 02, ... , 19 to Assign $c \leq 20$ Patients in Each Block, to $K \leq 20$ Treatments (A, B, C, ...), That Will Yield Samples of Sizes (n_A, n_B, n_C ...) in Each Block

First Permutation

	11	19	15	05	09	00	06	13	07	02	16	01	12	18	04	17	10	08	03	14
Plan 1	A	B	C	D	E	F	G	H	I	J	K	L	M	N	O	P	Q	R	S	T
Plan 2				A						A	B	B							C	
Plan 3	A	A	A	A	A	A	A	A	A	A	B	B	B	B	B	B	B	B	B	B
Plan 4				A											B				B	
Plan 5 (& 7)				A			A					A			A			B	B	A
Plan 7	A				B		B	A	B	A	A	A						B	B	A

Second Permutation

	14	12	00	01	19	08	07	17	11	18	02	15	05	09	04	16	10	06	13	03
Plan 1	A	B	C	D	E	F	G	H	I	J	K	L	M	N	O	P	Q	R	S	T
Plan 2													A		B	B				C
Plan 5 (& 7)		A		B		B							A		B					B
Plan 6			A	B	C	D	E	F	G	H	I	J	K	L	M	N	O	P	Q	R

Note: Adapted from Pocock, 1983, Table 5.4.

Consider that 40 patients are to take part in a trial designed to determine the relative efficacy of 20 treatments. The 40 patients are divided into $n = 2$ blocks of 20 (Block 1 consisting of the first 20 patients, and Block 2 the last 20 patients, to enter the trial), and one patient in each block will receive each treatment. With $K = 20$ treatments, labeled A, B, C, . . . , T (and listed in this order in the Plan 1 rows of Table 9.4), and blocks of size $c = 20$, and equal distribution of patients over treatments ($n_A = n_B = \ldots = n_T = 1$), each of the 2 permutations listed in Table 9.4 can be used to determine assignment of patients to treatments in a block, as illustrated in the rows labeled Plan 1 of Table 9.4. Thus Patient "11" in Block 1 would receive Treatment A, Patient "19" in Block 1 would receive Treatment B, and so forth; Patient "14" in Block 2 would receive Treatment A, Patient "12" would receive Treatment B, and so forth. If the patient "names" reflect the order in which they entered the trial within each block, then the 11th patient in Block 1 and the 14th patient in Block 2 would receive Treatment A, the 19th patient in Block 1 and the 12th in Block 2 would receive Treatment B, and so forth.

Plan 2: Number of Treatments = Block Size < Size of Tabled Permutation
($K = 3$, $c = 3$, $n = 2$, $n_A = n_B = n_C = 1$)
The principal difference between Plans 1 and 2 is that in Plan 2 the number of patients is smaller than 20, the size of the random permutations in Table 9.4. Use of the random permutations in Table 9.4 to determine treatment assignments for Plan 2 is justified because the expected relative frequency of any permutation of a subset of numbers (e.g., 01, 02, 03 written as 1, 2, 3, when leaving out the leading 0 digits) drawn from a larger set (e.g., 20 numbers) will not be affected by inclusion of the other numbers (e.g., the other 17 numbers) in the random permutations of the entire set of numbers. Thus, for example, the permutation (2, 1, 3), which would be expected to occur one sixth of the time (Table 9.3) in a table of random permutations of the integers 1, 2, 3, is also expected to occur one sixth of the time in a table of random permutations of the 20 numbers 00, 01, . . . , 19. Therefore, in general, a table of random permutations of 20 numbers can be used with blocks of size $c \le 20$, in order to obtain a random assignment of N patients that would result in any desired distribution of patients over treatments—that is, any desired values of n_A, n_B, n_C, . . . per block. In Plan 2, three patients (1, 2, 3) in each of 2 blocks are to be assigned to 3 treatments (A, B, C), with 1 patient per treatment per block. The random assignment of patients to treatments within blocks can be carried out by using the 1st permutation to determine treatment assignment of patients in Block 1, and the 2nd permutation to determine treatment assignments for patients in Block 2. First let the digit pairs 01, 02, and 03 identify corresponding patients (1, 2, 3). Then enter the treatment names (in alphabetical order) under these digit pairs: In Block 1, Patient 2 (the 2nd to enter the trial in Block 1) would receive Treatment A, Patient 1 would receive Treatment B, and Patient 3 would receive Treatment C. For Block 2, Patient 1 would receive Treatment A, Patient 2 would receive Treatment

B, and Patient 3 would receive Treatment C. Note that the 2 permutations from Pocock's table result in the permutations listed in Columns 3 (for Block 1) and 1 (for Block 2), respectively, of Table 9.3.

Plan 3: Two-Group Parallel RCT With Balancing ($K = 2$, $c = 20$, $n = 1$, $n_A = n_B = 10$)

Plans 1 and 2 involved assignment of only one patient to each treatment within each of two blocks. A more popular design involves (a) no partitioning of patients into blocks (or, equivalently, the use of a single block), (b) balancing, and (c) random assignment of more than 1 patient to each of two treatments. This design is often described as a balanced two-group parallel RCT: For example, consider that $K = 2$ (i.e., the number of treatments is 2) and that these treatments are called Treatment A and Treatment B, $c = 20$ (i.e., the block size is 20), and that $n_A = 10$ and $n_B = 10$ (i.e., 10 patients are assigned to each treatment). The Plan 3 row of Table 9.4 shows how patients could be assigned to treatments given the first random permutation selected from Pocock (1983): The name of each treatment would first be listed, as often as this treatment is to be administered, and the listing of treatment names could be in an alphabetical (or any other systematic) order: The Plan 3 row indicates that Patients 11, 19, . . . , 2 would receive Treatment A, and Patients 16, 1, . . . , 14 would receive Treatment B.

Plan 4: Two-Group Parallel RCT With Unequal Allocation of Patients to Treatments ($K = 2$, $c = 5$, $n = 1$, $n_A = 2$, $n_B = 3$)

Given a total of 5 patients, 2 of whom are to be assigned to Treatment A and 3 to Treatment B, random assignment would require equiprobability of all possible ways of assigning these patients so that $n_A = 2$ and $n_B = 3$. As in Plan 2, a randomly selected permutation of 20 numbers can be used to achieve this goal of Plan 4, by ignoring irrelevant digits: Match names of patients with paired digits in the first permutation listed in Table 9.4 and then list the treatments to which patients are to be assigned in alphabetical order (2 As and 3 Bs) as shown in the first permutation Plan 4 row of Table 9.4: Patients 5 and 2 would receive Treatment A, and Patients 1, 4, and 3 would receive Treatment B.

Plan 5: Two Blocks of $c = 6$, With Balancing in Each Block: $n_A = n_B = 3$

The general method of using tables of randomly permuted blocks that can be inferred from Plans 1 through 4 involves: (a) assigning one digit pair (from the permutations) to each patient "name" (ignoring digit pairs that have not been matched with patient names), (b) listing names of treatments (A, B, C . . .) in (say) alphabetical order under digit pairs that correspond to the patient names, where each treatment name is repeated as often as the treatment will be administered, and (c) determining treatment assignments by matching digit pairs (patient names) with treatment names. Using this method, with $K = 2$, $n_A = n_B = 3$, and the 1st and 2nd permutations in Table 9.4, results in Patients 5, 6, and 2 receiving Treatment A, and Patients 1, 4, and 3 receiving Treatment B in Block 1;

and Patients 1, 2, and 5 receiving Treatment A and Patients 4, 6, and 3 receiving Treatment B in Block 2.

1.2.2. CHOOSING BLOCK SIZES

The choice of block size (c) and number of blocks (n), given that $N = (c)(n)$ patients are included in a study, is not only important in (a) the control of imbalance, but also in (b) the determination of the efficiency and statistical power of the test of relative efficacy of treatments (see Myers, 1979, chap. 6) and (c) the control of the selection bias that may occur because of predictability (by the researcher) of treatment assignment to patients within blocks (see below). Concerning (b), the main factor that determines the optimal ratio of block size to number of blocks (when the blocking is based on the time or order of entry of patients in the trial) is the correlation of the response measure with the time (or order) of enrollment of patients in the trial (see Fleiss, 1986, p. 124; see also Myers, 1979, pp. 156–160). As noted by Fleiss (1986), this correlation may be high with diseases or disorders that vary systematically with the seasons of the year (e.g., asthma, psoriasis, depression).

1.2.3. CONTROLLING SELECTION BIAS IN RANDOMLY PERMUTED BLOCKS

Selection bias may occur, with randomly permuted blocks, when the researcher knows or can predict the order of administration of treatments within blocks. For example, suppose that a researcher must make a decision, as each patient enters the trial, about the patient's qualification for inclusion in the trial, and suppose that he or she knows that for a 6-patient block the 2nd, 5th, and 6th patients are to receive Treatment A, and that the 1st, 3rd, and 4th are to receive Treatment B. It is possible that this knowledge could (unconsciously) influence the researcher's decision about the eligibility of each entering patient, and that this might lead to nonequivalence of treatment groups on prognostic variables (see Hodges & Lehmann, 1970). Even if he or she does not know the exact match between order of entry and treatments, knowledge of what treatments had already been administered to some patients in the block would provide some information about likely treatment for later patients in that block. He or she could predict (better than chance) from knowledge of treatments received by the first X patients in a block what treatment would be assigned to the $(X + 1)$th patient: For the preceding example, knowing that $n_A = n_B$ and that of the first 5 patients, 2 received Treatment A and 3 received Treatment B, the researcher could infer that the 6th patient would receive Treatment A. Clearly, selection bias will be more of a problem with small than with large blocks, and in fact Lachin et al. (1988) recommend that "small block sizes, especially of size 2, should be avoided in favor of larger block sizes" (p. 372). However Lachin et al. (1988) note that this type of selection bias can be eliminated entirely (regardless of block size) by randomizing patients in a block as each block is filled rather than as patients arrive. Thus, in the preceding example the researcher would (for the first block) identify, as patients arrive, the first 6 eligible patients, and only then carry out the randomization.

Plan 6: Factorial Designs

Factorial designs involving multiple between-subject factors (e.g., race, gender of therapist, and interventions) can easily be handled by considering combinations of levels of the factors to be "treatments." For example, suppose that the factors are Gender (2 levels) and Race (say, 3 levels) and Psychosocial Interventions (say, 3 levels). There would be $(2)(3)(3) = 18$ combinations of levels of these three factors. Thus, for purposes of using the random assignment methods described earlier, let the 18 combinations be called A, B, C, . . . , R. Then if it is desired to have a completely balanced design with 1 patient per combination (per "treatment"), the assignment of patients would be as shown in the Plan 6 row of Table 9.4 (when using the 2nd random permutation). Patients could similarly be assigned to combinations of levels of two or more within-subject factors (see, e.g., Greenhouse and Meyer, 1991).

Plan 7: Single and N Subject Designs With Multiple Treatments per Subject

Edgington (1987) notes that random assignment in single-subject designs involves "random assignment of treatment times to treatments. For example, with 10 successive days on which treatments are to be administered to a subject, the 10 days may be randomly divided into two sets of 5 days each, with one set the days to receive one treatment [A] and the other set the days for the other treatment [B]" (p. 439). Matching days (1st , 2nd, . . . , 10th) with pairs of digits 01, 02, . . . , 10, in the 1st permutation of Table 9.4 results in the assignment shown in the Plan 7 row of the table. More generally, with N subjects, each exposed to n_A days of Treatment A, n_B days of Treatment B, and so forth, each subject can be viewed as a "block," and n randomly selected permutations, drawn from a table of random permutations, could be used to determine days on which each patient would receive each treatment. For example, for $n = 2$, $n_A = 3$, and $n_B = 3$, the Plan 5 (and 7) permutations in Table 9.4 imply that the first subject (see Permutation 1) would receive Treatment A on Days 5, 6, and 2 and Treatment B on Days 1, 4, and 3, and that the second subject (see Permutation 2) would receive Treatment A on Days 1, 2, and 5 and Treatment B on Days 4, 6, and 3.

■ Section 2. Randomization Methods Designed to Control Effects of Prognostic Factors: Randomly Permuted Blocks Within Strata

A *prognostic factor* can be defined as a variable (other than the treatments that are of interest to the researcher) that is related (often causally) to the outcome measure of interest to the researcher. Prognostic factors in medical and behavioral research can often be viewed as "risk factors." One of these factors that requires attention in most treatment efficacy studies is the initial severity of the patient at the start of the treatment; another is the presence or absence of problems (psychological or medical) other than the one for which the patient is seeking treatment. Serious threats to the validity of causal inferences drawn from comparative efficacy studies can occur when treatment groups are nonequivalent on important prognostic factors, especially if this nonequivalence is not recognized or if no attempt is made to take it into account in the data analysis (e.g., using analysis of covariance or multiple regression models). A limitation of all random assignment methods discussed earlier in this chapter is the possibility (in spite of random assignment) of serious nonequivalence of treatment groups on important prognostic factors. Even though a random assignment method can result in complete balance (equality of numbers of patients assigned to different treatments), this balance should not be equated with equivalence of treatment groups on prognostic factors (e.g., equality of means of prognostic factors across treatment groups—see Hsu, 1989). Permuted blocks within strata represent one (experimental design) way of preventing serious nonequivalence of treatment groups.

2.1. Stratification on a Single Prognostic Factor

Prognostic factors can be categorical, ordinal, interval, or ratio-scaled variables. A single level of a prognostic factor or, in the case of metric factors, a narrow range of values of the prognostic factor is often called a *stratum* of this prognostic factor (see, e.g., Pocock, 1979). Patients who belong to this stratum are homogeneous (or relatively homogeneous) with respect to this factor, whereas patients in different strata are heterogeneous across strata. When a single prognostic factor has been identified in a comparative efficacy study, patients can be stratified (classified into strata defined in terms of this factor) prior to the start of the study (prestratification). Then randomly permuted blocks can be generated within strata. Thus the random assignment of patients to treatments is carried out as described in Section 1.2., but it is done one stratum at a time. Poststratification (in which stratification is carried out posttreatment) can also yield statistically analyzable data as long as "it can be assumed that the covariate values are statistically independent of the treatment assignment" (Lachin et al., 1988, p. 369). However, as noted by Lachin et al. (1988), "this is a strong but untestable assumption" (p. 369). Another limitation of poststratification is lack of control for imbalance.

The stratification on the prognostic factor prior to the use of randomly permuted blocks (prestratification) (a) reduces nonequivalence of treatment groups on the prognostic factor, (b) increases efficiency by balancing and by allowing the separation of variability attributable to the prognostic factor from the error variance, (c) allows examination of possible interactions of this factor with treatments, and (d) permits assessment of relative efficacy of the treatments within levels of the prognostic factor. However Lachin et al. (1988) warn that "stratification [on prognostic covariates] is principally advantageous for a small trial and has negligible advantages in terms of power or efficiency in a large trial (say $N > 100$)" (p. 368).

2.2. Stratification Involving Multiple Prognostic Factors

When several prognostic factors are considered important, strata can be defined in terms of combinations of levels of these factors. For example, with two dichotomous prognostic factors there would be $2 \times 2 = 4$ strata. More generally, the maximum number of possible strata will be the product of the numbers of levels of the prognostic factors, a product that can easily be very large. To reduce the number of strata, similar levels of some prognostic factor may be combined, or prognostic variables with many levels may even be dichotomized (e.g., age can be rescaled to yield 10-year intervals, or dichotomized: e.g., over 30 years old, less than 30 years old). Then, before the trial begins, "a separate restricted randomization list is prepared for each of the patient strata . . . random permuted blocks being the usual approach" (Pocock, 1983, p. 82). The main problem with this method is that even with a small number of prognostic variables, the number of strata and strata-block combinations can easily become undesirably large. With many strata-block combinations an uneven distribution of patients over strata-block combinations, and very small or zero values of n for some strata are to be expected even when N is large. If interest is limited to the relative efficacy of treatments within specific strata (combinations of levels of prognostic factors) that have adequate numbers of patients, this may not be a problem. But if the researcher is interested in (a) disentangling effects of prognostic factors or (b) addressing questions about interactions involving prognostic, block, and/or treatment factors, the imbalance across strata may result in non-orthogonality and collinearity problems associated with the specific hypotheses that are of interest, and to both data analysis and interpretation problems. Most important, perhaps, is the fact that prognostic factors that are highly collinear with treatments may mask real treatment effects. Lachin et al. (1988) note that stratification on many covariates "remains controversial" (p. 368). Meier (1975) recommends "analysis based on some stratification on really major variables, but primary reliance on randomization" (p. 521). He notes that "insistence on stratification for every conceivable combination of baseline variables is not required by the canons of good science, nor is it generally effective in improving precision or clarifying our understanding" (p. 522). It is important to keep in mind that the extent to which problems are present with stratification on multiple covariates cannot be addressed independently of the hypotheses that are of interest to the researcher: The same experimental design might be perfectly acceptable to test one set of hypotheses and totally unacceptable to test another.

2.3 Stratification Involving Estimated Risks

Lee (1980) notes that "in order to reduce the effects of prognostic heterogeneity, the original cohort can be divided into subgroups, or strata, of members who are similar in prognostic expectation" (p. 403). As noted by Kalish and Begg (1985), this can be accomplished not only by defining strata in terms of combinations of levels of prognostic factors but also by stratifying on the basis of estimated risks, where the risks can be estimated from regression models applied to data of previous trials (see also Simon, 1979; Miettinen, 1976). The risk estimates would then constitute a single "prognostic factor," and random permuted blocks could then be used for assignment of patients to treatments within risk factor strata (as in Section 2.1.). This appears to be a promising, albeit seldom used, method of addressing some of the most serious problems described in Section 2.2.

■ **Section 3. Is Random Assignment Preceded by Random Sampling? Implications for Data Analysis and Interpretation**

The random assignment of N participants included in a comparative efficacy study refers to a method that involves random allocation of *all* of the the N patients to K treatments. This sample may (a) have been drawn at random from a much larger population of patients, or (b) not have been randomly sampled from such a population. In RCTs some form of random assignment is carried out (see Sections I and II) with both (a) and (b), but (a) involves *random sampling* prior to random assignment, whereas (b) simply involves random assignment of patients from what is often called a "sample of convenience" (Kazdin, 2003, p. 153). Because (a) and (b) have very important implications for the choice of significance or hypotheses tests and, more importantly, for the interpretation of results of these tests, it would be desirable to explicitly distinguish between these two type of RCTs, perhaps *random sampling RCTs* (RS-RCTs) and *sample of convenience RCTs* (SoC-RCTs). Ludbrook and Dudley (1998) recently provided information about the frequency of use of RS-RCTs and SoC-RCTs in medical research. In "a survey of 252 prospective, comparative studies reported in five, frequently cited biomedical journals . . . [they found that] experimental groups were constructed by randomization [without random sampling] in 96% of cases and by random sampling in only 4%" (p. 127). Lunneborg (2000) suggested that similar findings could be expected in psychological research.

With RS-RCTs, parametric (normal theory) statistical models can be used to obtain point and interval estimates of the population parameters, and to test hypotheses about these population parameters (e.g., population means and differences between population means), because the underlying assumption of random sampling, under which the parametric tests were derived, are met by the random sampling carried out as part of the experimental design. Thus the parametric statistical models allow generalizability of conclusions, in the sense that they allow inferences about parameters of populations from which the samples were randomly drawn (see Dallal, 1998; Lunneborg, 2000, 2001).

With SoC-RCTs, on the other hand, the experimental design does *not* satisfy the random sampling assumption of parametric tests. However, the randomization (random assignment) of the patients, which was part of the experimental design, meets the assumption of nonparametric tests, including permutation tests and randomization tests, and applications of these tests justify statistical inferences concerning relative efficacy of treatments *for the N patients included in the study* (Dallal, 1998). Lunneborg (2001) refers to the N patients in the sample of convenience as a "local population" (p. 402), in contrast to the populations associated with RS-RCTs, which he calls "global populations" (Lunneborg, 2000, p. 16); a similar distinction appears in Maxwell and Delaney (2004). With SoC-RCTs, nonparametric permutation tests permit statistical inferences about the local populations. However, permutation tests do *not* justify *statistical inferences* about any larger (global) population of patients (see Hsu, 2007).

In cases involving sufficiently large Ns, the null distributions of the nonparametric test statistics (including permutation test statistics) can often be well approximated by distributions of parametric test statistics (Box, Hunter, & Hunter, 1978; Maxwell & Delaney, 2004) so that in these cases parametric tests can legitimately be applied to data of randomized designs that involve only randomization and not random sampling. However, *when a parametric test provides a p value that is close to that of a permutation test, this correspondence of p values does not imply justifiability of inferences about efficacy of treatments beyond the N patients included in the study.*[3] As noted by Lunneborg (2001), "Using a t test [an example of a normal theory parametric test] for the statistical analysis does not provide justification for extending those statistical inferences to the response distribution for any larger population [than the local population consisting of patients included in the study]" (p. 411). Thus, as noted by Maxwell and Delaney (2004), "The generalization to a real population or to people in general that is likely of interest [must then be] made on *non-statistical* grounds [italics added]" (p. 50).

Furthermore, Lunneborg (2000) draws attention to the fact that

> the typical analysis of variance [a parametric test] yields more than P-values. Students, by their texts, and researchers, by their editorial reviewers, are encouraged to report not only estimates of contrasts among means but estimates, as well, of the standard errors (S.E.s) for these estimates and of confidence intervals (C.I.s) for the contrasts. The conventional estimates of S.E.s and C.I.s, those taught by our experimental design texts and incorporated into population statistical computing packages, assume random sampling from very large populations with response distributions that are homoscedastic and normal. The robustness of the P-value, however, does not carry over to these accuracy assessments. *The large population estimates of*

S.E.s and C.I.s are not appropriate to the randomized available case design [italics added]. (p. 17)

For small samples, parametric test distributions may not satisfactorily approximate exact distributions of the relevant nonparametric test statistics (see Edgington, 1995; Lunneborg, 2000, 2001, Ludbrook & Dudley, 1998; Reichardt & Gollob, 1999), in which case parametric tests are not an option for the analysis of SoC-RCT data. Ludbrook and Dudley (1998) provide information about software programs that are currently available for some of the most popular nonparametric tests used in RCTs. These programs include RANDIBM (from Edginton, 1995), R.T 2.1 (from Manly, 1997), and STATXACT (from Cytel Software Corp., 1995, Cambridge, MA). Maxwell and Delaney (2004) also note that "sets of command that allow one to carry out [randomization tests with SPSS and SAS] have been published for both of these packages (Chen & Dunlap, 1993; Hayes, 1998)" (p. 46). Lunneborg (2000, 2001) describes how Efron's nonparametric bootstrap may be used to analyze data collected in SoC-RCTs.

The APA Presidential Task Force on Evidence-Based Practice (Levant, 2005) described RCTs as the "standard for drawing causal inferences about the effects of interventions" (p. 186) and emphasized the need to establish the "*generalizability* and transportability of interventions shown to be efficacious in controlled research settings [italics added]" (p. 187). Relevant to this goal is the recommendation of Wilkinson and the APA Task Force on Statistical Inference (1999) that confidence intervals, and not just results of hypothesis tests, should be reported: "Interval estimates should be given . . . Confidence intervals are usually available in statistical software; otherwise, confidence intervals for basic statistics can be computed from typical output . . . Collecting intervals [i.e., confidence intervals] across studies also helps in constructing plausible regions for population parameters" (p. 599). Three caveats concerning these recommendations of the two APA task forces should be noted: (a) The vast majority of RCTs concerned with the efficacy of interventions are undoubtedly SoC-RCTs and *not* RS-RCTs, (b) statistical inferences that are justified with SoC-RCTs are limited to the "local population" consisting of a sample of convenience used in the trial, regardless of whether the data are legitimately analyzed with nonparametric permutation tests or with parametric (normal-theory) tests, and (c) when parametric tests are applied to data of RoC-RCTs (which is undoubtedly the rule rather than the exception—see, e.g., Ludbrook & Dudley, 1998), neither the reported standard errors nor the confidence intervals are interpretable.

The APA Task Force on Statistical Inference (Wilkinson et al., 1999) agrees with the APA Presidential Task Force on Evidence-Based Practice (Levant et al., 2005) about the value of random assignment: "Random assignment . . . allows for the strongest possible causal inferences free of extraneous assumptions" (Wilkinson et al., 1999, p. 595). But it is essential to recognize, in relation to inferences about the generalizability of findings of RCTs, that in the RCTs that are typically used to evaluate psychosocial interventions—namely, SoC-RCTs rather than RS-RCTs—the statistical inferences that support causal inferences are valid *only* for the sample of convenience used in the RCT, regardless of whether the preferable non-parametric permutation tests or the less preferable parametric models were used in the data analysis (see Dallal, 1998; Edgington, 1973, 1995; Lunneborg, 2000, 2001). This point is particularly important given the fact that (as noted earlier) samples used in comparative treatment efficacy studies are typically very small.

Notes

1. Several terms and phrases related to randomized designs are, unfortunately, defined in different ways in the different sources cited in this chapter. When these terms are used in this chapter, sources that define them in the same way as in this chapter will be noted.

2. Since patients tend to enter clinical trials sequentially, they are often "named" with integers that reflect the order in which they entered the trial; "blocking" on time of entry into the trial (unlike blocking on other factors) and generating randomly permuted blocks allow balancing of the trial at various points in time prior to the planned end of the trial.

3. This is not to say that inferences about global populations should not be drawn, but that "if the sample was not a random sample from some larger population, then generalizing beyond the trial is a matter of non-statistical judgement" (Dallal, 1998, p. 1). Lunneborg (2000), drawing attention to the work of Welsh (1938), points out that although it is not possible to draw statistical inferences about global populations in the case of SoC-RCTs, it may be possible to draw important "scientific inferences" (p. 13) from these trials: "The researcher may know enough about the science driving the research to argue successfully that the response difference caused by the differential treatment of these particular cases, e.g., water-deprived-mice in a San Francisco laboratory, hypertensive patients from a Cleveland clinic, English-speaking sophomores enrolled in a first course in psychology at a Minnesota college, could be reproduced among similar cases, in other places at other times, given the same treatments. That is, scientific inference about the generalizability of the results may be feasible where statistical generalizability is not" (p. 14). It is therefore clearly important in making these scientific (but nonstatistical) inferences that "extensive tabulations of baseline patient characteristics should be performed, both marginally and jointly, so as to provide a complete description of the [local] 'population' of patients studied" (Lachin et al., 1988, p. 369).

■ References

Box, G. E. P., Hunter, W. G., & Hunter, J. S. (1978). *Statistics for experimenters: An introduction to design, data analysis and model building.* New York: Wiley.

Chen, R. S., & Dunlap, W. P. (1993). SAS procedures for approximate randomization tests. *Behavior Research Methods, Instruments, and Computers, 25,* 406–409.

Cochran, W. G. (1963). *Sampling techniques.* New York, NY: Wiley.

Cohen, J. (1988). *Statistical power analysis for the behavioral sciences* (2nd ed.). Hillsdale, NJ: Erlbaum.

Dallal, G. (1998). *Random samples/randomization.* Retrieved from http://www.tufts.edu.gdallal/rand.htm

Edgington, E. S. (1973). The random-sampling assumption in "comment on component-randomization tests." *Psychological Bulletin, 80,* 84–85.

Edgington, E. S. (1987). Randomized single-subject experiments and statistical tests. *Journal of Counseling Psychology, 34,* 437–442.

Edgington, E. S. (1995). *Randomization tests* (3rd ed.). New York: Marcel Dekker.

Fleiss, J. L. (1986). *The design and analysis of clinical experiments.* New York: Wiley.

Greenhouse, J. B., & Meyer, M. M. (1991). A note on randomization and selection bias in maintenance therapy clinical trials. *Psychopharmacology Bulletin, 27,* 225–229.

Hayes, A. F. (1998). SPSS procedures for approximate randomization tests. *Behavioral Research Methods, Instruments, and Computers, 30,* 536–543.

Hodges, J. L., & Lehmann, E. L. (1970). *Basic concepts of probability and statistics* (2nd ed.). San Francisco: Holden-Day.

Hsu, L. M. (1989). Random sampling, randomization, and equivalence of contrasted groups in psychotherapy outcome research. *Journal of Consulting and Clinical Psychology, 57,* 131–137.

Hsu, L. M. (1993). Using Cohen's tables to determine the maximum power attainable in two- sample tests when one sample is limited in size. *Journal of Applied Psychology, 78,* 303–305.

Hsu, L. M. (1994). Unbalanced designs to maximize statistical power in psychotherapy efficacy studies. *Psychotherapy Research, 4,* 95–106.

Hsu, L. M. (2000). Effects of directionality of significance tests on the bias of accessible effect sizes. *Psychological Methods, 5,* 333–342.

Hsu, L. M. (2007). Fisher Exact Probability Test. In *Encyclopedia of measurement and statistics* (Vol. 1, pp. 354–359). Thousand Oaks, CA: Sage Publications.

Kalish, L. A., & Begg, C. B. (1985). Treatment allocation methods in clinical trials: A review. *Statistics in Medicine, 4,* 129–144.

Kazdin, A. E. (2003). *Research design in clinical psychology* (4th ed.). Boston: Allyn & Bacon.

Lachin, J. M., Matts, J. P., & Wei, L. J. (1988) . Randomization in clinical trials: Conclusions and recommendations. *Statistics in Medicine, 9,* 365–374.

Lee, E. T. (1980). *Statistical methods for survival analysis.* Belmont, CA: Lifetime Learning Publications.

Levant, R. F. (2005). *Report of the 2005 Presidential Task Force on Evidence-Based Practice.* Retrieved from http://www.apa.org/practice/ebpreport.pdf

Ludbrook, J., & Dudley, H. (1998). Why permutation tests are superior to t and F tests in biomedical research. *American Statistician, 52,* 127–132.

Lunneborg, C. E. (2000). *Random assignment of available cases: Let the inferences fit the design.* Retrieved from http://faculty.washington.edu/lunnebor/ Australia/randomiz.pdf

Lunneborg, C. E. (2001). Random assignment of available cases: Bootstrap standard errors and confidence intervals. *Psychological Methods, 6,* 402–412.

Maxwell, S. E., & Delaney, H. D. (2004). *Designing experiments and analyzing data* (2nd ed.). Mahwah, NJ: Erlbaum.

McClelland, G. H. (1997). Optimal design in psychological research. *Psychological Methods, 2,* 3–19.

Manly, B. F. J. (1997). Randomization, bootstrap and Monte Carlo methods in biology (2nd ed.). London: Chapman & Hall.

Meier, P. (1975). Statistics and medical experimentation. *Biometrics, 31,* 511–529.

Miettinen, O. S. (1976). Stratification by multivariate confounder score. *American Journal of Epidemiology, 104,* 609–620.

Moses, L. E., & Oakford, R. V. (1963). *Tables of random permutations.* Stanford, CA: Stanford University Press.

Myers, J. L. (1979). *Fundamentals of experimental design* (3rd ed.). Boston, MA: Allyn & Bacon.

Myers, J. L., & Well, A. D. (1995). *Research design and statistical analysis.* Hillsdale, NJ: Lawrence Erlbaum Associates.

Nam, J. M. (1973). Optimum sample sizes for the comparison of the control and treatment. *Biometrics, 29,* 101–108.

Pocock, S. J. (1979). Allocation of patients to treatment in clinical trials. *Biometrics, 35,* 183–197.

Pocock, S. J. (1983). *Clinical trials: A practical approach.* Chichester, England: Wiley.

Reichardt, C. S., & Gollob, H. F. (1999). Justifying the use and increasing the power of a t test for a randomized experiment with a convenience sample. *Psychological Methods, 4,* 117–128.

Shadish, W. R., Cook, T. D., & Campbell, D. T. (2002). *Experimental and quasi-experimental designs for generalized causal inference.* New York: Houghton Mifflin.

Shapiro, D. A., & Shapiro, D. (1983). Comparative therapy outcome research: Methodological implications of meta-analysis. *Journal of Consulting and Clinical Psychology, 51,* 42–53.

Simon, R. (1979). Restricted randomization designs in clinical trials. *Biometrics, 35,* 503–512.

Welsh, B. L. (1938). On the z-test in randomized blocks and Latin squares. *Biometrika, 29,* 21–52.

Wilkinson, L., and the Task Force on Statistical Inference. (1999). Statistical methods in psychology journals. *American Psychologist, 54,* 594–604.

Zelen, M. (1974). The randomization and stratification of patients to clinical trials. *Journal of Chronic Diseases, 27,* 365–375.

10. RESEARCH DESIGNS

Matthew K. Nock, Irene Belle Janis, and Michelle M. Wedig

This chapter reviews the primary questions addressed in treatment outcome research and the various randomized controlled trial (RCT) designs most appropriate to evaluate each question. We begin by describing the importance of RCTs to research on psychosocial interventions. We then review the primary questions for outcome research and discuss the RCT design options most appropriate to address each specific question. Examples of prior studies that have used each research design are described throughout the chapter to illustrate each design and to direct the interested reader toward relevant literature in each area. We conclude with practical recommendations for clinical scientists conducting research using RCTs.

■ The Importance of RCTs for Outcome Research

At the most basic level, clinical scientists are interested in demonstrating *correlations* among variables. Most often, it also is of interest to gain a deeper understanding of the nature of such relations, such as the direction or dependence of observed relations. For instance, if it can be shown that Variable A not only is associated with Variable B but also is temporally prior, then A is considered a *predictor* of, or *risk factor* for, B (see Kraemer et al., 1997; Kraemer, Stice, Kazdin, Offord, & Kupfer, 2001). Knowledge of risk factors is vital for understanding the development of psychopathology and for planning and guiding psychosocial interventions. It is notable, however, that not all risk factors are malleable (e.g., sex, ethnicity), and changing risk factors does not always change the outcome of interest. For instance, advanced parental age (Byrne, Agerbo, Ewald, Eaton, & Mortensen, 2003), urbanization (Sundquist, Frank, & Sundquist, 2004), and migration (Cantor-Graae, Zolkowska, & McNeil, 2005) are all risk factors for the development of schizophrenia. However, modifying these factors on a large scale (e.g., moving people out of the cities and restricting childbirth and migration) is not practical and may not alter schizophrenia risk. This distinction is well captured in the popular phrase "Correlation does not equal causation."

So what *does* equal causation? The requirements for demonstrating causality have been variously proposed by numerous scientists (Haynes, 1992; Hill, 1965; Hume, 1739; Kenny, 1979; Schlesselman, 1982; Shadish, Cook, & Campbell,

2001). Although the criteria suggested differ slightly across authors, there is a strong consensus among scientists that the use of a true experiment is necessary to provide convincing evidence of a causal relation between variables. In a true experiment, participants are randomly assigned (see chapter 9) either to an experimental condition in which they receive the manipulation or treatment or to some comparison condition in which they receive something else (what this is may vary and will be discussed in detail later) in order to rule out or "control for" potential sources of bias that may influence the dependent variable. A strong case for causality is made if participants in the different conditions are shown to be equivalent on all variables that may influence the dependent variables *except* exposure to the manipulation, and if introduction of the manipulation leads to large and immediate change in the dependent variables.

The inclusion of a comparison or control group is vital for ruling out alternative explanations for the observed results. For instance, if we administer treatment to only one group and observe change in that group, it is possible that the treatment caused any observed change, but it also is possible that factors such as historical events, maturation, repeated testing, and regression to the mean are the cause of the change (see Kazdin, 2003; Shadish et al., 2001). Randomization and the inclusion of a comparison condition allow the researcher to convincingly rule out such threats; both groups should experience the same level of change due to each of these factors, so any difference between groups can be attributed to the experimental manipulation. Although all RCTs include randomization and at least one comparison condition, variations on RCT design features provide opportunities to test a wide range of questions about psychosocial interventions.

Single-Case Research Designs

Before discussing between-group RCTs in greater detail, which is the primary focus of this chapter, it is important to acknowledge the usefulness of single-case research designs (SCRDs) and how they can complement RCTs in the evaluation of psychosocial intervention research. In SCRDs, a single individual (or more typically a series of individuals) alternates between *both* treatment and comparison conditions over time. Outcomes are assessed continuously (e.g., hourly, daily), and data are inspected to determine if behavior during the treatment condition differs from behavior during the comparison condition. To the extent to which all variables are held constant across conditions except for the administration and removal of treatment, observed behavior changes can be attributed to the treatment. As such, various SCRDs can demonstrate causal relations among treatment and outcome and represent a flexible and efficient method of testing the efficacy of an intervention. Notably, randomization may be used in SCRDs to assign a participant to an intervention condition or to determine the point in time at which a condition change occurs (Lall & Levin,

2004). Thus, randomization procedures have a place not only in between-group research designs but also in SCRDs.

Perhaps the greatest limitation of SCRDs, however, is in the restricted ability to generalize beyond the individuals studied. Given this limitation, and given the development of more sophisticated methodological and statistical procedures for evaluating clinical change over the past several decades, the majority of intervention research currently conducted uses between-group research designs to examine treatment efficacy and effectiveness. As such, the role of SCRDs has been largely diminished, and such designs are used most often to examine novel treatment approaches (e.g., Nock, 2002) and to provide preliminary tests of an intervention before conducting a larger between-group comparison (e.g., Moras, Telfer, & Barlow, 1993). The use of SCRDs before conducting a larger between-group test of a new intervention or even a smaller pilot study of the intervention is highly recommended. Indeed, SCRDs are efficient and flexible and allow one to test causal relations while making and testing modifications to the treatment and assessment procedures. Readers interested in learning more about SCRDs should consult sources covering these designs in greater detail (see Barlow & Hersen, 1984; Barlow, Nock, & Hersen, in press; Kazdin, 1982; Nock, Michel, & Photos, in press); the following sections focus on the use of different between-group research designs.

■ Questions Guiding Outcome Research and Recommended Designs

The primary goals of research on psychosocial interventions can be conceptualized as (a) demonstrating that interventions cause positive outcomes, (b) identifying the factors that influence treatment effects (i.e., moderators of change), and (c) identifying and understanding the processes through which clinical change occurs (i.e., mechanisms of change). There is a natural progression among these three goals. When a new treatment is developed, researchers and clinicians are first interested in learning whether or not it works, and subsequently *for whom* or under what conditions it works best, and ultimately *how* it works. To date, most uses of RCTs of psychosocial interventions have aimed at testing the efficacy of different treatment packages, and such studies have resulted in the creation of lists of evidence-based treatments (Chambless & Hollon, 1998; Kazdin & Weisz, 2003; Nathan & Gorman, 2002). Unfortunately, less research has focused on understanding the factors that influence treatment effects and how treatment actually works (Doss, 2004; Kazdin & Nock, 2003; Nock, 2003). Although RCTs have been used most often to address only the first goal, slight modifications in their design enable them to test moderators and mechanisms of clinical change as well. The more specific scientific questions guiding treatment research, and the RCT designs needed to answer each of these questions, are outlined in the following sections and summarized in Table 10.1.

TABLE 10.1
Primary Questions for Psychosocial Intervention Research and Associated Designs

Goal of research	Specific research question	Design strategy
Demonstrate causal relation between treatment and outcome	Is this treatment more efficacious than . . . ? (no treatment, wait-list, placebo, TAU, another treatment)	Treatment efficacy design
	Does the addition of this component increase treatment efficacy?	Additive/constructive design
	Does changing the parameters of treatment increase treatment efficacy?	Parametric design
Identify the factors that influence treatment effects	Does this pretreatment factor influence the strength or direction of treatment effects	Treatment moderator design
Identify the processes through which clinical change occurs	What components of this treatment are necessary and sufficient for maximum change?	Dismantling design/ component analysis
	Through what mechanism or processes does clinical change occur?	Treatment mechanism design

Note. Adapted from Kazdin (2000), Nock (2003).

■ Does Treatment Work?

Treatment Efficacy Designs

The first question addressed when evaluating a new or untested treatment typically is whether it is efficacious and thus is associated with favorable clinical change relative to a comparison condition. The most common research design used to test treatment efficacy is the *pretest-posttest comparison group design.* In such a design, all participants are assessed before receiving treatment (i.e., pretest) and after receiving treatment (i.e., posttest), and clinical change observed in the experimental condition is compared with that in the comparison condition. The same assessments are administered to participants in both conditions and at both time points. The inclusion of a pretest assessment conveys several important advantages, such as allowing one to (a) ensure between-group equivalence on key variables, (b) match participants on key variables and assign pairs of matched subjects randomly to conditions, (c) draw conclusions about the amount of change over the course of treatment, (d) examine potential moderators of treatment effects (as described later), and (e) examine factors that predict treatment attrition. Beyond deciding on the use of a pretest-posttest comparison group design, one must decide on the appropriate comparison group for a given study.

NO-TREATMENT COMPARISON DESIGN

Early studies of psychosocial interventions often have employed a no-treatment comparison design. The question addressed by this design is: "Is the experimental intervention more effective than no treatment?" Following the pretest-posttest design strategy, such a design can be diagrammed as follows (with R = random assignment to condition, O = observation/assessment, and X = treatment/intervention):

Experimental condition: R O_1 X O_2 O_3
No treatment condition: R O_4 O_5 O_6

In such a study, there are two groups, but only one receives the intervention. Following random assignment, individuals in both conditions are assessed on outcomes of interest at pretreatment (O_1 and O_4). Next, individuals in the experimental condition receive the intervention, whether it be 1 session (e.g., Ost, Alm, Brandberg, & Breitholtz, 2001), 12 sessions (e.g., Foa et al., 2005), or more than 100 sessions (e.g., Linehan, Armstrong, Suarez, Allmon, & Heard, 1991). Once the intervention period has ended, individuals in both conditions are assessed once again (O_2 and O_5). The efficacy of the intervention is examined by comparing change on the outcome measures for those in the experimental condition ($O_1 \rightarrow O_2$) with change for those in the no-treatment condition ($O_4 \rightarrow O_5$) (see section IV of this volume for a discussion of statistical analyses). It is always advisable to include a follow-up assessment (O_3 and O_6) to examine the extent to which treatment effects are maintained over time.

The inclusion of the comparison group allows one to rule out threats to the *internal validity* of the study, which refers to the extent to which the observed change can be attributed to the intervention rather than extraneous factors. However, such a design does not rule out potential threats to the *construct validity* of the study, which refers to the extent to which the intervention caused clinical change through the components and mechanisms proposed. Beyond demonstrating that an intervention is superior to no intervention, it is important to isolate the components and mechanisms through which an intervention has its effects. Several increasingly stringent design options allow the researcher to gain increasing clarity regarding the factors responsible for clinical change.

WAIT-LIST COMPARISON DESIGN

A large body of research has demonstrated the powerful change that can occur through hope and expectation of change (Frank & Frank, 1991; Snyder, Ilardi,

Michael, & Cheavens, 2000). Indeed, prior research on psychosocial interventions has shown that expectancies account for a significant portion of clinical change (Borkovec & Costello, 1993; Garfield, 1994; Kazdin & Wilcoxon, 1976), and that a substantial amount of clinical change occurs after treatment is scheduled but before it actually begins (Frank, Nash, Stone, & Imber, 1963) or as a result of participating in assessment alone (Paul, 1966). Despite the importance of hope and expectancies, many studies do not measure or account for the influence of these factors. One way to do so is through the use of a wait-list comparison design, in which all participants receive the experimental intervention, but those in the comparison condition do so after waiting until those in the experimental intervention have finished treatment. Such a design can be diagrammed as follows:

$$\begin{array}{llllllll} \text{Experimental condition:} & R & O_1 & X_1 & O_2 & & O_3 & \\ \text{Wait-list condition:} & R & O_4 & & O_5 & X_1 & O_6 & \quad O_7 \end{array}$$

In such a design, individuals in the comparison condition know they will receive the intervention when they are assessed at pretreatment (O_4), so the effectiveness of the intervention above and beyond the effect of hope and expectancies can be determined by comparing clinical change from $O_1 \rightarrow O_2$ with that from $O_4 \rightarrow O_5$. An added benefit of this design is that the extent of within-group clinical change due to the intervention can be determined by examining change from $O_1 \rightarrow O_2$ as well as from $O_5 \rightarrow O_6$, increasing the statistical power of this analysis. Here, too, it is advisable to include follow-up assessment (O_3 and O_7). It is also advisable to include assessment of treatment expectancies; several brief measures are available for this purpose (Devilly & Borkovecb, 2000; Nock, Ferriter, & Holmberg, in press; Nock & Kazdin, 2001).

ATTENTION/PLACEBO COMPARISON DESIGN

Beyond hope and expectancies, features associated with having weekly contact with a clinician may be responsible for much of the clinical change observed in psychosocial interventions. The amount of change due to specific treatment above and beyond nonspecific or unspecified factors such as attention, support, and therapeutic alliance can be tested using an attention or placebo comparison condition. Such a design can be diagrammed as follows:

$$\begin{array}{llllllll} \text{Experimental condition:} & R & O_1 & X_1 & O_2 & & O_3 \\ \text{Comparison condition:} & R & O_4 & X_2 & O_5 & & O_6 \end{array}$$

In such a design, X_2 represents an attention or placebo comparison condition in which individuals meet with a clinician for the same duration and frequency as those in the experimental condition, and they receive attention and support from the clinician, but not the aspects of the intervention believed active or most responsible for clinical change. Such a design is the psychosocial equivalent to a single-blind placebo-controlled study in medicine, in which those in the comparison condition meet with a clinician and receive medication, but unbeknownst to the patient the medication is inert and contains no active ingredient. An excellent example of an attention/placebo comparison design is one conducted by Brent and colleagues (1997) in which the investigators compared individual cognitive-behavioral therapy and individual nondirective supportive therapy as treatments for adolescent patients with major depressive disorder. Their findings demonstrated more rapid relief in interviewer-rated depression in cognitive behavior therapy than in individual nondirective supportive therapy. However, both treatments showed significant and similar reductions in suicidality and functional impairment. Thus, in this case, while cognitive behavior therapy might be suggested to provide some benefit over nondirective supportive therapy (the attention or placebo comparison condition) in the treatment of depressive symptoms, this study design shows that it does not provide significant benefit in reducing suicidality and functional impairment over and above that obtained through more unspecific attentional and supportive factors.

In such designs, the investigator should not assume that because an attention/placebo condition was included the condition adequately controlled for all associated factors. Indeed, it is important to assess alternative explanations beyond the difference in treatment content that could explain the findings. As an example, Brent and colleagues (1997) demonstrated that the different conditions did not vary in the number of sessions received, number of hours in contact with the clinician, years of experience of the clinicians, duration of treatment, or ratings of the credibility of treatment and their expectancies for change.

RELATIVE EFFICACY DESIGN

Often the primary research question is not whether a new treatment works at all, but whether it is superior to an existing standard of care. Here, too, one's research question should guide the decision about what comparison group to use. For instance, one may wish to test the efficacy of a newly developed treatment relative to an existing evidence-based or at least specified, manualized treatment. In such a relative efficacy design, one would use the same design as outlined in the previous section, but here X_2 would represent the active treatment comparison condition. As an example, the NIMH Treatment of Depression Collaborative Research Program compared the relative efficacy of cognitive behavior therapy, interpersonal therapy, imipramine hydrochloride plus clinical management, and placebo pill plus case management (Elkin et al., 1989). The results of this study demonstrated that each of the active treatment conditions was superior to placebo, but the differences between active treatments were relatively small. Many studies have performed secondary analyses of these data to test more specific hypotheses about the relative efficacy of these treatment conditions, highlighting the value of large-scale RCTs such as this one.

If an evidence-based treatment does not already exist, one may use treatment as usual (TAU) as the comparison condition. As an example, Linehan and colleagues (1991) conducted an RCT comparing dialectical behavior therapy (DBT) to TAU in the community. Findings showed that at most assessment points, patients who received DBT had fewer instances of self-injurious behavior, were more likely to stay in psychotherapy, and spent fewer days in inpatient psychiatric hospitals, suggesting that this innovative treatment resulted in considerable improvement in patient functioning over the treatment currently being provided in the community.

ADDITIVE/CONSTRUCTIVE TREATMENT DESIGN

Once an efficacious intervention is developed for a given psychological or behavioral problem, there often is interest in developing and testing the benefit of adding treatment components to the intervention. Additive or constructive treatment designs are those in which individuals in both the experimental and comparison conditions receive the same active intervention; however, those in the experimental condition also receive an additional intervention component. As a recent example, Nock and Kazdin (2005) used an additive treatment design to examine whether adding a brief participation enhancement intervention (PEI) to parent management training (PMT) would lead to increased treatment motivation, treatment attendance, and treatment adherence. All parents received PMT, but those randomly assigned to the experimental condition also received the brief PEI. They found that parents assigned to the experimental condition had significantly higher treatment motivation, attended more treatment sessions, and were more adherent to treatment procedures over the course of the study.

PARAMETRIC TREATMENT DESIGN

The efficacy of a given intervention also may be increased through modifications to the parameters of treatment, or in the way the intervention is delivered. In such studies, the content of the intervention is the same across conditions; however, conditions differ in factors such as the number, length, and duration of sessions, the use of group versus individual session, or variations in the treatment settings. Parametric treatment studies use the same design as the last diagram outlined here, with X_1 and X_2 representing versions of the same intervention that vary in a key parameter of interest. For example, Bastien, Morin, Ouellet, Blais, and Bouchard (2004) administered 8 weeks of cognitive-behavioral therapy (CBT) to participants with insomnia in group therapy format, in individual face-to-face therapy, and through brief individual telephone consultations. Participants in all three treatment modalities experienced similar improvements in their sleep habits. These findings indicate that the more cost-effective methods of group and telephone-based CBT are as effective as individual CBT at reducing symptoms of insomnia.

Like additive treatment studies, parametric treatment studies are useful for developing ways to enhance the efficacy of existing evidence-based treatments in order to determine the most efficacious method of delivering the intervention. Indeed, even the most powerful evidence-based treatments are not 100% effective for all individuals who receive them. Therefore, modifying existing interventions, rather than developing and testing alternative interventions, is a valuable way to maximize the efficacy and efficiency of care.

■ What Factors Influence Treatment Effects?

Treatment Moderator Design

A treatment moderator is a variable measured at pretreatment that influences the strength or direction of the relation between treatment and outcome (Baron & Kenny, 1986; Holmbeck, 1997; Kraemer, Wilson, Fairburn, & Agras, 2002). Knowledge of factors that moderate intervention effects will enhance understanding of for whom and under what conditions treatment is most efficacious. Such information could be used to triage patients to the interventions likely to be most effective and could also provide clues about how interventions actually work. Unfortunately, tests of treatment moderators have been fairly uncommon in the psychosocial intervention literature. When performed, they often have focused on testing variables of convenience, such as those measured for other purposes in the study but now available for tests of moderation (e.g., sociodemographic and diagnostic factors). Of course, such studies provide useful information about potential treatment moderators; however, future research on factors that influence treatment effects will progress much more rapidly if investigators build tests of theoretically derived moderators (e.g., expectancies, motivation) into their study design from the start.

Many different factors may moderate the effects of psychosocial interventions; however, testing most of these factors will involve using the same research design, which is one that makes only a minor modification to the treatment efficacy design and thus is quite economical. Factors that may moderate intervention effects can be examined by simply including an assessment of the potential moderator at the pretreatment assessment of outcomes (see the following, where M = potential moderator) and testing whether scores on the potential moderator at pretreatment are associated with the strength or direction of clinical change overall or within treatment conditions.

Experimental condition: R   O/M$_1$ X$_1$ O$_2$ O$_3$
Comparison condition: R   O/M$_4$ X$_2$ O$_5$ O$_6$

As an example, Dawson-McClure, Sandler, Wolchik, and Millsap (2004) evaluated the long-term effects of two preventive interventions for children from divorced families and examined whether the outcomes were moderated by baseline levels of risk. Analyses indicated that the programs were effective and attenuated the relation between risk and adolescent internalizing and externalizing problems, competence, and mental disorder, but moderational analyses showed that program effects were generally greater for children with higher baseline risk scores.

■ How Does Treatment Work?

Clinical researchers have developed an impressive armamentarium of evidence-based psychosocial interventions over the past several decades, and current progress suggests such advancement will continue. Although researchers and clinicians have many theories about the mechanisms through which these interventions have their effects, the sobering truth is that we do not yet know how any of these interventions actually work. There are at least two types of research designs that will be useful to clinical researchers in (a) isolating the active components of efficacious interventions, and (b) examining the mechanisms or processes through which these components lead to clinical change.

DISMANTLING TREATMENT DESIGN

Dismantling studies, also known as *component analyses,* use a between-group design to compare the relative efficacy of the different components of a treatment package in order to determine which components are necessary and sufficient for maximum clinical change. Most psychosocial interventions contain numerous components, many of which may be unnecessary. Therefore, isolating the active components can result in more efficient and potentially more effective treatments, as one could increase the proportion of treatment time devoted to the active components. For instance, most forms of cognitive-behavioral therapy contain psychoeducation, behavioral activation, and cognitive restructuring, among other things. Similarly, dialectical behavior therapy (Linehan et al., 1991), one of the few evidence-based treatments for self-injurious behaviors, is composed of four core skills modules (mindfulness, emotion regulation, distress tolerance, and interpersonal effectiveness) taught during weekly group sessions, but it also includes weekly individual sessions in which clinicians aid clients in learning and practicing these and other psychosocial skills and are also available at all times via a pager. Although such multifaceted treatments have shown impressive efficacy, it is not clear which of the many components included are necessary and sufficient for clinical change. Dismantling studies are aimed at testing such questions, and can be diagrammed as follows:

Experimental condition:	R	O_1	X_1	O_2	O_3
Experimental condition:	R	O_4	X_2	O_5	O_6
Comparison condition:	R	O_7	X_3	O_8	O_9

Here, X_3 represents the full treatment package, and X_1 and X_2 represent individual components that are also included together in X_3. An excellent example of a dismantling study is provided by Jacobson and colleagues' (1996) study of the efficacy of CBT for depression. In this study, participants with major depression were randomly assigned to receive either treatment based on only the behavioral activation (BA) component of CBT, a treatment that involved both BA and skills training to change automatic thoughts (AT), but excluding the components of CBT focused on core schema, or the full CBT. Each component treatment was as effective as the full CBT at reducing symptoms of depression and negative thoughts. This suggests that not all of the components of traditional CBT are necessary for clinical change.

TREATMENT MECHANISM DESIGN

Beyond isolating the active components of psychosocial interventions, a key goal for research is to identify the actual mechanisms or processes through which change occurs. Doing so will serve many very important purposes. First, identifying mechanisms of change will help bring parsimony to the many treatments that currently exist. More than 500 different psychosocial interventions are currently in use (Kazdin, 2000), and it is highly unlikely that they all operate via different change mechanisms. Identifying common mechanisms will help eliminate overlap among treatments and will streamline both research and clinical efforts. Second, understanding mechanisms of change will increase the efficiency and efficacy of psychosocial interventions. If research identifies how change occurs, interventions can be modified to include more of that mechanism or process. Third, obtaining a firmer grasp on the actual mechanisms through which people change during psychosocial interventions will illuminate behavior change processes more generally and thus has implications that reach far beyond treatment research.

Although the benefits are clear, the procedures necessary for demonstrating the operation of mechanisms of change are more complex. Many studies attempting to identify mechanisms of change in psychosocial interventions have drawn from the valuable work on testing statistical mediation outlined 20 years ago by Baron and Kenny (1986). They suggest that to demonstrate statistical mediation one must demonstrate that treatment condition (T) is associated with some outcome of interest (O); that T is associated with the proposed mechanism (M); that M is associated with O; and when T and M are both covaried with O, M continues to be associated with O, but the relation between T and O is diminished (see Figure 10.1). This pattern of relations provides evidence that T is associated with O through its relation with M (Baron & Kenny, 1986; Holmbeck, 1997; MacKinnon, Lockwood, Hoffman, West, & Sheets, 2002).

Although useful for testing whether statistical mediation has occurred, such an approach does not provide sufficient evidence for the operation of a mecha-

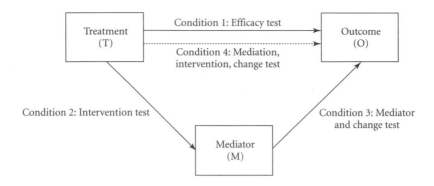

FIGURE 10.1. Four conditions to test statistical mediation among three therapy variables: the treatment (T), the proposed mediator (M), and outcome (O).
Note: Solid lines refer to tests of univariate relations between variables. Dashed line refers to test of relation between T and O while statistically controlling for M, as outlined in the text.

nism of change. Indeed, just as correlation does not equal causation, mediation does not equal mechanism. The more stringent criteria for demonstrating the operation of a mechanism of change in psychosocial interventions have been outlined in detail elsewhere (Kazdin & Nock, 2003; Nock, in press). These criteria, summarized in Table10.2, require showing strong associations between treatment, mechanism, and outcome, as in the statistical mediation approach. However, the case for the operation of a mechanism of change is strengthened if one can show specificity of the proposed mechanism, a gradient or dose-response relation between constructs, that the mechanism changes prior to change in the outcome, that there is a causal relation between the mechanism and outcome, and that the observed findings are reliable, plausible, and coherent. Taken together, these criteria synthesize the requirements for demonstrating statistical mediation with those for demonstrating causal relations—which includes conducting an RCT.

The use of one of the RCT designs outlined here is necessary but not sufficient to meet the criteria for testing a mechanism of change. Given the importance of showing temporal precedence of change in the proposed mechanism relative to change in the outcome, it is necessary to modify traditional, pretreatment-posttreatment designs so that assessment of both mechanism and outcome occurs as frequently as possible. Such a design may be diagrammed as follows, where M = assessment of the proposed mechanism:

Experimental condition: R O/M_1 X_1 O/M_2 X_1 O/M_3 X_1 O/M_4 X_1 O/M_5 X_1 O/M_6
Comparison condition: R O/M_7 X_2 O/M_8 X_2 O/M_9 X_2 O/M_{10} X_2 O/M_{11} X_2 O/M_{12}

In addition to performing assessments frequently, it is preferred to do so early in the course of treatment given that significant change often occurs within the first few weeks of the intervention (Ilardi & Craighead, 1994) and in many

TABLE 10.2
Criteria for Demonstrating Mechanisms of Change

Criteria	Specific requirement
Strong association	Demonstration of a significant association among treatment (T), proposed mechanism (M), and outcome (O).
Specificity	Demonstration that T is uniquely related to change in M, and that change in M is uniquely related to change in O.
Gradient	Demonstration of dose-response relation between T, M, and O.
Temporal relation	Demonstration that change in M temporally precedes change in O.
Consistency	Replication of observed results across samples, settings, and researchers.
Experiment	Use of a true experimental design, such as a randomized clinical trial.
Plausibility	Findings must be credible and reasonable.
Coherence	Findings should fit logically with broader scientific knowledge.

cases before the intervention even begins (Howard, Kopta, Krause, & Orlinsky, 1986). Comprehensive assessment of multiple, theoretically derived mechanisms is also recommended in order to maximize the yield of each study, especially given the time and resources required to conduct any given trial and the dearth of information on mechanisms of change currently available (Nock, in press).

Although no studies of psychosocial interventions have met all these criteria, several model studies are notable. Barber, Connolly, Crits-Christoph, Gladis, and Siqueland (2000) conducted an investigation in which they examined the relations among therapeutic alliance, outcome, and early symptom improvement in a group of patients with psychiatric illness who received supportive-expressive dynamic psychotherapy. Their results showed that alliance at all sessions significantly predicted subsequent change in depression, when prior change in depression was parceled out, suggesting that therapeutic alliance plays a causal role in patient outcome. An additional study by Huey, Henggeler, Brondino, and Pickrel (2000) examined the mechanisms through which multisystemic therapy (MST) decreased delinquent behavior in juvenile offenders. They assessed not only delinquent behavior in the adolescents at multiple time points but also therapist adherence to the MST protocol, as well as measures of family relations (family cohesion, family functioning, and parent monitoring) and delinquent peer affiliation. Their results showed that therapist adherence to the MST protocol was associated with improved family relations and decreased delinquent peer affiliation, which, in turn, were associated with decreased delinquent behavior. The findings from these example studies highlight the importance of identifying central change mechanisms in determining more specifically how complex treatments such as MST as well as therapy relationships more generally contribute to ultimate outcomes.

■ Conclusions

Designing and conducting an RCT requires significant time and resources. It is important that, before beginning, one has carefully thought through the primary theoretical question and the specific hypotheses that will be tested, and that one has designed the study in a way that will provide the appropriate test of the key hypotheses. It is recommended that those designing an RCT consider the three goals of research on psychosocial interventions outlined in this chapter, and the more specific questions that follow from these goals (see Table 10.1). Perhaps the greatest consideration in addressing the first goal is in selecting the appropriate comparison condition or conditions. Doing so requires reflection on the current state of research on the intervention under examination. Once this decision is made, it is strongly recommended that attention is given to testing potential moderators and mechanisms of clinical change. Testing moderators of change requires simply thinking of what factors are most likely to influence the strength and direction of treatment effects, and adding measurement of such factors to the pretreatment assessment battery. Testing mechanisms of change requires significant modifications to one's treatment design, but we believe it is well worth the effort. If major modifications, such as the inclusion of frequent assessment of outcomes and proposed mechanisms, are not possible, one may consider simply adding measures of proposed mechanisms to the pre- and posttreatment assessment batteries in order to test whether such factors statistically mediate treatment effects. Indeed, multiple studies are needed to address each question, as any one study will be insufficient to do so satisfactorily. Nevertheless, careful consideration of theories of change and the use of rigorous and creative research design strategies, such as those outlined in this chapter, will aid the researcher in answering the relevant research question and in advancing scientific and practical understanding of clinical change resulting from psychosocial interventions.

■ Acknowledgment

Completion of this work was facilitated by a grant from the National Institute of Mental Health (MH076047) awarded to Matthew K. Nock.

■ References

Barber, J. P., Connolly, M. B., Crits-Christoph, P., Gladis, L., & Siqueland, L. (2000). Alliance predicts patients' outcome beyond in-treatment change in symptoms. *Journal of Consulting and Clinical Psychology, 68,* 1027–1032.

Barlow, D. H., & Hersen, M. (1984). *Single case experimental designs: Strategies for studying behavior change* (2nd ed.). New York: Pergamon.

Barlow, D. H., Nock, M. K., & Hersen, M. (in press). *Single-case experimental designs: Strategies for studying behavior change* (3rd ed.). Boston: Allyn & Bacon.

Baron, R. M., & Kenny, D. A. (1986). The moderator-mediator variable distinction in social psychological research: Conceptual, strategic, and statistical considerations. *Journal of Personality and Social Psychology, 51,* 1173–1182.

Bastien, C. H., Morin, C. M., Ouellet, M. C., Blais, F. C., & Bouchard, S. (2004). Cognitive-behavioral therapy for insomnia: Comparison of individual therapy, group therapy, and telephone consultations. *Journal of Consulting and Clinical Psychology, 72,* 653–659.

Borkovec, T. D., & Costello, E. (1993). Efficacy of applied relaxation and cognitive-behavioral therapy in the treatment of generalized anxiety disorder. *Journal of Consulting and Clinical Psychology, 61,* 611–619.

Brent, D. A., Holder, D., Kolko, D., Birmaher, B., Baugher, M., Roth, C., et al. (1997). A clinical psychotherapy trial for adolescent depression comparing cognitive, family, and supportive therapy. *Archives of General Psychiatry, 54,* 877–885.

Byrne, M., Agerbo, E., Ewald, H., Eaton, W. W., & Mortensen, P. B. (2003). Parental age and risk of schizophrenia: A case-control study. *Archives of General Psychiatry, 60,* 673–678.

Cantor-Graae, E., Zolkowska, K., & McNeil, T. F. (2005). Increased risk of psychotic disorder among immigrants in Malmo: A 3-year first-contact study. *Psychological Medicine, 35,* 1155–1163.

Chambless, D. L., & Hollon, S. D. (1998). Defining empirically supported therapies. *Journal of Consulting and Clinical Psychology, 66,* 7–18.

Dawson-McClure, S. R., Sandler, I. N., Wolchik, S. A., & Millsap, R. E. (2004). Risk as a moderator of the effects of prevention programs for children from divorced families: A six-year longitudinal study. *Journal of Abnormal Child Psychology, 32,* 175–190.

Devilly, G. J., & Borkovecb, T. D. (2000). Psychometric properties of the credibility/expectancy questionnaire. *Journal of Behavior Therapy and Experimental Psychiatry, 31,* 73–86.

Doss, B. D. (2004). Changing the way we study change in psychotherapy. *Clinical Psychology: Science and Practice, 11,* 368–386.

Elkin, I., Shea, M. T., Watkins, J. T., Imber, S. D., Sotsky, S. M., Collins, J. F., et al. (1989). National Institute of Mental Health Treatment of Depression Collaborative Research Program: General effectiveness of treatments. *Archives of General Psychiatry, 46,* 971–982; discussion 983.

Foa, E. B., Hembree, E. A., Cahill, S. P., Rauch, S. A., Riggs, D. S., Feeny, N. C., et al. (2005). Randomized trial of prolonged exposure for posttraumatic stress disorder with and without cognitive restructuring: Outcome at academic and community clinics. *Journal of Consulting and Clinical Psychology, 73,* 953–964.

Frank, J. D., & Frank, J. B. (1991). *Persuasion and healing* (3rd ed.). Baltimore: Johns Hopkins University Press.

Frank, J. D., Nash, E. H., Stone, A. R., & Imber, S. D. (1963). Immediate and long-term symptomatic course of psychiatric outpatients. *American Journal of Psychiatry, 120,* 429–439.

Garfield, S. L. (1994). Research on client variables in psychotherapy. In A. E. Bergin & S. L. Garfield (Eds.), *Handbook of psychotherapy and behavior change* (4th ed., pp. 190–228). New York: Wiley.

Haynes, S. N. (1992). *Models of causality in psychopathology: Toward dynamic, synthetic, and nonlinear models of behavior disorders.* Needham Heights, MA: Allyn & Bacon.

Hill, A. B. (1965). The environment and disease: Association or causation? *Proceedings of the Royal Society of Medicine, 58,* 295–300.

Holmbeck, G. N. (1997). Toward terminological, conceptual, and statistical clarity in the study of mediators and moderators: Examples from the child-clinical and pediatric psychology literatures. *Journal of Consulting and Clinical Psychology, 65,* 599–610.

Howard, K. I., Kopta, S. M., Krause, M. S., & Orlinsky, D. E. (1986). The dose-effect relationship in psychotherapy. *American Psychologist, 41,* 159–164.

Huey, S. J., Jr., Henggeler, S. W., Brondino, M. J., & Pickrel, S. G. (2000). Mechanisms of change in multisystemic therapy: Reducing delinquent behavior through therapist adherence and improved family and peer functioning. *Journal of Consulting and Clinical Psychology, 68,* 451–467.

Hume, D. (1739). *A treatise of human nature: Being an attempt to introduce the experimental method of reasoning.* London: Printed for J. Noon.

Ilardi, S. S., & Craighead, W. E. (1994). The role of nonspecific factors in cognitive-behavior therapy for depression. *Clinical Psychology: Science and Practice, 1,* 138–156.

Jacobson, N. S., Dobson, K. S., Truax, P. A., Addis, M. E., Koerner, K., Gollan, J. K., et al. (1996). A component analysis of cognitive-behavioral treatment for depression. *Journal of Consulting and Clinical Psychology, 64,* 295–304.

Kazdin, A. E. (1982). *Single-case research designs: Methods for clinical and applied settings.* New York: Oxford University Press.

Kazdin, A. E. (2000). *Psychotherapy for children and adolescents: Directions for research and practice.* New York: Oxford University Press.

Kazdin, A. E. (2003). *Research design in clinical psychology* (4th ed.). Boston Allyn & Bacon.

Kazdin, A. E., & Nock, M. K. (2003). Delineating mechanisms of change in child and adolescent therapy: Methodological issues and research recommendations. *Journal of Child Psychology and Psychiatry, 44,* 1116–1129.

Kazdin, A. E., & Weisz, J. R. (Eds.). (2003). *Evidence-based psychotherapies for children and adolescents.* New York: Guilford.

Kazdin, A. E., & Wilcoxon, L. A. (1976). Systematic desensitization and nonspecific treatment effects: A methodological evaluation. *Psychological Bulletin, 83,* 729–758.

Kenny, D. A. (1979). *Correlation and causality.* New York: Wiley.

Kraemer, H. C., Kazdin, A. E., Offord, D. R., Kessler, R. C., Jensen, P. S., & Kupfer, D. J. (1997). Coming to terms with the terms of risk. *Archives of General Psychiatry, 54,* 337–343.

Kraemer, H. C., Stice, E., Kazdin, A., Offord, D., & Kupfer, D. (2001). How do risk factors work together? Mediators, moderators, and independent, overlapping, and proxy risk factors. *American Journal of Psychiatry, 158,* 848–856.

Kraemer, H. C., Wilson, G. T., Fairburn, C. G., & Agras, W. S. (2002). Mediators and moderators of treatment effects in randomized clinical trials. *Archives of General Psychiatry, 59,* 877–883.

Lall, V. F., & Levin, J. R. (2004). An empirical investigation of the statistical properties of generalized single-case randomization tests. *Journal of School Psychology, 42,* 61–86.

Linehan, M. M., Armstrong, H. E., Suarez, A., Allmon, D., & Heard, H. L. (1991). Cognitive-behavioral treatment of chronically parasuicidal borderline patients. *Archives of General Psychiatry, 48,* 1060–1064.

MacKinnon, D. P., Lockwood, C. M., Hoffman, J. M., West, S. G., & Sheets, V. (2002). A comparison of methods to test mediation and other intervening variable effects. *Psychological Methods, 7,* 83–104.

Moras, K., Telfer, L. A., & Barlow, D. H. (1993). Efficacy and specific effects data on new treatments: A case study strategy with mixed anxiety-depression. *Journal of Consulting and Clinical Psychology, 61,* 412–420.

Nathan, P. E., & Gorman, J. M. (Eds.). (2002). *Treatments that work* (2nd ed.). New York: Oxford University Press.

Nock, M. K. (2002). A multiple-baseline evaluation of the treatment of food phobia in a young boy. *Journal of Behavior Therapy and Experimental Psychiatry, 33,* 217–225.

Nock, M. K. (2003). Progress review of the psychosocial treatment of child conduct problems. *Clinical Psychology: Science and Practice, 10,* 1–28.

Nock, M. K. (in press). Conceptual and design essentials for evaluating mechanisms of change. *Alcoholism: Clinical and Experimental Research.*

Nock, M. K., Ferriter, C., & Holmberg, E. (2007). Parent beliefs about treatment credibility and expectancies for improvement: Assessment and relation to treatment adherence. *Journal of Child and Family Studies, 16,* 27–38.

Nock, M. K., & Kazdin, A. E. (2001). Parent expectancies for child therapy: Assessment and relation to participation in treatment. *Journal of Child and Family Studies, 10,* 155–180.

Nock, M. K., & Kazdin, A. E. (2005). Randomized controlled trial of a brief intervention for increasing participation in parent management training. *Journal of Consulting and Clinical Psychology, 73,* 872–879.

Nock, M. K., Michel, B. D., & Photos, V. (in press). Single-case research designs. In D. McKay (Ed.), *Handbook of research methods in abnormal and clinical psychology.* Thousand Oaks, CA: Sage.

Ost, L. G., Alm, T., Brandberg, M., & Breitholtz, E. (2001). One vs. five sessions of exposure and five sessions of cognitive therapy in the treatment of claustrophobia. *Behaviour Research and Therapy, 39,* 167–183.

Paul, G. L. (1966). *Insight versus desensitization in psychotherapy: An experiment in anxiety reduction.* Stanford, CA: Stanford University Press.

Schlesselman, J. J. (1982). *Case-control studies: Design, conduct, and analysis.* New York: Oxford University Press.

Shadish, W. R., Cook, T. D., & Campbell, D. T. (2001). *Experimental and quasi-experimental designs for generalized causal inference.* Boston: Houghton Mifflin.

Snyder, C. R., Ilardi, S. S., Michael, S. T., & Cheavens, J. (2000). Hope theory: Updating a common process for psychological change. In C. R. Snyder & R. E. Ingram (Eds.), *Handbook of psychological change: Psychotherapy processes and practices for the 21st century* (pp. 128–153). New York: Wiley.

Sundquist, K., Frank, G., & Sundquist, J. (2004). Urbanisation and incidence of psychosis and depression: Follow-up study of 4.4 million women and men in Sweden. *British Journal of Psychiatry, 184,* 293–298.

11. EFFICACY AND EFFECTIVENESS IN DEVELOPING TREATMENT MANUALS

Kathleen M. Carroll and Bruce J. Rounsaville

The development of treatment manuals, which specify various psychotherapies and provide guidelines for their implementation, has both revolutionized psychotherapy research (Luborsky & DeRubeis, 1984) and provoked remarkable controversy around their roles and value in clinical practice. On one hand, manuals are now virtual requirements in treatment efficacy research (Chambless & Hollon, 1998; Chambless & Ollendick, 2001; Westen, Novotney, & Thompson-Brenner, 2004) and are more frequently being used as a basis for training clinicians in a range of programs and disciplines (Crits-Christoph, Frank, Chambless, Brody, & Karp, 1995; Vakoch & Strupp, 2000; Weissman et al., 2006). Although manuals are increasingly present in clinical practice as changes in the health care system exert greater pressure on clinicians to define and evaluate the effectiveness of services they provide (Addis, Wade, & Hatgis, 1999), they are still met with resistance and strong criticism by clinicians. Although this chapter appears in a volume describing key design and methodological issues in randomized clinical trials of psychosocial interventions and hence focuses on the essential features of manual development for efficacy research, it is important for clinical researchers to develop manuals and treatment programs recognizing they may be eventually used in clinical practice with more heterogeneous populations and implemented by more heterogeneous clinicians (Carroll & Rounsaville, 2003). Thus, this chapter will review the roles of treatment manuals in efficacy research, the challenges inherent in moving a manual from research to clinical practice, and review strategies for developing treatment manuals throughout the phases of development, evaluation, and dissemination of a treatment (Carroll & Nuro, 2002).

■ Roles of Manuals in Clinical Research

That manuals have become an essential feature of randomized clinical trials of psychosocial interventions underscores their multiple roles in clinical efficacy research. These include, primarily, specification of the independent (treatment) variable in clinical trials. The level of specification can range from a minimal blueprint of treatment, akin to how a medication would be formulated in a pharmacotherapy trial (e.g., dose, content, agent, putative active ingredients) to a fully elaborated description of all aspects of the therapy. The optimal level of specification should be driven by the design and research questions asked in the trial. For example, a therapy that is "added on" to a standard clinical approach (addressing the question, "Does Treatment X improve outcomes when added to standard treatment?") may require a somewhat less detailed description than a psychotherapy that is compared with another active psychotherapy (e.g., "Is Treatment X more effective than Treatment Y under these conditions?"). In the latter case, it would be important that the respective manuals not only clearly describe the two approaches but also clearly convey the specific features that distinguish the two approaches (e.g., any intervention or feature that should not overlap or be present in both interventions), as well as clarify techniques, processes, or procedures that the two approaches may have in common. Manuals for comparative studies might also specify whether the same clinicians could deliver both approaches (e.g., whether therapists can be crossed or should be nested within conditions), which again depends on the research questions being addressed and the nature of the treatments studied. Similarly, manuals for component analysis studies (e.g., Jacobson et al., 1996) must specify the nature of the specific components to be compared (e.g., if cognitive versus behavioral aspects of a treatment were contrasted, the manuals must clearly isolate and specify each of those components—not only which of the myriad techniques would be considered "cognitive" or "behavioral" but also how the clinician is to handle a wide range of problems with a purely cognitive approach). A crucial point that emerges from these examples is that in clinical treatment research, the nature, level of specification, and content of the manual(s) used are predicated on the specific research questions being addressed and the nature of the treatments, or conditions, being compared. Similarly, the manual might complement the protocol by articulating each of the key aspects of the treatment necessary to address the questions asked (these might include, but are not limited to, theoretical foundations of the treatment, mechanism of action of the treatment, essential components or processes of the approach, strategies at key change points, stance toward alternative approaches, training and monitoring of the clinicians, and so forth). The many complexities of selecting appropriate control conditions for psychotherapy efficacy research (Wampold & Bhati, 2004) are discussed in chapter 10 of this volume.

A second key role of manuals is to provide definitions of standards and criteria for evaluating adherence and competence in delivering the treatment.

Adherence has been defined as the extent to which the therapist used techniques, interventions, and processes described in the manual and avoided those interventions proscribed by the manual (see Waltz, Addis, Koerner, & Jacobson, 1993; and chapter 13 in this volume). *Competence* is generally defined as the skill with which the clinician delivered those interventions, that is, took into account the status of the patient, appreciated the timing and context of the intervention, and delivered it effectively. Waltz et al. (1993) note that "competence presupposes adherence, but adherence does not necessarily imply competence" (p. 620). Again, the specific issues to be addressed through process analyses must be dictated by the research design and questions; however, if those process elements are not defined in the manual, it is less likely that they will be evident in the treatment as delivered and detectable in process analysis (Ablon & Jones, 2002). For example, if the treatment development intends the treatment to have high levels of structure but does not provide an operational definition of *structure* for that treatment or concretize what the therapist should do to achieve the appropriate level of structure, structure may vary widely across clinicians and patients. Many empirically validated therapies are "structured," but they may achieve their structure through very different means. Thus, a simple rule of thumb in treatment development is that all intended adherence/competence items should be explicitly defined in the manual. Waltz et al. (1993) elaborated this further to suggest four general types of items for adherence/competence ratings: (a) interventions that are both unique and essential to the treatment, (b) interventions that are essential to the treatment but not necessarily unique to it, (c) behaviors that are compatible with the therapy but not unique or essential to it, and (d) behaviors that are proscribed, or not part of the therapy. This final element is important but frequently overlooked by manual developers; we note that it is often very clarifying to describe a therapy in terms of *what it is not* as well as what it is. Proscribed behaviors may be prohibited because they are distinctive of an alternate therapy but also because they reflect behaviors characteristic of ineffective implementation of a therapy (e.g., direct advice giving or closed-ended questions in motivational approaches).

A third role of manuals is in facilitating training of therapists and reducing variability in their delivery of treatments. Although manuals are clearly not sufficient, by themselves, to train therapists to deliver treatments competently (Davis et al., 1999; Miller, Yahne, Moyers, Martinez, & Pirritano, 2004; Sholomskas et al., 2005), by defining the treatment and articulating standards for its delivery, they are essential for therapist training in clinical trials. By demarking the boundaries of the treatment, the treatment manual typically serves as the cornerstone of therapist training (Dobson & Shaw, 1993). As described in more detail in chapter 12 of this volume, training of therapists for clinical trials typically involves detailed review of the manual, followed by viewing of tapes of effective implementation of the therapy, role plays, and then supervised practice and supervision, all with frequent reference to the manual. Thus, to facilitate this process, manuals may provide specific guidelines and standards for therapist training. A fairly recent but important component of many manuals is clear description of competence standards for therapists, with checklists and self-monitoring tools (Carroll, Nich, & Rounsaville, 1998) that can be used by therapist trainees and their supervisors to evaluate their performance (Weissman et al., 2006).

A fourth role of manuals is to provide quality assurance standards. Thus, manuals are used as the basis for developing competency and certification standards for the treatment. Although many clinicians and programs assert they routinely use a range of evidence-based practices, it is very difficult to ascertain whether they are actually doing so without reviewing their clinical work. Thus, review of session audiotapes or videotapes for minimal levels of fidelity and adherence/competence is increasingly becoming a standard in both research and clinical practice (Weissman et al., 2006).

A fifth major role of treatment manuals is to facilitate replication of studies. Criteria for determining whether a therapy is empirically validated requires independent replication of a treatment's efficacy (Chambless & Hollon, 1998) by investigators other than the treatment's originators (Luborsky et al., 1999). However, since seemingly minor changes may alter a treatment's efficacy, a well-defined, detailed, and clear treatment manual is necessary to foster valid replication research.

A sixth major function of manuals is to foster dissemination and transfer of effective therapies to clinical practice. As noted earlier, a well-crafted manual is a necessary but by no means sufficient component in moving a treatment from clinical research to clinical practice. A treatment's utility in clinical practice often depends on its being implemented as efficiently as possible; thus, the inclusion in the manual on what are seen as essential "active ingredients" or change strategies may further foster its adoption in clinical practice. Similarly, clarity regarding what elements are seen as "essential" to achieve fidelity to the manual versus what elements are "optional" may also be more attractive to clinicians.

■ Criticisms of Manuals and Strategies to Address Those Criticisms

Then anyone who leaves behind him a written manual, and likewise anyone who receives it, in the belief that such writing will be clear and certain, must be exceedingly simple-minded.
—PLATO, *Phaedrus*

Despite their many advantages, many psychotherapy manuals, including those that specify psychotherapies with extensive levels of empirical support, have been met with only mixed enthusiasm and acceptance by the clinical community.

Existing treatment manuals have been criticized on several grounds, including (a) limited applicability to the wide range of populations and complex problems regularly encountered in clinical practice (Abrahamson, 1999; Henry, 1998; Schulte & Eifert, 2002; Westen et al., 2004); (b) excessive emphasis on technique with inadequate focus on the working alliance and other important common elements of treatment (Dobson & Shaw, 1993; Henry, Strupp, Butler, Schacht, & Binder, 1993; Vakoch & Strupp, 2000); (c) restriction of clinical innovation and the clinical expertise of the therapist (Castonguay, Schut, Constantino, & Halperin, 1999; Wampold & Bhati, 2004; Wolfe, 1999); (d) emphasis on technique over theory (Mahrer, 2005; Silverman, 1996; Vakoch & Strupp, 2000); (e) overemphasis on adherence may reduce therapist competence (Henry et al., 1993; Mahrer, 2005); and (f) feasibility when the manual is implemented by clinicians of great diversity regarding experience, discipline, and clinical expertise (Addis et al., 1999).

Clearly, the failure of many scientifically validated treatments to find their way into clinical practice is not entirely due to shortcomings of the manuals themselves. For example, even a highly flexible and sophisticated manual is not likely to be adopted by clinicians if the treatment it describes is not feasible, cost-effective, or acceptable to the clinical community. Conversely, however, assuming that a novel treatment is practical and appealing to clinicians, a well-written manual may facilitate its acceptance.

One strategy for addressing some of these criticisms and encouraging broader use of treatment manuals in clinical practice might be to view manual development not as a single event but as a series of progressive stages, with each successive stage addressing more complex clinical issues. A major recent innovation in behavioral therapies development was the articulation of a "stage model" of behavioral therapies development (Onken, Blaine, & Battjes, 1997). This sequence of research on new treatments was conceived to facilitate an orderly progression of behavioral therapies research to allow a comparatively rapid and systematic development of promising treatments from the point where they are merely "good ideas" to one where they are capable of being disseminated to the clinical field as validated, effective, well-defined treatments with guidelines for choosing the patients, providers, and settings most associated with optimal outcomes (Rounsaville, Carroll, & Onken, 2001). Stage I consists of pilot/feasibility testing, initial manual writing, training program development, and adherence/competence measure development for new and untested treatments. Stage II consists principally of controlled clinical trials to evaluate efficacy of manualized and pilot tested treatments that have shown promise or efficacy in earlier studies. Studies in this stage may also be devoted to evaluating mechanisms of action or effective components of treatment. Stage III consists of studies to evaluate transportability of treatments (e.g., efficacy of the treatment in diverse populations, means of training therapists, cost-effectiveness) whose efficacy has been demonstrated in at least two Stage II trials (Carroll & Rounsaville, 2003; Rounsaville et al., 2001).

To offer a conceptual model for addressing many criticisms of manuals and developing manuals that are useful in both clinical research and clinical practice, we have proposed a parallel stage model for the development of treatment manuals (Carroll & Nuro, 2002). This model posits that the apparent disconnect between researchers and clinicians regarding manuals (see Addis & Krasnow, 2000) may reflect in part that treatment researchers tend to develop and disseminate manuals appropriate for Stage I and Stage II research, while what is needed to facilitate broader dissemination of effective treatments and thus be most appropriate for clinicians are all-too-rare Stage III manuals. This model recognizes that the purposes and roles, and therefore content, of manuals should evolve with the stage of development of a given treatment. The development of many manuals essentially stops at Stage I or early Stage II—the level of manual development that is appropriate for clinical efficacy studies—while effective dissemination to the clinical community is likely to require ongoing efforts involving the synthesis of process and outcome data from several trials to enhance, elaborate, and extend the manual in order to be of use to clinicians applying the treatment to broader populations and settings. In the following sections we suggest guidelines for the content of manuals at the various stages of development, as well as strategies for developing "clinician-friendly" manuals at all stages to facilitate greater use of scientifically validated treatments in clinical practice (see Street, Niederehe, & Lebowitz, 2000).

■ Evolving Roles of Manuals

As noted earlier, the fundamental purpose of a psychotherapy manual is to specify a treatment and provide guidelines to therapists for its implementation. However, manuals have been described as having myriad potential roles; these include providing a means for objective comparisons of different psychotherapies, setting standards for training and evaluation of therapists, providing a means of linking treatment process to outcome, defining treatment goals, establishing clinical care standards, fostering replication of clinical trials, facilitating transfer of promising treatments from research to clinical settings, reducing variability in outcome due to therapist effects, and many more (Castonguay et al., 1999; Crits-Christoph et al., 1991; Kazdin, 1995; Luborsky & DeRubeis, 1984; Moras, 1993; Rounsaville, O'Malley, Foley, & Weissman, 1988).

A psychotherapy researcher in the nascent stages of developing a novel therapy would be overwhelmed with this daunting list, particularly if he or she failed to recognize that what a given manual can do depends very much on the current level of empirical support for the treatment it describes. That is, manuals serve very different functions as the level of development of a treatment moves from Stage I (where the critical role of the manual is to define the treatment in broad strokes for preliminary evaluation of feasibility and efficacy) to

Stage II (where the manual is used as the basis for training therapists, reducing the magnitude of therapist effects in clinical efficacy trials, sharpening the distinction between therapies, dismantling of treatment elements, and linking process to outcome) to Stage III (where the manual may be used to evaluate the treatment when used by diverse clinicians and applied to diverse patient populations, as well as in fostering replications of clinical trials in other settings) and ultimately to broad dissemination to the clinical community (providing clinical care standards, providing practice guidelines, serving as the basis for training of clinicians). Table 11.1 provides an overview of the roles of manuals across the various stages, evolving from the essential "bare bones" of Stage I to a highly detailed, elaborate, clinically sophisticated version in Stage III and beyond. This "stage model" of psychotherapy manual development conceives of manuals as being enriched over time with accumulated clinical experience, but more important, with process and outcome data.

This model is not, however, predicated solely on widespread acceptance of the stage model of therapy development. We have merely attempted to codify what is, or should be, a logical sequence of manual development and to drive home that treatment manual development should not stop with the versions of manuals used in Stage II efficacy trials. Nevertheless, just as an important benefit of the stage model of treatment development is that it has fostered support for treatment development and pilot studies in Stage I and dissemination studies in Stage III (Onken et al., 1997), articulation of a parallel model for manual development may foster greater recognition of the need to support the development of "Stage III" manuals as a strategy to foster broader use of manuals in clinical practice.

Guidelines for a Stage I Treatment Manual

The overall goals of the initial stage of treatment development are to specify the treatment and provide an initial evaluation of its feasibility and efficacy. Thus, at this stage, the treatment developer often has in mind only a general outline of the treatment and a rough conception of the major contents of sessions. Table 11.2 provides a general outline for a Stage I manual that would define the boundaries, basic structure, and preliminary contents of a treatment at a level that would be minimally sufficient for a preliminary pilot study aimed at evaluating its feasibility and efficacy. Although it may not be necessary or appropriate to include lengthy descriptions for each of these topics in any single manual, treatment developers may find it helpful to consider each of these issues in order to more thoroughly define their treatment.

Very briefly, a "bare-bones" Stage I–level manual should cover issues such as the overview, description, and theoretical justification of the treatment; a conception of the nature of the disorder or problem the treatment targets; the theoretical mechanisms of change; the goals of the treatment; a description of how the treatment may be similar to or different from other existing treatments

TABLE 11.1
Overview of Roles of Manuals by Stage of Treatment Development

Stage	Purpose	Focus	Principal roles of treatment manual
I	Preliminary evaluation of feasibility and efficacy	Pilot/feasibility trials	Initial specification of treatment techniques, goals, and format Initial specification of theoretical "active ingredients"
II	Randomized clinical trials	Efficacy trials	Specifications of standards for training and supervision of therapists Specification of unique versus common elements Discrimination from comparison/control approaches Discrimination from other approaches for the disorder Evaluation of treatment process
III	Transportability and dissemination to clinical community	Effectiveness trials	Provide detailed guidelines for implementation of the treatment with diverse patient groups and in a range of clinical settings Provide guidelines for tailoring treatment to different patient subgroups Explicate limits of treatments effectiveness

Note. Adapted from Carroll & Nuro (2002). Reprinted with permission from Blackwell Publishing, © 2002.

TABLE 11.2
General Outline for a Stage I Manual

Section	Content area	Issues to be addressed
I. Overview, description, and rationale	A. General description of the approach	Overview of treatment and goals
	B. Background and rationale for the treatment	• Theoretical rationale • Empirical underpinnings of treatment • Rationale for application of this treatment to this population
	C. Theoretical mechanism of action	Brief summary of hypothesized mechanisms of action, critical "active ingredients"
II. Conception of the disorder or problem	A. Etiological factors	Summary of treatments' conception of the forces or factors that lead to the development of the disorder in a particular individual
	B. Factors believed to be associated with behavior change	According to treatment/theory, what factors or processes are thought to be associated with change or improvement in the problem or disorder?
	C. Agent of change (e.g., patient, therapist, group affiliation)	What is the hypothesized agent of change? Who, or what, is thought to be responsible for change in the disorder?
	D. Case formulation	What is the conceptual framework around which cases are formulated and understood?
	E. How is the disorder/symptoms assessed by the therapist?	Therapist strategy for assessment of the disorder/problem Specification of any standardized assessment to be used
III. Treatment goals	A. Specification and determination of treatment goals	Specification of principal treatment goals Determination of primary versus secondary goals Strategies for prioritization of goals, goal setting with patient
	B. Evaluation of patient goals	Strategies the therapist uses to identify and evaluate patient goals

(continued)

227

TABLE 11.2 *(continued)*

Section	Content area	Issues to be addressed
	C. Identification of other target behaviors and goals	Clarification of other problem areas that can be targeted as secondary goals of the treatment versus those that must be handled outside of the treatment
	D. Negotiation of change in goals	Strategies for renegotiation of goals as treatment progresses
IV. Contrast to other approaches	A. Similar approaches	What are the available treatments for the disorder or problem that are most similar to this treatment? How do these differ from this treatment?
	B. Dissimilar approaches	What treatments for the disorder or problem are most dissimilar to this approach?
V. Specification of defining interventions	A. Unique and essential elements	What are the specific active ingredients, which are unique and essential to this treatment?
	B. Essential but not unique elements	What interventions are essential to this treatment but not unique?
	C. Recommended elements	What interventions or processes are recommended but not essential or unique?
	D. Proscribed elements	• What interventions or processes are prohibited or not characteristic of this treatment? • What interventions may be harmful or countertherapeutic in the context of this treatment?
VI. Session content	Explication of unique and essential elements	Where appropriate, detailed, session-by-session content with examples and vignettes

VI. General format

A. Format for delivery
- Individual, group, family, mixed
- If group, closed- or open-ended format?

B. Frequency and intensity of sessions
- How often do sessions occur? How long are sessions?
- How many sessions should be delivered over what period of time?

C. Flexibility in content
- Are there essential versus "elective" content areas?
- Is there flexibility in sequencing session content areas?

D. Session format
- Length of sessions
- Guidelines for within-session structure

E. Level of structure
- Does the therapist set an agenda for each session? Is this done collaboratively?
- How structured are the sessions? What determines the level of structure in this treatment?
- Who (therapist or patient) talks more?

F. Extra-session tasks
- Are extra-session (e.g., homework) tasks a part of this treatment?
- What is the purpose of extra-session tasks?
- How are specific tasks or assignments selected?
- How does the therapist present a rationale for the tasks?
- How does the therapist assess patient implementation of tasks?
- How does the therapist respond to the patient's completion of an assignment? How is it integrated into the work of therapy?
- How does the therapist respond to the patient's failure to complete an assignment?

Note. Adapted from Carroll & Nuro (2002). Reprinted with permission from Blackwell Publishing, © 2002.

for the disorder (as a means of highlighting its unique elements); and some specification of the treatment's defining characteristics.

Other elements critical to a Stage I–level manual include defining the treatment in terms of its overall structure, including duration, format (e.g., group vs. individual), intensity (number and length of sessions in a given week), level of flexibility versus structure, session format, and so on. Detailed guidelines for the conduct and goals of sessions as well as major content areas to be conveyed to the patient should also be provided. Special attention should be devoted to clarifying and defining those elements of the treatment that are anticipated to distinguish it from the control or comparison approach to which it will be contrasted in an initial pilot feasibility/efficacy study.

The model described by Waltz and colleagues (1993) for delineating treatments in terms of four defining characteristics (its unique and essential elements, essential but not unique elements, recommended elements, and proscribed elements) is an excellent one for defining psychotherapies at all stages. This model is valuable in helping treatment developers sharpen the distinctive features of a given treatment, in training therapists by highlighting the essential defining elements of the approach, and in developing efficient adherence/competence rating systems.

Guidelines for a Stage II Manual

At this stage, the treatment researcher has typically gained some experience with the treatment through one or more pilot studies. Thus, experience with the training and supervision of therapists to conduct the treatment, review of session tapes, and analysis of process and outcome data can be used to expand and elaborate the content areas laid out in Stage I, but also to address additional areas that would have been difficult to articulate without substantial clinical experience with the treatment. Thus, a Stage II–level manual is conceived as one that would be sufficiently comprehensive to serve as the basis of a larger randomized controlled trial. Table 11.3 outlines additional topics to be included at this stage. These include guidelines for troubleshooting, that is, strategies for managing clinical problems that commonly arise in the course of treatment, such as missed sessions, low motivation for treatment, and exacerbation of symptoms, as well as strategies for managing major transitions or clinical choice points in the treatment. Stage II–level manuals should also include a description of the role of nonspecific (common) elements of treatment, their importance to the nature of the treatment, and their relationship to unique or specific aspects of the treatment, with particular emphasis on the role and importance of the therapeutic alliance. Manuals at this stage of development should also address the compatibility of the treatment with other commonly used approaches, including permissible adjunctive treatments (see Rounsaville, Weiss, & Carroll, 1999). Again, clear differentiation of the treatment from the control or comparison conditions to which it may be compared in a Stage II (efficacy) trial is essential.

TABLE 11.3
General Outline of Additional Areas to Be Addressed in a Stage II Manual

Section	Content area	Issues to be addressed
I. Elaborated rationale	Empirical evidence supporting the effectiveness of this approach	• Summary of data on effectiveness of this population, process findings
	Variations by subgroups	• Did preliminary or pilot studies suggest variability in outcome across different patient groups?
II. Troubleshooting	Strategies for dealing with common clinical problems	• Specific guidelines for therapist handling of common issues such as patient lateness, missed sessions, recurrent crises, poor motivation, relapse, intoxication, failure to implement extra-session tasks
		• Are these strategies "generic" or highly specific to this type of treatment?
III. Managing transitions	Guidelines for clinical decision making through stages of treatment	• How does the therapist assess the patient's readiness to move on to a new stage of the treatment?
		• How does the therapist determine whether to repeat/review old material or move on?
		• How does the therapist deal with an apparent clinical impasse?
		• How does the therapist assess core issues to be targeted during treatment?
		• How are shifts in the treatment introduced?
		• How does the therapist handle issues related to termination, including determination of readiness for termination?
IV. Nonspecific or common aspects of treatment	A. Patient-therapist relationship	• What is the ideal therapist role in this treatment (educator, collaborator, teacher, peer, adviser)? What is the patient's role?
		• What is the nature of the optimal or ideal patient-therapist relationship?

(continued)

TABLE 11.3 (*continued*)

Section	Content area	Issues to be addressed
		• How important is the therapeutic relationship to the outcome of the treatment?
		• How important are relationship issues relative to other aspects of the therapy?
		• Strategies the therapist uses to develop desired relationship
		• Strategies the therapist uses to address poor or weak therapeutic relationship
	B. Relationship of common and unique elements	• What is the nature of the relationship between unique and common elements?
		• What characterizes a "good" session of this treatment from a poor one?
V. Compatibility with other treatments	A. Permissibility and limits of adjunctive treatments	• What adjunctive treatments (e.g., medications, family therapy, case management) are permitted, encouraged, or even prohibited?
		• For permitted treatment adjuncts, are there limits on their frequency or intensity?
	B. Role of self-help groups	• Especially for substance abuse treatments, or those where peer- or community-based alternatives are available, how are these handled within the treatment (e.g., neutrally, supportively)?
VI. Therapist selection, training, supervision	A. Therapist selection	• Educational, training, credentialing, and experience requirements for therapists
		• Ideal personal characteristics of therapists
	B. Therapist training	• Components and goals of training, training materials available
		• Issues to be covered in didactic training

	• Number, nature of training cases required
	• Standards for therapist initial certification
	• Common problems encountered in training
	• Standards for determination of therapist adherence and competence
	• Explication of ratings systems and assessments of therapist adherence and competence
C. Therapist supervision	• Educational, credentialing, experience, training requirements of supervisors
	• Recommendations for frequency, type (group, individual), goals, content, and intensity of supervision
	• Strategies to address therapist drift in treatment delivery
	• Strategies to help therapists balance adherence and competence
	• Strategies for supervision sessions; use of videotapes and rating systems
VIII. Clinical care standards	Specification of guidelines for managing clinical issues • How does the therapist assess symptoms that may have occurred since the last session?
	• How does the therapist assess treatment progress?
	• How does the therapist respond to lack of progress or clinical deterioration?
	• How does the therapist assess and respond to expressions of suicidal or homicidal ideation?
	• How does the therapist respond to a contradiction between a patient's self-report of symptoms and a collateral source?

Note. Adapted from Carroll & Nuro (2002). Reprinted with permission from Blackwell Publishing, © 2002.

A particularly crucial component of a Stage II manual is explication of procedures and standards for therapist selection, training, and supervision. These include definition of the level of training and expertise of clinicians who are seen as likely to be competent to implement the treatment. The manual should also describe the minimal training standards for the therapists, for example, the didactic and experiential training each therapist will be required to complete before treating patients in a clinical trial, as well as the goals, intensity, and format of the supervision to be provided. Also essential is clarification of the process by which the therapists' adherence and competence in delivering the treatment are evaluated, for example, through an objective rating system (Barber, Krakauer, Calvo, Badgio, & Faude, 1997; DeRubeis, Hollon, Evans, & Bemis, 1982; Hill, O'Grady, & Elkin, 1992).

Guidelines for a Stage III Treatment Manual

Ideally, prior to the development of a Stage III–level manual, several efficacy trials will have been completed that have evaluated the treatment among diverse clinical samples. Thus, the treatment developer will be in a far better position to articulate how the treatment should, or should not, vary when applied to different populations. Process and outcome data will be available that may inform guidelines regarding the limits of the applicability of the treatment to some patient groups, that is, whether the effectiveness of the treatment varies across clinical subtypes and whether the treatment should not be applied to individuals with specific characteristics (e.g., through patient profiling; see Beutler, 1999). Detailed guidelines regarding how the use of assessment instruments may help clinicians tailor the treatment to the specific patient subgroups may also be provided (see Beutler, 1999).

The treatment may have been evaluated using a wider range of therapists than in the Stage I or early Stage II trials, and the treatment developer may have a sense of what additional training and supervision may be required if more diverse, less experienced, or less committed clinicians are to implement the treatment adequately.

Thus, a Stage III–level manual would be viable only after the completion of several clinical trials and the resultant accumulation of a great deal of process and outcome data for a variety of patient populations. Such a manual would require that treatment guidelines be, essentially, translated from the "ideal conditions" of research to the "reality" of clinical work (Wolfe, 1999). As suggested in Table 11.4, a Stage III manual would provide empirically informed guidance to therapists regarding how the treatment may be adapted to meet the varied needs of patients typically encountered in clinical settings, the limits on the flexibility therapists may use in tailoring the treatment to meet individual patient needs, and strategies for tailoring the treatment to be implemented in different settings, formats, and intensities.

TABLE 11.4
General Outline of Additional Areas to Be Addressed in a Stage III Manual

Section	Content area	Issues to be addressed
I. Issues related to patient diversity	Specification of variations in the treatment for managing different types of patient groups, including LIMITS of the treatment with particular groups	• Managing patients with comorbid disorders, including (as appropriate) depression, anxiety and post–traumatic stress disorders, antisocial personality disorder, concurrent substance use, psychotic disorders, cognitive impairments • Managing patients who have concurrent medical problems • Managing patients who are homeless, have few psychosocial supports • Managing patients who are mandated for treatment • Managing patients who are not motivated for treatment • Managing patients from different cultures, ethnic backgrounds • Managing other patient types commonly encountered in this population
II. Program diversity	Variability of resources	• Delivering treatment in a range of settings, time frames • Managing issues such as imposed length of treatment, number of sessions, and so on • Managed care and third-party reimbursement issues • Managing delivery of treatment in a range of treatment frameworks
III. Implementation by therapists with diverse range of disciplines and experience	Training and supervision	• Common problems involved in training novice therapists to use this approach • Common problems encountered in training experienced therapists to use this approach • Common problems encountered in training therapists with a commitment to a particular orientation to treatment, or conversely to a more eclectic approach • Strategies to help avoid therapist "drift" from adherence to jargon and active ingredients of the treatment • Learning tools available (e.g., training videotapes, suggested background reading in theoretical basis of treatment)

Note. Adapted from Carroll & Nuro (2002). Reprinted with permission from Blackwell Publishing, © 2002.

A critical component of Stage III–level manuals is attention to how the manual may be used by clinicians of greater diversity than those who typically deliver treatment in randomized efficacy trials. Thus, while assumption of basic psychotherapy skills, extensive experience with the patient population, and familiarity with the theoretical basis of a given treatment might be assumed when therapies are implemented solely by highly selected and trained therapists in efficacy trials, it is likely that Stage III manuals will have the burden of articulating, or at least setting minimal standards for, these basics of therapy. Similarly, manuals can, and should, be developed that are appropriate for and address a wider range of patient populations (Munoz & Mendelson, 2005).

■ Developing "Therapist-Friendly" Manuals

Any treatment manual represents at best a detailed guideline, or set of instructions, for a highly complex task. Thus, the clearer, more specific, and more detailed those instructions, the more likely the treatment as practiced will reflect the intention of the treatment's originators and foster greater consistency in treatment delivery and quality across therapists and settings. Therapists may be more accepting of manuals and feel more comfortable and competent in delivering a treatment if they believe the manual can enhance, rather than limit, their clinical expertise (Addis, 1997; Addis & Krasnow, 2000). The following recommendations do not address all the criticisms commonly made of manuals, but they are intended to help treatment researchers developing manuals at all stages develop more "clinician-friendly" manuals by anticipating at least some of these common criticisms.

Anticipate "Real-World" Problems

Treatment manuals sometimes describe theoretically compelling and elegant approaches that bog down quickly in the complex realities of treating challenging patients who present with multiple problems. Some manuals, particularly at those Stages I and II, are written as if for "ideal patients" without comorbid psychopathology or concurrent problems. Clearly, manuals geared only to ideal or uncomplicated patients are likely to be of limited clinical utility. Moreover, although therapist adherence is likely to be high with comparatively "easy" or uncomplicated patients, adherence is likely to be poorer with more impaired, symptomatic, challenging patients who often (directly or indirectly) pressure therapists to deviate from manual guidelines (Foley, O'Malley, & Rounsaville, 1987). Manuals that anticipate that some patients will be challenging, poorly motivated, ambivalent, resistant, inarticulate, or cognitively impaired and that provide explicit guidance for addressing these issues are more likely to foster adherence, consistency, and perhaps even greater effectiveness than manuals that do not address these issues (Carroll & Nuro, 2002).

Provide Troubleshooting Guidelines

In research and clinical practice, few treatments proceed without at least some problems and difficulties along the way. Because therapists may be more likely to deviate from manual guidelines and "borrow" from other familiar approaches when they encounter clinical challenges, clinician-friendly manuals anticipate and provide guidance around handling a range of common clinical problems encountered in treatment. Ideally, guidelines should be provided for handling these common problems in a manner that is consistent with the theoretical background and goals of the treatment. Issues where specific guidelines are particularly likely to be helpful include guidelines for handling lateness to sessions, missed sessions, patients whose lives are so consumed by crises that the work of the therapy may be hampered, patients with low levels of motivation to change or to engage in treatment, and so on. Furthermore, manuals should also provide guidelines for determining when these problems have eclipsed the benefits the treatment might provide, that is, when it is time to refer the patient to another type or more intensive form of treatment.

Don't Ignore the Basics

Therapists frequently have a variety of misconceptions about manuals (Addis et al., 1999; Addis & Krasnow, 2000). Rather than viewing manuals as detailed "blueprints" that define the treatment and guide the therapist, some therapists perceive them as therapeutic straitjackets. Many clinicians are concerned that manuals put too much emphasis on technique, thereby negatively impacting the therapeutic alliance, and that manuals are not flexible enough to meet the needs of patients with comorbid disorders (Addis et al., 1999). It should be noted that while some studies have found evidence to suggest that use of manuals in some therapies may reduce therapist skill (Henry et al., 1993), other studies suggest the opposite (Vinnars, Barber, Noren, Gallop, & Weinrieb, 2005).

Therapists' anxieties usually abate during training as they become more confident in the treatment and their own experience, but manuals themselves can attempt to directly confront this apprehension by clarifying how adherence is to be balanced with clinical judgment. For example, it would be unusual and inappropriate, in any therapy, for a therapist to plunge into difficult therapeutic tasks without first establishing rapport, formulating the case, agreeing on treatment goals, or building a working alliance. However, some manuals (particularly those at Stage I or early Stage II) fail to explicitly point out the importance of these more fundamental tasks of treatment as a prerequisite for moving ahead to other, treatment-specific tasks and instead tend to emphasize specific techniques over competent delivery of those techniques in the context of a positive therapeutic relationship. Although it is clearly easier to specify technique than competence in manuals, the crucial importance of clinical competence should not be ignored when developing treatment manuals. There is emerging consensus that adherence can be enhanced through the use of manuals, but whether manuals can adequately teach, or even convey, competence is much less clear.

Thus, a "clinician-friendly" manual should attempt to articulate definitions of therapist competence (in addition to adherence) in the conduct of the treatment; specify the role of common elements of treatment and how they are to be balanced with treatment-specific techniques; define the fundamental requirements and indicators of progress that must be present before each new stage or technique is undertaken; and provide strategies for addressing difficulties in the therapeutic alliance. Addis and colleagues (1999) point out that articulating and emphasizing the techniques that may play a role in building or strengthening the therapeutic alliance is a potential strategy for countering perceptions that manual-guided treatments undervalue the role of the alliance at the price of effectiveness.

Clarify Choice Points

Therapists conducting manual-guided treatments are frequently faced with a wide array of possible interventions and strategies, often with comparatively little guidance about which intervention to select at different phases of treatment. Clinician-friendly manuals should define important transition points in therapy (e.g., managing transitions between early to middle stages of treatment or from a treatment focused solely on a single principal goal to greater focus on secondary problems) and provide direction to therapists for managing them. Decision trees for determining a patient's stage in treatment and readiness to move on may also be helpful to therapists and may minimize excessive drift or overly aggressive interventions. Provision of clinical rules of thumb, or general strategies the therapist can use to organize complex treatments and maintain appropriate treatment goals, is likely to enhance the usefulness of a manual. An excellent example of this approach is the use of the Core Conflictual Relationship Theme method (Luborsky & Crits-Christoph, 1990) to focus dynamically oriented therapies.

Build in Flexibility and Clarity Regarding Required Versus Optional Elements

Some manuals may give the impression that "all interventions are created equal," that key interventions should be delivered in an invariant format and order in all sessions, regardless of the patient's readiness or individual needs. This is, in fact, rarely so. Treatment developers usually expect that some interventions be present in all sessions and some in only selected sessions, depending on the needs of each patient.

Therapist-friendly manuals have built-in flexibility and clarify the essential, key, active ingredients of the therapy that must be delivered in some or all sessions versus those that are optional or indicated only for specific patients or in particular circumstances. Again, the classification developed by Waltz and colleagues (1993) for defining treatments is an excellent framework for describing the expected salience and intensity of various interventions.

Specification of the strategies the therapist may use to tailor the treatment to meet the needs of different patient types is critical in developing clinician-friendly manuals. Examples include the distinction between "core" versus "elective" sessions in the cognitive-behavioral treatment in Project MATCH (Kadden et al., 1992), the four problem types of interpersonal psychotherapy (IPT; Klerman, Weissman, Rounsaville, & Chevron, 1984), or the personality types in Beck's schema-based approach for personality disorders (Beck & Freeman, 1990).

Furthermore, therapist-friendly manuals make it clear which interventions or behaviors are proscribed in the therapy and, more important, provide feasible "substitutes." That is, if a commonly used therapeutic intervention is proscribed within a treatment manual, manual developers should provide an alternate intervention to be used as a substitute for the commonly used but proscribed one. Finally, clarity regarding possible negative effects or countertherapeutic interventions is likely to enhance the helpfulness of a manual to therapists (Moras, 1993). Clarity regarding countertherapeutic interventions is a critical aspect of treatment definition and is particularly important if a treatment is to be used by relatively novice therapists.

Include Summaries and Outlines

Given the many complex and sometimes competing demands on therapists during the therapy hour, therapists may find it helpful to refer to brief session summaries or outlines to remind them of a few key points to be conveyed. This may be particularly useful in treatments with a more didactic focus, where a number of issues are to be covered in a given session. Similarly, treatment outlines to which therapists may refer just before a session may be extremely helpful in cueing them to key elements to convey during the session (Carroll & Nuro, 2002). We have also found it useful to provide therapists with detailed therapist checklists, which are essentially a therapist self-report version of our adherence/competence ratings systems (Carroll et al., 1998; Carroll et al., 2000). Therapist checklists may encourage clinicians to self-monitor their delivery of key features of the treatment, as well as provide a useful strategy for reminding therapists of critical defining strategies of a given treatment and thus prevent drift in treatment implementation over time.

■ Summary

The limited use of manual-driven, empirically validated treatment in clinical practice is a complex issue and clearly will require much more than clinician-friendly manuals to surmount. Some challenges are inherent in the nature of manuals themselves, which systematize, codify, and often reduce flexibility in a process that is, by nature, complex and highly variable. However, some of these issues might be addressed in part by greater adoption of the stage model of treatment manual development proposed here, which underscores the need for treatment manuals to evolve from meeting the needs of therapists implementing the treatment in highly controlled efficacy trials to the needs of clinicians implementing the treatment in diverse clinical settings. Recognition that a "one-size-fits-all" approach is inappropriate for psychotherapies as well as psychotherapy manuals may be an important step in bridging the divide between research and practice.

■ Acknowledgments

Support was provided by National Institute on Drug Abuse grants P50-DA09241 and K05-DA00457 (KMC), and the U.S. Department of Veterans Affairs VISN 1 Mental Illness Research, Education and Clinical Center (MIRECC). Sections of this chapter first appeared in Carroll and Nuro (2002).

■ References

Ablon, J. S., & Jones, E. E. (2002). Validity of controlled clinical trials of psychotherapy: Findings from the NIMH Treatment of Depression Collaborative Research Program. *American Journal of Psychiatry, 159,* 775–783.

Abrahamson, D. J. (1999). Outcomes, guidelines, and manuals: On leading horses to water. *Clinical Psychology: Science and Practice, 6,* 467–471.

Addis, M. E. (1997). Evaluating the treatment manual as a means of disseminating empirically validated psychotherapies. *Clinical Psychology: Science and Practice, 4,* 1–11.

Addis, M. E., & Krasnow, A. D. (2000). A national survey of practicing psychologists' attitudes toward psychotherapy treatment manuals. *Journal of Consulting and Clinical Psychology, 68,* 430–441.

Addis, M. E., Wade, W. A., & Hatgis, C. (1999). Barriers to dissemination of evidence-based practices: Addressing practitioners' concerns about manual-based psychotherapies. *Clinical Psychology: Science and Practice, 6,* 430–441.

Barber, J. P., Krakauer, I., Calvo, N., Badgio, P. C., & Faude, J. (1997). Measuring adherence and competence of dynamic therapists in the treatment of cocaine dependence. *Psychotherapy Practice and Research, 6,* 12–24.

Beck, A. T., & Freeman, A. (1990). *Cognitive therapy of personality disorders.* New York: Guilford.

Beutler, L. E. (1999). Manualizing flexibility: The training of eclectic therapists. *Journal of Clinical Psychology, 55,* 399–404.

Carroll, K. M., Nich, C., & Rounsaville, B. J. (1998). Use of observer and therapist ratings to monitor delivery of coping skills treatment for cocaine abusers: Utility of therapist session checklists. *Psychotherapy Research, 8,* 307–320.

Carroll, K. M., Nich, C., Sifry, R., Frankforter, T., Nuro, K. F., Ball, S. A., et al. (2000). A general system for evaluating therapist adherence and competence in psychotherapy research in the addictions. *Drug and Alcohol Dependence, 57,* 225–238.

Carroll, K. M., & Nuro, K. F. (2002). One size can't fit all: A stage model for psychotherapy manual development. *Clinical Psychology: Science and Practice, 9,* 396–406.

Carroll, K. M., & Rounsaville, B. J. (2003). Bridging the gap between research and practice in substance abuse treatment: A hybrid model linking efficacy and effectiveness research. *Psychiatric Services, 54,* 333–339.

Castonguay, L. G., Schut, A. J., Constantino, M. J., & Halperin, G. S. (1999). Assessing the role of treatment manuals: Have they become necessary but nonsufficient ingredients of change? *Clinical Psychology: Science and Practice, 6,* 449–455.

Chambless, D. L., & Hollon, S. D. (1998). Defining empirically supported therapies. *Journal of Consulting and Clinical Psychology, 66,* 7–18.

Chambless, D. L., & Ollendick, T. H. (2001). Empirically supported psychological interventions: Controversies and evidence. *Annual Review of Psychology, 52,* 685–716.

Crits-Christoph, P., Baranackie, K., Kurcias, J., Beck, A. T., Carroll, K. M., Perry, K., et al. (1991). Meta-analysis of therapist effects in psychotherapy outcome studies. *Psychotherapy Research, 1,* 81–91.

Crits-Christoph, P., Frank, E., Chambless, D. L., Brody, C., & Karp, J. F. (1995). Training in empirically validated therapies: What are clinical psychology students learning? *Professional Psychology: Research and Practice, 26,* 514–522.

Davis, D. D., O'Brien, M. A., Freemantle, N., Wolf, F. M., Mazmanian, P., & Taylor-Vaisey, A. (1999). Impact of formal continuing medical education: Do conferences, workshops, rounds and other traditional continuing education activities change physician behavior or health care outcomes? *Journal of the American Medical Association, 282,* 867–874.

DeRubeis, R. J., Hollon, S. D., Evans, M. D., & Bemis, K. M. (1982). Can psychotherapies for depression be discriminated? A systematic evaluation of cognitive therapy and interpersonal psychotherapy. *Journal of Consulting and Clinical Psychology, 50,* 744–756.

Dobson, K. S., & Shaw, B. F. (1993). The training of cognitive therapists: What have we learned from treatment manuals? *Psychotherapy, 30,* 573–577.

Foley, S. H., O'Malley, S. S., & Rounsaville, B. J. (1987). The relationship between patient difficulty and therapist performance in interpersonal psychotherapy. *Journal of Affective Disorders, 12,* 207–217.

Henry, W. P. (1998). Science, politics, and the politics of science: The use and misuse of empirically validated treatment research. *Psychotherapy Research, 8,* 126–140.

Henry, W. P., Strupp, H. H., Butler, S. F., Schacht, T. E., & Binder, J. L. (1993). Effects of training in time-limited dynamic psychotherapy: Changes in therapist behavior. *Journal of Consulting and Clinical Psychology, 61,* 434–440.

Hill, C. E., O'Grady, K. E., & Elkin, I. (1992). Applying the Collaborative Study Psychotherapy Rating Scale to rate therapist adherence in cognitive-behavioral therapy, interpersonal therapy, and clinical management. *Journal of Consulting and Clinical Psychology, 60,* 73–79.

Jacobson, N. S., Dobson, K. S., Truax, P. A., Addis, M. E., Koerner, K., Gollan, J. K., et al. (1996). A component analysis of cognitive-behavioral treatment for depression. *Journal of Consulting and Clinical Psychology, 64,* 295–304.

Kadden, R., Carroll, K. M., Donovan, D., Cooney, J. L., Monti, P., Abrams, D., et al. (1992). *Cognitive-behavioral coping skills therapy manual: A clinical research guide for therapists treating individuals with alcohol abuse and dependence.* NIAAA Project MATCH Monograph Series, Vol. 3. DHHS Pub. No. (ADM)92-1895. Rockville, MD: National Institute on Alcohol Abuse and Alcoholism.

Kazdin, A. E. (1995). Methods of psychotherapy research. In B. M. Bongar & L. E. Beutler (Eds.), *Comprehensive textbook of psychotherapy: Theory and practice* (pp. 405–433). New York: Oxford University Press.

Klerman, G. L., Weissman, M. M., Rounsaville, B. J., & Chevron, E. S. (1984). *Interpersonal psychotherapy of depression.* New York: Guilford.

Luborsky, L., & Crits-Christoph, P. (1990). *Understanding transference: The core conflictual relationship theme method.* New York: Basic Books.

Luborsky, L., & DeRubeis, R. J. (1984). The use of psychotherapy treatment manuals: A small revolution in psychotherapy research style. *Clinical Psychology Review, 4,* 5–15.

Luborsky, L., Diguer, L., Seligman, D. A., Rosenthal, R., Krause, E. D., Johnson, S., et al. (1999). The researcher's own therapy allegiances: A "wild card" in comparison of treatment efficacy. *Clinical Psychology: Science and Practice, 6,* 95–106.

Mahrer, A. R. (2005). Empirically supported therapies and therapy relationships: What are the serious problems and plausible alternatives? *Journal of Contemporary Psychotherapy, 35,* 3–25.

Miller, W. R., Yahne, C. E., Moyers, T. B., Martinez, J., & Pirritano, M. (2004). A randomized trial of methods to help clinicians learn motivation interviewing. *Journal of Consulting and Clinical Psychology, 72,* 1050–1062.

Moras, K. (1993). The use of treatment manuals to train psychotherapists: Observations and recommendations. *Psychotherapy, 30,* 44–57.

Munoz, R. F., & Mendelson, T. (2005). Toward evidence-based interventions for diverse populations: The San Francisco General Hospital prevention and treatment manuals. *Journal of Consulting and Clinical Psychology, 73,* 790–799.

Onken, L. S., Blaine, J. D., & Battjes, R. (1997). Behavioral therapy research: A conceptualization of a process. In S. W. Hennegler & R. Amentos (Eds.), *Innovative approaches for difficult to treat populations* (pp. 477–485). Washington, DC: American Psychiatric Press.

Rounsaville, B. J., Carroll, K. M., & Onken, L. S. (2001). A stage model of behavioral therapies research: Getting started and moving on from Stage I. *Clinical Psychology: Science and Practice, 8,* 133–142.

Rounsaville, B. J., O'Malley, S. S., Foley, S., & Weissman, M. M. (1988). Role of manual-guided training in the conduct and efficacy of interpersonal psychotherapy for depression. *Journal of Consulting and Clinical Psychology, 56,* 681–688.

Rounsaville, B. J., Weiss, R. D., & Carroll, K. M. (1999). Options for managing psychotropic medications in drug-abusing patients participating in behavioral therapies clinical trials. *American Journal on Addictions, 8,* 178–189.

Schulte, D., & Eifert, G. H. (2002). What to do when manuals fail: The dual model of psychotherapy. *Clinical Psychology: Science and Practice, 9,* 312–328.

Sholomskas, D., Syracuse, G., Ball, S. A., Nuro, K. F., Rounsaville, B. J., & Carroll, K. M. (2005). We don't train in vain: A dissemination trial of three strategies for training clinicians in cognitive behavioral therapy. *Journal of Consulting and Clinical Psychology, 73,* 106–115.

Silverman, W. H. (1996). Cookbooks, manuals, and paint-by-numbers: Psychotherapy in the 90's. *Psychotherapy, 33,* 207–215.

Street, L. L., Niederehe, G., & Lebowitz, B. D. (2000). Toward greater public health relevance for psychotherapeutic intervention research: An NIMH workshop report. *Clinical Psychology: Science and Practice, 7,* 127–137.

Vakoch, D. A., & Strupp, H. H. (2000). The evolution of psychotherapy training: Reflections on manual-based learning and future activities. *Journal of Clinical Psychology, 56,* 309–318.

Vinnars, B., Barber, J. P., Noren, K., Gallop, R., & Weinrieb, R. M. (2005). Manualized supportive-expressive psychotherapy versus nonmanualized community-delivered psychodynamic therapy for patients with personality disorders: Bridging efficacy and effectiveness. *American Journal of Psychiatry, 162,* 1933–1940.

Waltz, J., Addis, M. E., Koerner, K., & Jacobson, N. S. (1993). Testing the integrity of a psychotherapy protocol: Assessment of adherence and competence. *Journal of Consulting and Clinical Psychology, 61,* 620–630.

Wampold, B. E., & Bhati, K. S. (2004). Attending to the omissions: A historical examination of evidence-based practice movements. *Professional Psychology: Research and Practice, 35,* 563–570.

Weissman, M. M., Verdeli, H., Gameroff, M. J., Bledsoe, S. E., Betts, K., Mufson, L., et al. (2006). National survey of psychotherapy training in psychiatry, psychology, and social work. *Archives of General Psychiatry, 63,* 925–934.

Westen, D., Novotney, C. M., & Thompson-Brenner, H. (2004). The empirical status of empirically supported psychotherapies: Assumptions, findings, and reporting in controlled clinical trials. *Psychological Bulletin, 130,* 631–663.

Wolfe, J. (1999). Overcoming barriers to evidence-based practice: Lessons from medical practitioners. *Clinical Psychology: Science and Practice, 6,* 445–448.

12. SELECTING, TRAINING, AND SUPERVISING THERAPISTS

Cory F. Newman and Judith S. Beck

In order to test the efficacy of a given psychosocial treatment, it is necessary to employ therapists who will be capable of delivering the particular therapy in the manner in which it was intended. That is to say, the therapists will need to be good practitioners in general, knowledgeable about the specific treatment modality (or modalities) being evaluated, conscientious about following the manual and protocol, and motivated to work as a team with fellow therapists and supervisors. This is a tall order, but it is important to strive for a high standard of treatment delivery in order to test the positive limits of what a psychosocial approach can achieve. Thus, investigator(s) will need to be thoughtful and diligent about whom to recruit for the trial, how to train them to a reasonably common standard of competence, and in what ways to supervise their work most effectively. Further, because problems are inherent in any major project of this sort, the investigator(s) will also need to have mechanisms in place to handle the complications and crises that periodically affect protocol therapists and their study clients. The ideal goal is to prevent clinical harm, while maintaining the integrity of the study design.

To ensure that therapists are appropriately selected, trained, and supervised, it is essential that investigators allocate sufficient resources to support these vital aspects of the study. Investigators must be aware, too, that resources may be required not only for an initial set of therapists but also for one or more replacements, if original therapists leave the study before the conclusion of the treatment phase. If the study is underfunded, the investigators risk facing limited options for employing a representative clinical team. Further, the time allotted for training, supervision, and even providing the treatment itself may be insufficient, thus weakening the study.

■ Selection of Therapists

There are a number of factors to consider when recruiting and selecting therapists for participation in a clinical trial. First, regardless of the psychosocial modality being studied, it is essential that therapists are selected for their general interpersonal skills. These are exemplified by their tactful style of communication with clients and colleagues alike, their ability to make their clients feel listened to and understood, and their propensity for demonstrating grace under pressure, such as when their clients are making complaints or threats. Therapists who possess these all-important capabilities will be in the best position to skillfully manage the myriad problems in real-life practice that often interfere with the process of therapy (e.g., when clients are mistrustful of the therapist's intentions). Such skills represent a measure of clinical competence that transcends theoretical orientation, thus serving as a boon to the implementation of any manualized treatment.

Second, prospective protocol therapists should be chosen on the basis of their reliability in meeting clinical responsibilities and their proficiency in keeping accurate data (e.g., administering questionnaires at the correct intervals; promptly and thoroughly recording therapy notes; transmitting data to the project director). Therapists who consistently and punctually attend their supervisory and clinical appointments, keep their charts (and/or computerized databases) up to date, well organized, and well safeguarded, and demonstrate good organizational skills will succeed in maintaining a level of professionalism that assists the study at every level (including reducing potential liability).

Conducting a randomized controlled trial of a psychosocial treatment is a complicated undertaking even under the best of circumstances; therefore, investigators need to be practical in their selection of therapists. They should consider a number of factors in therapist selection, including:

- The therapists' level of experience (e.g., advanced graduate students; postdoctoral fellows; seasoned, licensed therapists; combinations of these)
- Their proximity to training and supervision sites (e.g., employed at the site itself; based in the surrounding community; in a distant office)
- Their familiarity with the model of therapy they will be using in the study (e.g., predominantly trained in the study modality; having some familiarity with the study modality; being new to the modality)

It is often desirable, other factors being constant, to use qualified therapists who are on-site and who have already been trained in the treatment modality being studied. There are both advantages and disadvantages to using skilled novice therapists, depending on the study hypotheses. One potential drawback is that they may not have sufficient clinical experience to deliver the treatment competently across a range of cases. On the other hand, beginning therapists may have a steep enough learning curve; they are often enthusiastic, embrace the model, and welcome supervision. Additionally, their performance may more closely model the real world, where expert therapists are the exception and not the rule. In any event, investigators will need to address the issue of generalizability of findings, whether the therapists are venerable experts, new initiates, or some combination thereof.

Prospective therapists should also be evaluated as to their receptivity to supervisory input. Experienced therapists who have been engaged in independent practice for many years may be unaccustomed to having their work so closely scrutinized and critiqued (e.g., via ratings of the session tapes). It is important that study therapists be open to such feedback and to the learning of new methods with which they may not yet be optimally familiar. With less experienced therapists, it may also be advisable to obtain written recommendations from former supervisors who can attest not only to the therapist's skill in delivering the treatment modality being studied but also to his or her "coachability." With all candidates, it is recommended that investigators obtain a work sample—most often an audiotape or videotape, complete with confirmation of signed consent from the client who was taped—to go along with a general interview, plus documentation of the therapist's training background.

Because clinical trials often take a number of years to execute, it is also desirable for therapists to make a good-faith commitment to remain in the study for its entirety (life-altering events notwithstanding). Continuity of clinical staff is an asset, especially because the recruitment and training of replacement therapists can be labor-intensive and time-consuming. This issue will be discussed further in a later section.

■ Selection of Supervisors

The number of supervisors employed depends on the scope of the study, including its budget. In some situations, the primary investigator serves as the sole clinical supervisor. In other cases, the primary investigator may be part of the supervision team, or may be one of a number of protocol therapists who serve as peer supervisors for each other. In still other instances, the investigator hires outside supervisors whose chief job it is to oversee and evaluate the ongoing clinical work of the protocol therapists.

When investigators recruit prospective supervisors, they typically seek individuals whose professional identity is strongly associated with the treatment model in question, who have extensive experience as clinical supervisors and instructors, and who have developed a reputation for high professional standards of behavior (Weissman, Rounsaville, & Chevron, 1982). Further, it is preferable that supervisors in a randomized controlled trial have an active familiarity with and appreciation of the rigors of an experimental design. Supervisors will need to model fidelity to the treatment approach to their supervisees, and they will be charged with the responsibility of documenting and rating the performance and progress of the therapists. This requires high levels of reliability, diligence, timeliness, and organizational skills. Clinicians who do not possess these qualities—no matter how stellar their reputations in other ways—probably should not be chosen as supervisors in a research protocol.

It is also preferable for the supervisors to commit to participate in the study until its completion. However, if they do not also serve as therapists (and thus do not have any direct contact with clients), it may not be particularly disruptive to the study if they drop out. When this occurs, the other supervisors bear the burden of an increased load, but this is often manageable, especially if their monetary compensation is increased.

■ Initial Training

Prior to initiating the clinical operations of the study, it is advisable to assemble all the therapists and supervisors for an intensive set of meetings, such as a workshop. Ideally, the workshop should span several days, though practical constraints may limit the meetings to 1 or 2 days. Here, the purpose is literally to get everyone on the same page. Participants should be required to read the treatment protocol/manual prior to the initial training meetings, so that they are ready to discuss the material at a sophisticated level. Investigators often give lectures that emphasize the central and most difficult aspects of the protocol. Further, video demonstrations and role-playing of the treatment methods also reinforce the clinicians' understanding of their responsibilities. Ideally, therapists will pick up their training cases promptly, so that they can begin applying what they have learned from the manual and initial training session right away, while the information is most fresh and vivid in their minds.

Workshops alone have not been found to have an enduring effect on the way that clinicians practice (Miller & Mount, 2001). This is why ongoing, regular supervision is vital to the project. However, there is merit in these workshops— both at the start of the study and at various intervals during the course of the study (e.g., every 6 to 12 months)—as a means by which to clarify the responsibilities of the participants, to gauge the flexibility of the manual's mandates, to minimize clinician "drift" (Liese, 1998), and to increase enthusiasm for the research project during the course of the study.

■   Supervision of Practice

Following initial intensive workshop training, therapists should start treating clients using the study protocol. These clients should be similar to those they will later treat in the study itself. It is important for supervisors to review entire audiotapes or videotapes of therapists' sessions before the supervision session itself and to recognize that therapists are often unable, especially initially, to accurately recognize, conceptualize, and report difficulties.

Supervisors must conceptualize what is most important for therapists to learn and plan supervision sessions accordingly, taking into consideration both learning factors (e.g., How much can the therapist absorb? Which supervision techniques—such as case discussion, didactic instruction, description of techniques, role-playing—will be most effective?), and psychological factors (e.g., How should the supervisor approach the therapist? Is the therapist likely to be relatively open to correction, or will he or she be defensive or resistant?). Setting goals with therapists is useful (e.g., "Let's talk about the level we hope you'll achieve by the end of this practice period"). It is important not only to provide clear expectations of supervisors' and therapists' roles vis-à-vis supervision but also to elicit and respond to therapists' reactions to these expectations.

Therapists' learning is enhanced when they believe that their supervisor is respectful, knowledgeable, and collaborative. Therapists, especially those who are inexperienced at following a treatment protocol, may have dysfunctional thinking that can get in the way of providing effective treatment or receiving adequate supervision. Therefore, supervisors should take care to alleviate therapists' undue anxiety by reassuring them, for example, that they have reasonable expectations of the therapists and that the purpose of seeing practice cases is for them to become proficient in carrying out the treatment protocol by the *end* of this practice period.

Supervisors may choose to utilize measures of therapist competency and adherence to the given treatment model even at this early stage of training. Although it may be premature to expect that the protocol therapists will have mastered the details and nuances of the treatment in question during the practice case phase, it is reasonable to expect that the therapists are working toward approximation of this goal. By using rating scales of the therapists' delivery of the treatment, supervisors will be able to assist therapists in bolstering areas of weakness, as well as give positive feedback when the therapists are approaching the necessary standards of competency and adherence.

Often, the categorical items on the measure serve as a "checklist" for *adherence* (e.g., "Is the therapist addressing each of the mandated areas of session structure, clinical assessment, and intervention?"), whereas the level of *competency* is assessed by evaluating how the therapists handled each of the checkpoints (e.g., the proficiency scores on each of the categorical items). If therapists skip important points altogether, the use of a rating scale will alert the supervisor to bring such omissions to the therapists' attention for remediation in upcoming sessions with the practice cases.

A comprehensive listing of the extant measures of competency and adherence in delivering a wide range of psychosocial interventions goes well beyond the scope of a short review chapter on training and supervision; however, the following are a few examples. The Penn Adherence-Competence Scale for Supportive-Expressive therapy (PAC-SE; Barber & Crits-Christoph, 1996) employs a 7-point Likert scale for each of 45 criterion items in terms of both *frequency* and *competency*. The Fidelity of Implementation Rating System (Forgatch, Patterson, & DeGarmo, 2005) is a "measure of competent adherence" to the Oregon Model of Parent Management Training. The Vanderbilt Therapeutic Strategies Scale (VTSS; Butler, Henry, & Strupp, 1995) is a measure of adherence to the tenets of time-limited dynamic psychotherapy (TLDP). A treatment adherence measure was developed for Attachment-Based Family Therapy (ABFT) for depressed adolescents by Diamond, Reis, Diamond, Siqueland, and Isaacs (2002). The Group Sessions Rating Scale (GSRS; Kaminer, Blitz, Burleson, Kadden, & Rounsaville, 1998) is a group therapy measure for substance abuse treatment that includes a check for therapist adherence. The Adherence and Competence Scale for Addiction Counseling (Mercer, Calvo, Krakauer, & Barber, 1994) was developed as a measure of therapist delivery of individualized drug counseling in a multisite study of psychosocial treatments for cocaine addiction (Crits-Christoph et al., 1998).

Protocols involving cognitive therapy often employ instruments such as the Cognitive Therapy Scale (CTS; Young & Beck, 1980). This kind of instrument can help supervisors recognize areas of relative strength, for which they can plan to positively reinforce therapists, and areas of relative weakness, which supervisors will need to point out and help the therapist correct. As an illustration, an audiotaped session may reveal that a cognitive therapist omitted reviewing last week's *homework,* and neglected to ask the client for *feedback* about the session (italicized items indicate that they are on the CTS "checklist" of required elements of cognitive therapy). These would be two subareas of nonadherence to the treatment protocol. At the same time, the therapist may have emphasized *focusing on key cognitions and behaviors,* perhaps succeeding greatly in bringing the client's problematic automatic thoughts to his or her attention. Likewise, on the item *cognitive and behavioral techniques,* the therapist may have implemented a skillful and educative role-playing exercise with the client that merits a high score. This would indicate both adherence and potentially high competency on these items. Similarly, the therapist may have demonstrated a high level of *interpersonal effectiveness* and *understanding* by being able to elicit the client's automatic thoughts in an accurate, accepting, nonshaming fashion, to the point where the client shifted from being reluctant to being eager to do more self-assessment. In sum, the use of the rating scale assists in the process of training and supervision, all the while giving the supervisor an indication of the therapist's readiness for actual study cases.

Guidance is often enhanced when the supervisor structures the supervision session, collaboratively determines what is important to discuss, and elicits feedback from the therapist at the end of the session (Beck, Sarnat, & Barenstein, in press). By doing so, the supervisor will succeed in using training time efficiently, will facilitate a positive working relationship with the therapist-in-training, and will model an approach that can be emulated when working with clients. No matter what the treatment modality, being structured, well organized, and collaborative in supervision will set the tone for therapists to use the training manual and protocol in a faithful way.

■ Ongoing Supervision of Study Cases

Depending on the personnel resources available, a study may opt to employ a format of individual supervision, group supervision, or both. In the individual supervision model, there is a clear role division between therapist and supervisor, whereas in group supervision the roles may be more flexible. For example, group meetings may entail having one supervisor preside over the work of a number of therapists, or they may involve a number of therapists acting as peer supervisors for each other. Whether the supervision is in individual or group format, the participants have the option of meeting in person or communicating by distance media (still achieved most frequently by phone at the time of the writing of this chapter). In our experience, it is possible to conduct group supervision by conference call, if necessary, though there are disadvantages associated with this method. One or more therapists may be able to "hide" on a conference call without participating in an optimal fashion, while others (lacking visual and nonverbal cues from each other) may often talk over each other and cause a decrement of learning for everyone. However, when therapists are scattered geographically, and the number of supervisors is limited, this method becomes a more practical option. If supervision is held long-distance, it is usually more desirable for one therapist to speak by phone on a regular basis with one ongoing supervisor.

Meeting for supervision in person is usually the best option. When therapists can be assembled without too much time, money, and effort being expended, face-to-face contact should be the norm. Aside from the benefits of improving communication, in-person meetings can allow for the review of taped session material in the supervision sessions themselves. It is almost always preferable for a supervisor to review therapy tapes in their entirety before the supervision session, whether the supervisor meets in person or by phone with the therapist. Of course this prospective review of tapes is more practical in the beginning stages of a trial, when only the first few cases have been randomized into treatment. Under these conditions, both individual and group supervisors can give a great deal of attention to the protocol therapist's pressing concerns about his or her new case. Further, there is ample time to illustrate the particular issues the therapist is describing by observing sections of videotape that the therapist has cued to in advance of the meeting. However, as the study progresses and more clients have entered treatment, such individualized attention may be prohibitively time-intensive, though it is still important for supervisors to review therapy tapes regularly. The supervisor and therapist will have to prioritize the most pressing matters for discussion, and some cases may get only fleeting coverage or review.

Reviewing Tapes

Observing therapists' performance in actual sessions is one of the best ways to determine if they are adhering to the treatment protocol (Waltz, Addis, Koerner, & Jacobson, 1993) and allows supervisors the most direct means by which to give corrective feedback. Ideally, session tapes should be reviewed in their entirety so the content and process of treatment can be assessed and understood as a coherent whole. In practice, however, it is often the case that tapes are reviewed in supervision sessions only; in this circumstance, supervisors generally listen to or watch just small sections of a tape so there is time for a lengthy discussion of the case. There are pros and cons to this approach. The advantages include (a) allowing more time for supervisory (individual or group) input into the case, (b) leaving time for the viewing of more than one tape in a given meeting, and (c) being time-effective in terms of focusing specifically on one problematic point in a session where the therapist requests feedback from the clinical team. Drawbacks of this approach include (a) giving the therapist redundant feedback (e.g., the team recommends a course of action that the therapist has already taken, and which perhaps appears in the session minutes after the point at which the tape was stopped), (b) the supervision participants jumping to conclusions about the client's cognitive and behavioral patterns, based on insufficient data, (c) missing the opportunity to learn from watching the natural unfolding of a session, as conducted by a therapist who has been chosen for participation in the study for his or her clinical acumen, and (d) giving off-the-mark advice because important aspects of the session were not played.

Time in supervision seems always to be at a premium, thus making it impractical to implement the sort of supervisory procedures that might maximize the advantages alluded to previously, while minimizing the drawbacks. For example, in an optimal situation where the study therapists and supervisors have extra time to review videotapes between group supervision meetings, it would be advantageous if all the clinicians could view the same tape in its entirety, taking notes and making ratings (e.g., on the CTS if the treatment is cognitive therapy) along the way. Later, when they assemble for supervision, each person could discuss his or her respective observations, hypotheses, evaluations, and recommendations. In this manner, the session in question would have been viewed as a coherent whole, and the therapist's choices of interventions would be understood within a more complete context. In group supervision, each clinician would benefit from seeing the manner in which his or her colleagues perform the treatment, and would gain a better conceptual grasp of the client's problems. Each therapist could submit a tape in rotating fashion, or, alternatively, tapes could be chosen by the team leader based on clinical necessity (e.g., to help a therapist whose confidence is flagging, to provide extra supervision in the case of an acutely suicidal client, to address a particular topic such as homework problems).

In practice, this method typically is not implemented in group supervision. However, it is more likely that tapes can be reviewed in their entirety prior to one-on-one supervision sessions. It is best if multiple supervisors work on the project, because just one or two supervisors will be hard-pressed to find the time to listen to numerous session tapes *and* meet with a number of therapists. In the end, each protocol is funded and/or staffed in such a way that resources need to be utilized optimally but not overtaxed. One of the important challenges for a primary investigator of a clinical trial is to determine the supervisory methods and procedures that will best meet the clinical needs of the clients, the training needs of the therapists, and the specifications for adhering to the protocol, given the time and personnel available. The exact figures may differ, depending on the nature of the study. For example, a primary investigator may determine that a given protocol therapist may be able to treat as many as 10 clients at a given time in a treatment-of-depression study, and still receive adequate supervision and emergency coverage (e.g., DeRubeis et al, 2005; Hollon et al., 2005). On the other hand, the primary investigator may "cap" each therapist at 3 clients at a given time, such as when the disorder under investigation is characterized by frequent clinical crises (e.g., Brown, Newman, Charlesworth, Crits-Christoph, & Beck, 2004).

Feedback

Regardless of whether supervision is conducted on an individual or group basis (or both), it is important for therapists to receive feedback on their performance, both in terms of their general professionalism and specific to the treatment modality they are conducting. General professionalism refers to such factors as the therapist's clinical judgment, regular availability to see clients, consistent attendance for supervision, receptivity to supervisory feedback, investment in the well-being of clients, awareness of the importance of interdisciplinary collaboration and consultation, sensitivity to cross-cultural issues in treatment, dedication to continuing education and professional development, proficiency in keeping documentation up to date, and overall ethical behavior. These criteria are quite similar to the "foundational competencies" (those competencies that cut across the "functional competencies" of assessment, treatment, science-based practice, etc.) identified and promulgated by the American Board of Professional Psychology (n.d.).

One of the ways to maximize the chances that these important professional standards will be achieved and maintained is to select therapists into the study who have already established positive reputations in this regard. By choosing study therapists who have a track record for being responsible, reliable, and thorough, and who maintain good rapport with colleagues, investigators and their supervisors can focus more on the nuts and bolts of the treatment protocol, and less on issues that distract and detract from the central purpose of the research. Further, when study therapists adhere to high standards of professionalism as a matter of routine, the chances that clients or their family members will file official complaints with the institutional review board (IRB) will be reduced.

Investigators and supervisors also must give their therapists ongoing procedural and conceptual feedback that is specific to their delivery of the treatment package. As noted, this objective is most readily achieved via the review of session audiotapes or videotapes because the progress of clients is not always a sufficient indicator of the effectiveness of the therapist.

Procedural feedback pertains to the implementation of manual-based directives. For example, a typical cognitive therapy protocol will instruct therapists to include such procedures as performing a mood check, creating and following an agenda, reviewing and assigning homework, focusing on important client behaviors and cognitions, and exchanging constructive summaries and feedback with the client in each session. When cognitive therapists omit any of these procedural components, supervisors (individual or peer) can readily point out the missing pieces, suggesting to the therapists how and where they can find opportunities to include these central aspects of cognitive therapy during the course of a given session. Supervision can include doing role-playing of these procedures, so therapists can practice the requisite skills. Role-playing becomes quite important when clients engage in therapy-interfering behaviors such as skipping sessions or arriving late to sessions.

Conceptual feedback is important regardless of the degree to which therapists are effectively implementing the procedural aspects of the protocol. In fact, formulating a case accurately is an essential part of planning treatment. Additionally, therapists need to learn how to conceptualize and strategize when roadblocks arise in session, often with the assistance of the supervision team.

For example, consider the case in which a cognitive therapy client is cooperating with the treatment and appears quite eager to do homework. Nevertheless, he is not showing signs of improvement on objective measures of affect or cognition. The therapist is stymied and discusses the case in group supervision, saying, "My client and I are both doing everything we're supposed to be doing, but his condition is not improving!" The group watches sections of a videotape, and each participant proceeds to pose a number of conceptual hypotheses. One peer supervisor offers that the client seemed so eager to please the therapist that he went along with anything the therapist said and did not wish to rock the boat by reporting his doubts or difficulties with any of the interventions or homework. Another peer supervisor asks the therapist about some of the details of the client's everyday life, which helps the therapist recognize that she does not have a clear picture of her client's life outside of therapy—and the group discusses ways for her to collect these missing data to discover what real-life factors may be interfering with treatment (e.g., use the Daily Activity Schedule for homework; see Beck, 1995). Collectively, this feedback allows the therapist to go into the next session prepared to alter the typical agenda, including such items as discussing the client's daily activities in greater depth and assuring the client that it is important for him to provide honest feedback rather than feel obliged always to appear agreeable in session.

Emergency Coverage

Supervision also entails the management of after-hours emergency coverage. The following are some options:

1. The simplest, "bare-bones" model is where the therapists inform each client that they are to proceed to the emergency room—either at their nearest hospital or at a designated hospital affiliated with the study—in the event of a clinical emergency between sessions. If this model is chosen, it is best if the investigators create a formal liaison with the emergency room associated with the research site, so that communication is facilitated.

2. In a more labor-intensive model of supervision, therapists and clients are instructed in how to page the rotating supervisor on call. Upon notification of a crisis, the supervisor becomes responsible (ideally in consultation with the therapist) for determining whether hospitalization is warranted. Clearly, it is vital for supervisors and therapists to maintain a complete and updated list of client addresses and phone numbers, along with a signed consent for study personnel to get in touch with an emergency contact, whose name and phone numbers the client provided upon enrollment in the study. In a recent study on cognitive therapy for borderline personality disorder (Brown et al., 2004), the supervisor on call also obtained the phone numbers of the *district police headquarters* in the towns where clients lived. Therapists should also be encouraged to contact their supervisors directly when an emergent situation requires prompt consultation that cannot wait until the next scheduled supervision meeting.

3. Yet another method of between-sessions and/or after-hours supervisory coverage employs the administrative team (e.g., the scheduling assistants) as contact persons in case of emergency. These personnel will have had prior direct contact with the clients (e.g., in recruitment, calling to make appointments for blind assessments) and will be able to contact and inform the client's therapist, supervisor, or the police.

4. In some instances, a study will mandate that each therapist be responsible for and accessible to his or her clients at all times (with backup coverage being provided when the therapist is ill or away). However, this is not an attractive

prospect for most therapists because it creates the potential for problematic boundary intrusions. The use of a rotating on-call clinician/supervisor as a buffer between the clients and their therapists after hours is typically preferred by the clinical staff as a whole. A possible exception to this policy may be for clients who, in the therapist's and supervisor's judgment are at high risk and are completely unwilling to call anyone else in a time of true suicidal or homicidal crisis.

■ Special Problems and Considerations

In spite of the word *control* indicated in *randomized controlled trial,* the study of psychotherapies is subject to any number of threats to internal validity. Although some of these threats cannot be eliminated without risking violating ethical guidelines for the treatment of human subjects, they often can be avoided or minimized. Therapists who take part in clinical trials have to be trained and supervised to handle (and seek supervisory consultation for) situations in which the genuine needs of the client may conflict with the study protocol. Additionally, investigators may, from time to time, need to replace study therapists who leave the program or are deemed unsuitable to continue, as described next.

Replacing a Study Therapist

Although infrequent, there are times when study therapists (who were assessed as competent at the end of the training period with practice clients) are unable to maintain an adequate level of competence when working with study clients. Even less commonly, they may behave in a manner detrimental to clients and the study. In these cases, the study team needs to assess whether additional training and supervision are likely to help the therapist improve sufficiently or whether the therapist should be replaced. If the therapists in question are able to achieve consistent competency and professional behavior once again through more intensive supervision, investigators can maintain them as study therapists. If they cannot do so, investigators may replace them at once or taper off their participation in the study, ceasing to assign them new cases (but continuing to provide the necessary level of supervision until all their current patients have terminated). Investigators and supervisors will need to be open and honest with therapists (in a sensitive, nonshaming manner) to elicit optimal cooperation and appropriate professionalism.

When a given study therapist is no longer available, investigators who had not previously made contingency plans may have difficulty recruiting an additional appropriate therapist. Sometimes study supervisors can become study therapists, receiving peer supervision to oversee their clinical work. Performing both roles does not generally pose problems if the study team works in a collaborative and congenial manner, roles are defined in terms of tasks rather than status, and the primary goal is the optimal execution of the clinical trial.

It may be more desirable to arrange from the outset to have a backup therapist who has received the same training and supervision as the other therapists, and who uses the protocol on practice cases, but who does not submit client data to be included in the study. These backup therapists may highly value the opportunity to promote their professional development, even if they ultimately are not included in the formal trial.

Problems in the Therapeutic Relationship

Although a positive therapeutic relationship in and of itself is insufficient to ensure therapeutic improvement in clients, it is a vitally important part of almost any psychosocial treatment. Problems in the therapeutic relationship, if left unaddressed, can compromise the treatment as a whole. Thus, study therapists will need to be mindful of stresses and strains in the therapeutic relationship, perhaps delegating other tasks and goals to secondary status during times when collaboration and mutual understanding need to be improved. Some therapists feel torn between focusing on repairing the therapeutic relationship and remaining focused on the task, but this is a false dichotomy. An important part of training and supervision involves demonstrating and reinforcing how therapists can give concerted attention to the therapeutic relationship while still conceptualizing the problems in the alliance in terms that are consistent with the treatment modality.

In fact, a key indicator of the therapist's general professionalism may be his or her ability to identify, address, and manage a strain in the therapeutic alliance. If therapists can be skillful, empathic, and artful in managing problems in the therapeutic relationship and yet remain grounded in the tenets and procedures of the treatment being investigated, this may be a strong criterion for the therapist's competency in the given model per se (Newman, 2007). In cognitive therapy, there is evidence that this sort of hybrid skill is associated with favorable outcome in the treatment of "difficult-to-engage" clients (Trepka, Rees, Shapiro, Hardy, & Barkham, 2004), the likes of whom may take up much of the time in supervisory discussions of cases.

Though not very common, there are times when problems in the therapeutic relationship cannot be resolved. When investigators and supervisors have determined that therapists are unable to preserve the therapeutic relationship, they may choose to reassign the client to a new protocol therapist. In real-life practice, clients do in fact switch from one therapist to another when they have the sense that they might work more effectively or comfortably with someone new. Sometimes making this change helps the client break through to make progress.

A Client Becomes Acutely Suicidal

When clients pose a risk to themselves, hospitalization may be indicated. From a research standpoint, this additional intervention may add "noise" to the interpretation of the data if the client returns to the outpatient treatment protocol, especially if additional medications have been prescribed and taken. When there is a conflict between maintaining the strict integrity of the research protocol and providing for the safety of a client at high, acute risk, safety must be the higher priority.

If clients are hospitalized, the study team must decide what to do at discharge. The team needs to assess the extent to which clients will be able to resume treatment within the study protocol. If it appears that they will not be able to do so, or that further emergency measures will need to be taken, clients' participation in the study should be discontinued. An exception to this guideline is when the target population being studied is usually characterized by suicidal crises. Here, therapists will need to be trained and supervised to handle such situations as part of the protocol, and to be prepared to resume treatment with clients upon discharge from hospital (see Ramsay & Newman, 2005).

Clients Are Distressed When Termination Approaches

Some clients become quite fearful or even angry when their treatment approaches its conclusion. Therapists can minimize clients' distress in several ways. First, if there is a set number (or range) of sessions, therapists should provide a rationale for the fixed length of treatment in the first session. Second, they should indicate the session number each time they meet, as well as the number of sessions that remain (e.g., "Today is our fifth session, so we have seven left"). Third, therapists must take care to discuss issues pertinent to termination well in advance of its occurrence. Despite these measures, some clients will still be upset. Supervision sessions should place strong emphasis on the therapists' management of the clients' concerns about termination. This involves examining the clients' data (e.g., scores on mood inventories), conceptualizing the clients' beliefs, feelings, and actions pertinent to the anticipated termination, and practicing ways of discussing the issues surrounding the clients' self-care goals following the end of therapy. Additionally, the team of investigator(s), supervisor, and therapist needs to give itself sufficient time to make an informed decision about the actual need to extend the client's treatment beyond the planned termination date, in light of any threats to the client's safety. At times, the study design may incorporate a period of additional treatment as deemed appropriate in individual cases, to allow for a more gradual transition from treatment phase to follow-up phase.

Clients Desire Different Treatment During the Follow-Up Phase

Most studies, in the process of obtaining informed consent, ask clients to refrain from receiving outside treatment for a period of time following termination from the study in order to determine maintenance of protocol therapy gains. Therapists must understand that clients have a right to pursue alternative treatments, their signed consent notwithstanding. When clients raise the issue, therapists can discuss the pros and cons of going through a treatment-free follow-up period (e.g., gaining self-efficacy vs. feeling apprehensive), as well as the pros and cons of seeking additional treatment elsewhere (e.g., engaging in a familiar process vs. missing an opportunity to independently practice skills learned in the treatment study). Supervision sessions can utilize techniques such as role-playing in order to prepare for such discussions with clients who imply that they may seek outside treatment.

The Involvement of Clients' Family Members

Another special issue has to do with problematic communications from clients' immediate family members. For example, one therapist frequently received complaints (via e-mail and voice mail) from the wife of one of her protocol clients in a depression study. The wife's messages railed against the study for not producing better results for her husband and actually accused the treatment team of making her husband's condition worse. The therapist obtained consultation and supervision to learn how she could respond in an ethical, appropriate, constructive way. First, she informed the client of these extratherapy communications, stating that his wife was very disconcerted by his poor condition. The therapist gave the client the option of inviting his wife to a session, so that they could discuss their respective views about his level of depression and the treatment plan. The client agreed, and they held a series of conjoint sessions. The client's wife's concerns were addressed, and individual treatment resumed anew.

As this section on special problems and considerations illustrates, it is sometimes desirable to bend the protocol to address a problem that is interfering with the delivery of the intended treatment. Such extraprotocol maneuvers must of course be documented and described in the eventual writing up of the study results. Also, the issues described here warrant the attention of the investigator(s) and the full treatment team because they are often tied to mandates set forth by the IRB, while also providing opportunities for interesting group supervision discussions. Because therapists are on the front line, they must have a working familiarity with handling such situations and must actively conceptualize what is going on with their clients before providing options or definitive answers to the clients' concerns.

■ Summary

Depending on the size and scope of the study, the investigator(s) will have to address some of the following questions:

- How many therapists and supervisors do I need to handle the expected number of clients (taking into consideration their prior expertise and the difficulty of the clinical problem area being treated)? Do I have the resources to hire backup therapists?
- Do I need therapists who are generally experienced? How much experience do they need in the specific treatment modality? Do I need less expert community therapists? Will skilled novices suffice?
- What are the practical constraints in working with therapists? Do they live and work nearby so that convening for training and supervision is logistically manageable? Are they located in places that make it easy for the study clients to attend their therapy sessions and periodic assessments?
- Should supervision be performed individually, in group format, or both? Should the supervisor(s) also serve as therapist(s)? Will supervision involve a hierarchy of authority, or will it be among peers? Will supervision sessions be held in person or via telephone or Internet?
- How frequently should training sessions be held, and how lengthy should those sessions be? How many practice cases are needed (and available) to adequately prepare therapists for the trial?
- How flexible is the training manual, and what are some teachable examples of instances in which the protocol can be stretched to accommodate special circumstances?
- How much time can be allotted to the review and rating of audiotapes or videotapes of sessions? How will therapist competence be assessed?
- How will emergency coverage for clients in crisis be arranged and managed?
- How much training and supervision time will need to be devoted to special problems and considerations in balancing the more extraordinary needs of clients with the goal of maintaining the integrity of the study design? Should this be done at the initial training, or in ongoing supervision as the problems arise, or both?

As this chapter has indicated, the answers to the preceding questions require careful weighing of advantages and disadvantages of a variety of choices, with an overarching goal of maximizing resources and minimizing unpreparedness for problems. The training and supervision of study therapists represent a fluid process, in that participants in a study do not have uniform backgrounds, life situations, or clinical needs, the latter of which may change at any time. The most straightforward and obvious point that can be made is that a clinical trial requires ongoing vigilance and steadfast attention to detail. Establishing set routines for the team of supervisors and therapists can go a long way toward helping them treat their clients effectively, collect data properly, and solve problems promptly.

As a footnote, it is worth noting that participation as a supervisor and/or therapist in a treatment study is the sort of enterprise that creates a sense of bonding among the group members. This is a valuable and enjoyable experience, which—coupled with the professional growth that occurs when striving toward high goals—can make the demands, stresses, and strains of such a project more than worthwhile.

■ References

American Board of Professional Psychology. (n.d.). *The standards manual.* Retrieved October 30, 2006, from http://www.ABPP.org

Barber, J. P., & Crits-Christoph, P. (1996). Development of a therapist adherence/competence rating scale for supportive-expressive dynamic psychotherapy: A preliminary report. *Psychotherapy Research, 6,* 79–92.

Beck, J. S. (1995). *Cognitive therapy: Basics and beyond.* New York: Guilford.

Beck, J. S., Sarnat, J., & Barenstein V. (in press). Psychotherapy-based approaches to supervision. In C. Falendar & E. Shafransky (Eds.), *Casebook for clinical supervision: A competency based-approach.* Washington, DC: American Psychological Association.

Brown, G. K., Newman, C. F., Charlesworth, S. E., Crits-Christoph, P., & Beck, A. T. (2004). An open trial of cognitive therapy for borderline personality disorder. *Journal of Personality Disorders, 18,* 257–271.

Butler, S. F., Henry, W. P., & Strupp, H. H. (1995). Measuring adherence in time-limited dynamic psychotherapy. *Psychotherapy: Theory, Research, Practice, and Training, 32,* 629–638.

Crits-Christoph, P., Siqueland, L., Chittams, J., Barber, J. P., Beck, A.T., Frank, A., et al. (1998). Training in cognitive, supportive expressive, and drug counseling therapies for cocaine dependence. *Journal of Consulting and Clinical Psychology, 66,* 484–492.

DeRubeis, R. J., Hollon, D., Amsterdam, J. D., Shelton, R. C., Young, P. R., Salomon, R. N., et al. (2005). Cognitive therapy vs. medications in the treatment of moderate to severe depression. *Archives of General Psychiatry, 62,* 409–416.

Diamond, G. S., Reis, B. F., Diamond, G. M., Siqueland, L., & Isaacs, L. (2002). Attachment-based family therapy for depressed adolescents: A treatment development study. *Journal of the American Academy of Child and Adolescent Psychiatry, 41,* 1190–1196.

Forgatch, M. S., Patterson, G. R., & DeGarmo, D. S. (2005). Evaluating fidelity: Predictive validity for a measure of competent adherence to the Oregon Model of Parent Management Training. *Behavior Therapy, 36*(1), 3–13.

Hollon, S. D., DeRubeis, R. J., Shelton, R. C., Amsterdam, J. D., Salomon, R. M., O'Reardon, J. P., et al. (2005). Prevention of relapse following cognitive therapy vs. medications in moderate to severe depression. *Archives of General Psychiatry, 62,* 417–422.

Kaminer, Y., Blitz, C., Burleson, J. A., Kadden, R. M., & Rounsaville, B. J. (1998). Measuring treatment process in cognitive-behavioral and interactional therapies for adolescent substance abusers. *Journal of Nervous and Mental Disease, 186,* 407–413.

Liese, B. S. (1998). New developments, advances, and possibilities in cognitive therapy. *Clinical Supervisor, 17*(1), 115–124.

Mercer, D., Calvo, N., Krakauer, I. D., & Barber, J. P. (1994). *Adherence/Competence Scale for Individual Drug Counseling for Cocaine Dependence.* Unpublished measure, Center for Psychotherapy Research, Department of Psychiatry, University of Pennsylvania.

Miller, W. R., & Mount, K. A. (2001). A small study of training in motivational interviewing: Does one workshop change clinician and client behavior? *Behavioural and Cognitive Psychotherapy, 29,* 457–471.

Newman, C. F. (2007). The therapeutic relationship in cognitive therapy with difficult-to-engage clients. In P. Gilbert & R. L. Leahy (Eds.), *The therapeutic relationship in* the cognitive-behavioral psychotherapies (pp. 165–184). London: Routledge-Brunner.

Ramsay, J. R., & Newman, C. F. (2005). After the attempt: Repairing the therapeutic alliance following a serious suicide attempt by a patient. *Suicide and Life-Threatening Behavior, 35,* 413–424.

Trepka, C., Rees, A., Shapiro, D. A., Hardy, G. E., & Barkham, M. (2004). Therapist competence and outcome of cognitive therapy for depression. *Cognitive Therapy and Research, 28,* 143–157.

Waltz, J., Addis, M. E., Koerner, K., & Jacobson, N. S. (1993). Testing the integrity of a psychotherapy protocol: Assessment of adherence and competence. *Journal of Consulting and Clinical Psychology, 61,* 620–630.

Weissman, M. M, Rounsaville, B. J., & Chevron, E. (1982). Training psychotherapists to participate in psychotherapy outcome studies. *American Journal of Psychiatry, 139,* 1442–1446.

Young, J., & Beck, A. T. (1980). *Cognitive therapy rating scale manual.* Unpublished manuscript, University of Pennsylvania.

13. ENSURING TREATMENT INTEGRITY

Arthur M. Nezu and Christine Maguth Nezu

Also referred to in the psychotherapy outcome literature as treatment fidelity, treatment integrity essentially focuses on the assurance that any therapy intervention under investigation was actually implemented in a competent manner in accord with the theoretical and procedural elements of the related underlying conceptual model, usually delineated in a treatment manual (Nezu & Nezu, in press; Vermilyea, Barlow, & O'Brien, 1984). Without documentation to determine whether the intervention was provided to study participants according to such a protocol, the ultimate findings remain vulnerable to alternative interpretations. In other words, in addition to controlling for other threats to internal validity, the principal investigator (PI) must ask two crucial questions: (a) Was the therapy (or therapies) being studied carried out by the providers in keeping with the recommendations prescribed by the treatment manual? and (b) Was it implemented in a competent manner? (Waltz, Addis, Koerner, & Jacobson, 1993). The first question addresses the concern of *therapist adherence*, whereas the second focuses on *therapist competence*. If two or more therapies are being evaluated within the context of the same study, a related issue involves *treatment differentiation*, or the ability to tell the difference between or among treatment protocols.

In this chapter, we define and describe the concepts of therapist adherence and competence, as well as provide examples of various measures previously developed to assess these constructs specific to certain types of clinical interventions (e.g., cognitive therapy, multisystemic family therapy). We also address the issue of whether enhanced adherence and competence predict improved patient outcome. The final section provides a set of guidelines for researchers interested in developing treatment integrity measures for their outcome studies.

■ Treatment Adherence

The first aspect of treatment integrity within the context of a randomized controlled trial (RCT) is the valid *implementation* of a specific therapeutic protocol. For investigations assessing the efficacy of a particular biological agent (e.g., antidepressant medication), this would involve, in part, ensuring that the correct amount of the active ingredient is actually contained in the medication (e.g., a pill). In such a study, it is likely that the pharmaceutical company manufacturing and providing study medications would have already addressed this issue of quality control. Unfortunately, psychotherapy researchers seeking to test the efficacy of a particular psychosocial intervention do not have this luxury—in other words, they cannot assume that even highly trained treatment providers will be able to consistently and reliably adhere to the therapy manual at hand. Differences can potentially occur concerning the levels of treatment adherence among therapists, as well as for the same therapist across study patients. Especially when an investigation is conducted over the course of several years, as is often the case in large RCTs, therapists are vulnerable to "drift," that is, changing the manner in which they conduct therapy due to, for example, boredom, lowered diligence, increased competence due to experience, or actual patient change.

If a psychosocial intervention is not delivered as originally intended by the principal investigator, thereby potentially changing the dosage or actual nature of the intervention, outcome results can be vulnerable to alternative explanations. For example, consider if at the end of an RCT no differences are found between Treatment A and a no-treatment control condition with regard to reductions in anxiety symptomatology. One possible interpretation is that Treatment A is not efficacious as a treatment for anxiety. However, an equally plausible interpretation is that Treatment A, in fact, was not delivered properly; rather, a diluted or "distorted" version of Treatment A was actually implemented. As such, this version of Treatment A would not be expected to reduce anxiety in a significant manner because it did not contain a sufficient dose of the prescribed active ingredients hypothesized to be effective in addressing anxiety.

Similar alternative interpretations are possible regarding the opposite scenario, where Treatment A *is* found to be associated with statistically significant differences in outcome as compared with a control condition. Unfortunately, if there is no quality control protocol (i.e., treatment adherence check) included in the RCT that allows the PI to determine the degree to which the implemented treatment was done in accord with the treatment manual, one cannot be certain that what actually led to such differences was in fact Treatment A. Poor adherence to Treatment A in this case does not necessarily equal ineffective therapy. It is possible, for example, that Treatment A can be highly effective but not for the reasons inherent in the investigator's hypotheses. Overall, then, limited treatment adherence can be seen to potentially impact negatively on a study's internal validity, external validity, construct validity, and statistical conclusion validity (Moncher & Prinz, 1991; Nezu & Nezu, in press).

Developing a well-articulated and operationally defined therapy manual can increase substantially the probability that therapists will adhere more diligently to a treatment protocol. That is, the better that therapists' behaviors are operationally defined, for example, the more probable a treatment provider is able to perform such behaviors. However, consider the old adage—"The proof of the pudding is in the eating." In other words, actual documentation of the degree to which therapists actually adhere to a manual is required. Therefore, a standard aspect of any RCT should be the inclusion of a therapist adherence assessment protocol (Nezu, 2001).

Treatment Adherence Measures

An example of a measure to assess treatment adherence was originally developed by Hollon et al. (1988) for the National Institute of Mental Health (NIMH) Treatment of Depression Collaborative Research Program (TDCRP; Elkin, Parloff, Hadley, & Autry, 1985) and called the Collaborative Study Psychotherapy Rating Scale (CSPRS). The final version of this scale contains 96 items and includes three modality-specific scales addressing each of three different treatments for depression evaluated in the TDCRP (i.e., cognitive-behavioral therapy, interpersonal therapy, clinical management), as well as several additional scales that assess generic therapeutic behaviors (e.g., facilitation, directiveness). Each of the three modality-specific scales contains several relevant subscales. For example, the cognitive-behavioral therapy (CBT) scale contains the following six subscales: cognitive rationale, assessing cognitive processes, evaluating and changing beliefs, behavioral focus, homework, and collaborative structure. The CSPRS was initially found to have acceptable psychometric properties, as well as being able to distinguish among the three treatments during the initial pilot and training phases of this multicenter research endeavor.

Using this scale, Hill, O'Grady, and Elkin (1992) assessed therapist adherence to the three treatment approaches as represented by four sessions from 180 patients who participated in the TDCRP treatment phase. Results from their investigation found the CSPRS to be able to reliably discriminate among the three treatments, with interrater reliability in rating adherence being high.

Markowitz, Spielman, Scarvalone, and Perry (2000) developed a revised version of the CSPRS to be specifically applicable to assess therapist adherence for providers treating depressed HIV-positive patients. The RCT was designed to compare four different interventions—cognitive-behavioral therapy, interpersonal psychotherapy, and supportive psychotherapy alone or with imipramine. The scale was found to reliably discriminate among the four treatments, with each scoring highest on its own scale.

Another example of this type of assessment tool is the 26-item Therapist Adherence Measure (Henggeler & Borduin, 1992), developed with specific regard to the family-based intervention known as multisystemic therapy (MST; Borduin, 1999). A factor analysis conducted by Henggeler, Melton, Brodino, Scherer, and Hanley (1997) yielded the following six factors: therapist adherence to the MST principles, the degree to which a session was nonproductive, efforts extended by the family and therapist to solve problems, therapist attempts to change the family's interactions, lack of therapeutic direction in a session, and degree of family-therapist consensus.

Additional formal measures of treatment adherence specific to a particular evidence-based therapy approach also exist, but as part of larger integrity protocols developed to assess both therapist adherence and competence. These will be described later in the section addressing competence.

Is Adherence Related to Outcome?

Although ensuring that treatment providers adhere to the prescribed intervention protocol fosters improved internal validity of an RCT, it has also been hypothesized that enhanced adherence should lead to improved patient outcome (Yeaton & Sechrest, 1981). Unfortunately, the literature overall provides equivocal support for this assumption (Perepletchikova & Kazdin, 2005). For example, on the negative side of the coin, although the CSPRS described earlier in this chapter was able to reliably discriminate among the three treatments included in the NIMH TD-CRP study, and that adherence was found to be high across interventions, treatment adherence was *not* found to be related to the outcome of either the cognitive-behavioral or interpersonal treatment conditions (Elkin, 1999).

DeRubeis and Feeley (1990), in evaluating the relationship between therapist adherence to the methods of cognitive therapy and depression outcome, found that adherence to "abstract" discussions did not predict improvement, although therapist adherence to "concrete," symptom-focused methods of cognitive therapy was associated with patient outcome.

In addition, in a study by Barber, Crits-Christoph, and Luborsky (1996) that examined the relationship between adherence and depressive symptom change regarding supportive-expressive dynamic psychotherapy, initial results indicated that adherence regarding both supportive and expressive techniques was not predictive of changes in depression as measured from session 3 to posttreatment. However, the reverse was true—that is, early improvement in patient symptomatology (i.e., between intake and session 2) predicted enhanced therapist adherence. In other words, it appeared that the more that patients benefited initially from treatment, the easier it was for therapists to adhere to the treatment manual.

Not only has adherence been found to be unrelated to patient outcome, but in a study by Castonguay, Goldfried, Wiser, Raue, and Hayes (1996), increased adherence to one aspect of cognitive therapy for depression (i.e., focus on the impact of distorted thoughts on depressive symptoms) was actually found to be *negatively* correlated with posttreatment outcome. In fact, results indicated that when cognitive therapists increased their adherence to cognitive rationales and techniques to correct problems in the therapeutic alliance (i.e., the quality of the patient-therapist interaction), such an increased focus actually *worsened* this alliance, thereby impacting negatively on treatment gains.

CHAPTER 13: Ensuring Treatment Integrity   **267**

In support of the positive predictive relationship between adherence and outcome, Bright, Baker, and Neimeyer (1999) found that therapist adherence to two different manual-based treatments (i.e., cognitive-behavioral therapy, mutual support) was found to be significantly associated with greater improvement in clinician-rated depressive symptoms in both conditions.

In addition, Henggeler et al. (1997) found therapist adherence to MST for violent and chronic juvenile offenders and their families to be significantly related to outcome. In a related investigation, this one focusing on substance-abusing delinquents, adherence to MST was found to be associated with decreased criminal activity and out-of-home placements (Henggeler, Pickrel, & Brondino, 1999). In another study conducted by members of the same team, therapist adherence to the MST protocol was found to be associated with improved family relations, as well as decreased delinquent peer affiliation, which, in turn, was related to decreased delinquent behavior (Huey, Henggeler, Brondino, & Pickrel, 2000).

More recently, Barber et al. (2006) found a curvilinear relationship between therapist adherence and patient outcome with regard to the National Institute on Drug Abuse Collaborative Cocaine Treatment Study, as well as an interaction between this effect and therapeutic alliance early in treatment. Specifically, for patients who reported a strong therapeutic alliance with their counselor, provider adherence to the treatment protocol was found to be irrelevant to treatment outcome. In contrast, when the alliance was weaker, a moderate level of counselor adherence was associated with better outcome. These findings suggest that adherence may not be related to outcome in a straightforward manner; rather, adherence and the patient-therapist relationship may influence each other in important ways as they impact on patient change (see also Castonguay et al., 1996).

■ Therapist Competence

The second major dimension of treatment integrity involves therapist or provider competence. Essentially, good adherence does not necessarily equal high competence. It is possible that a given therapist can adhere very closely to the prescriptions contained in the treatment manual but does so in a less than competent manner. In other words, therapist adherence refers to the occurrence or nonoccurrence of a given set of provider behaviors (e.g., "provides empathetic response when patients describe initial reasons why they decided to enter the research study"), but it does not capture the notion of the *quality* of such adherence. Thus, in order to accurately assess the impact of a given intervention, it is important that the treatment is conducted as prescribed in a competent manner. Otherwise, once again, it is difficult to state with any confidence that the treatment that was implemented was actually the one that was *intended* to be implemented. This generally requires that the individuals providing protocol therapy in an RCT are well trained, in terms of both the therapy process in general and the intervention(s) under investigation in particular. However, even if substantial previous experience is required and significant training in the protocol intervention occurs, without a formal assessment of this dimension, the assumption that the treatment implemented was done so in a competent manner remains untested. Therefore, along with an evaluation of therapist adherence, provider competence should also be assessed formally in any RCT (Nezu & Nezu, 2005).

Measures of Therapist Competence

An example of a measure of therapist competence is the Cognitive Therapy Scale (CTS), developed by Young and Beck (1980), which consists of 11 items divided into two conceptually defined subscales—general therapeutic skills and specific cognitive therapy skills. The general skills subscale contains 6 items (i.e., agenda, feedback, understanding, interpersonal effectiveness, collaboration, pacing), whereas the specific skills subscale includes 5 items (i.e., guided discovery, focus on key cognitions/behaviors, strategy for change, application of cognitive-behavioral techniques, homework).

Based in part on mixed findings regarding the psychometric properties of the CTS (e.g., Dobson, Shaw, and Vallis [1985] found this scale to have high internal consistency and high interrater reliability, whereas studies by Jacobson et al. [1996] and Crits-Christoph et al. [1998] found interrater reliability to be low), Liese, Barber, and Beck (1995) developed a subsequent measure of treatment integrity specific to cognitive therapy, the Cognitive Therapy Adherence and Competence Scale (CTACS). This scale consists of 25 items and is divided into five sections—cognitive therapy structure, development of a collaborative therapeutic relationship, development and application of the case conceptualization, cognitive and behavioral techniques, and overall performance. Barber, Liese, and Abrams (2003) assessed the psychometric properties of the revised 21-item CTACS and found interrater reliabilities to be acceptable for both the adherence and competence measures. In addition, the relationship between adherence and competence was found to be very high, and the ability to distinguish between cognitive therapy and two other treatment modalities was also found to be strong.

Additional measures of competence in conducting cognitive therapy have been developed. Milne, Claydon, Blackburn, James, and Sheikh (2001), for example, revised the CTS to include new items (i.e., "facilitation of emotional expression," "general facilitation around the experiential cycle," "charisma and flair") in order to take into account a patient's experiential learning or emotion expression. Two additional measures were developed to assess treatment integrity when conducting cognitive therapy for patients with psychotic features (Haddock et al., 2001; Startup, Jackson, & Pearce, 2002).

Another example of a formal system to measure therapist adherence and competence emanates from the National Institute on Drug Abuse (NIDA) Collaborative Cocaine Treatment Study referred to earlier. The multicenter project was essentially designed to evaluate the efficacy of four psychosocial-based interventions: cognitive therapy plus group drug counseling (GDC), supportive-expressive (SE) psychotherapy plus GDC, individual drug counseling, and GDC alone (Crits-Christoph et al. 1999). In order to adequately assess treatment integrity issues in this large project, several specific measures of adherence and competence were developed. For the individual drug counseling (IDC) component, Barber, Mercer, Krakauer, and Calvo (1996) developed the Adherence/Competence Scale for IDC for Cocaine Dependence that includes 43 items. Members of this same team also developed the Adherence/Competence Scale for SE for Cocaine Dependence (Barber, Krakauer, Calvo, Badgio, & Faude, 1997) to assess the integrity of the supportive-expressive intervention. This latter scale consists of three major subscales—supportive (13 items), expressive (31 items), and cocaine abuse (11 items). The CTACS (Liese et al., 1995) described earlier was used to assess fidelity in the project with regard to the cognitive therapy component.

A recent investigation focusing specifically on treatment integrity in this NIDA study by Barber, Foltz, Crits-Christoph, and Chittams (2004) found that both therapists' adherence and competence for all three major treatments (CT, SE, IDC) were rated reliably during early and late sessions and that treatment providers did make use of the techniques contained in the respective manuals rather than those from differing manuals. As a consequence, judges were able to also reliably discriminate among the three treatments.

Another example of a formal system that measures treatment integrity involves the Yale Adherence and Competence Scale (YACS) that was developed specifically with regard to behavioral interventions for substance use disorders (Carroll et al., 2000). This measure includes three scales that assess general aspects of drug abuse treatment (i.e., assessment, general support, treatment goals), as well as three scales that measure conceptually critical elements of three treatments that are often implemented as comparison or control conditions in RCT research in the addictions—clinical management, 12-step facilitation, and cognitive-behavioral therapy. An evaluation of its psychometric properties found it to have strong reliability, factor structure, and concurrent and discriminant validity. Additionally, the correlations between adherence and competence scores were in the moderate range, suggesting that they are assessing independent constructs. An example of an item from the General Support scale, as rated for both quantity (i.e., adherence) and quality (i.e., competence), is as follows: "To what extent did the therapist communicate confidence that patient efforts will yield success in the future?" Quantity is rated along a 5-point Likert scale, where 1 = "not at all" and 5 = "extensively," whereas quality is judged along a similar scale using similar anchor points.

Several measures have also been developed during the past several years that address treatment integrity concerns as a function of the increased popularity of motivational interviewing (MI). MI is a directive client-centered strategy for eliciting behavior change via helping clients to explore and resolve ambivalence (Miller & Rollnick, 2002). Although MI is showing promise as an effective intervention for a variety of behaviors (e.g., Burke, Arkowitz, & Menchola, 2003), significant variability has been identified among investigations with regard to how descriptions of training, supervision, and monitoring of MI therapists are described (Madson, Campbell, Barrett, Brondino, & Melchert, 2005). Therefore, the need to formally assess fidelity dimensions becomes increasingly important (Madson & Campbell, 2006). Such measures include the Motivational Interviewing Skill Code (Miller, 2000), the Motivational Interviewing Process Code (Barsky & Coleman, 2001), the Motivational Interviewing Treatment Integrity Scale (Moyers, Martin, Manual, Hendrickson, & Miller, 2005), and the Motivational Interviewing Supervision and Training Scale (Madson et al., 2005). In their review of these measures, Madson and Campbell (2006) note some problems with reliability and validity across assessment procedures and call for further evaluation and refinement of these inventories.

Is Therapist Competence Related to Outcome?

Similar to the literature addressing the relationship between therapist adherence and patient outcome, studies focusing on the association between therapist competence and treatment outcome have also yielded somewhat conflicting results. For example, using the data focusing only on the cognitive therapy arm of the NIMH TDCRP, Shaw et al. (1999), after controlling for therapist adherence and certain "facilitative factors," found that provider competence did predict patient improvement, but only with regard to the clinician rating of depression, and not for the self-report measures included in the study. In addition, the component of competence that was found to be the most highly correlated with treatment outcome involved a provider's ability to structure the treatment (e.g., setting an agenda, pacing, and homework assignment and review), as compared with a therapist's general or CBT-specific skill levels.

Contrary to the Shaw et al. (1999) study, Trepka, Rees, Shapiro, Hardy, and Barkham (2004) reported that competency ratings of therapists providing cognitive therapy to depressed patients were a significant predictor of decreases in depression as measured by a self-report measure of depression. Moreover, this association was found to be stronger with regard to those patients who completed treatment as compared with those who did not.

Adding to this picture of conflicting results, Weisman et al. (2002) evaluated the association between therapist adherence and competence and treatment outcome regarding a family-focused intervention for patients with bipolar disorder and their relatives. No significant findings between treatment integrity ratings and outcome were found. Moreover, in direct contradiction to the investigation's hypotheses, patients who eventually relapsed and had to be hospitalized were seen by therapists who were actually rated as *more* competent in their ability to conduct certain aspects of the family therapy protocol.

In another study that evaluated the efficacy of cognitive therapy (Davidson et al., 2004), therapist competence at a 6-month follow-up was found to be associated only with observer-rated depression, and not other self-ratings and observer ratings of functioning, self-harm, and anxiety. At the 12-month follow-up, therapist competence was found to significantly predict all the observer ratings, but not with regard to self-report measures. Moreover, therapist competence was not related to the frequency of self-harm episodes.

Finally, in an investigation that involved the treatment of personality problems via schema-focused therapy, Hoffart, Sexton, Nordahl, and Stiles (2005) found that therapist competence was associated with reductions in maladaptive schemas as measured from pre- to posttreatment, but was unrelated to across-session changes. In this study, competence influenced outcome independent of the construct of "connection," which was defined as the intimacy and mutual engagement between a patient and therapist.

■ Treatment Differentiation

The ability to differentiate between two or more treatments becomes an issue of treatment integrity in those RCTs that include more than one intervention that is being evaluated. On an initial level, this requires that the therapy manuals are distinct enough such that little overlap among the various treatments exists. Conceptually, it is rather easy, for instance, to distinguish between a treatment that primarily involves training in relaxation skills as a means of reducing anxiety as compared with an intervention that emphasizes verbal interactions between the therapist and study patient where the therapist creates a therapeutic environment of "normalizing the anxiety." However, if two therapies are compared and they involve differing "talk therapies," it becomes crucial to develop the manuals in such a manner as to underscore their differences. If not, although the therapies may be conceptually distinct, such differences may disappear in their implementation (Kazdin, 1986).

This becomes especially crucial in studies where the same therapist provides the differing treatments. Inadvertently, or deliberately, two therapies may become indistinguishable because a given therapist combines the different approaches. Having formal mechanisms to assess therapist adherence and competence can also allow for a test of this question. As noted previously, such measures have been developed and used to successfully differentiate among various therapies including in a given RCT (e.g., Burke et al., 2004; Hill et al., 1992).

■ Developing and Implementing a Treatment Integrity Protocol:
Suggested Guidelines

In this final section, we draw heavily from Nezu and Nezu (in press) in offering
practical guidelines for researchers interested in developing and implementing
a treatment fidelity component when designing and conducting an RCT. Only
in cases where one is interested in replicating previous studies that have been
found to be efficacious and did include a treatment integrity assessment can
one use the same fidelity protocol. Obvious examples include the evaluation of
an evidence-based psychotherapy protocol, such as cognitive therapy for depression, that is associated with an agreed-upon treatment manual. However,
although various forms of psychotherapy, including cognitive therapy, have
been found to be highly efficacious for various psychological disorders, one
cannot simply use the same treatment manual (and the same integrity assessment protocol) when applying it to different populations, such as patients with
differing comorbidities, or other demographic dissimilarities from the patient
population that was the included in the initial efficacy studies, such as gender,
age, sexual orientation, ethnicity, or cultural or socioeconomic status (Nezu,
Nezu, & Lombardo, 2004). As such, treatment manuals, as well as treatment fidelity protocols, even if previously found to be efficacious, need to be revised
with specific relevance to the population to be studied.

1. *Do include a treatment integrity protocol.* For all the reasons highlighted
throughout this chapter, we view it as imperative that all RCTs include measures
of treatment adherence and therapist competence (Nezu, 2001). Unfortunately,
formal reviews of the literature have indicated that psychotherapy outcome researchers have been amiss when addressing treatment integrity issues (e.g.,
Armstrong, Ehrhardt, Cool, & Poling, 1997; Billingsley, White, & Munson, 1980;
Gresham, MacMillan, Beebe-Frankenberger, & Bocian, 2000; Moncher & Prinz,
1991). For example, we recently conducted a survey of cognitive-behavioral outcome studies that were published between 1991 and 2000 in two journals—
Behavior Therapy (*BT*) and the *Journal of Consulting and Clinical Psychology*
(*JCCP*; Wilkins, Nezu, & Nezu, 2001). In *BT* during this period, 56 outcome investigations were identified. Of these articles, 21.4% conducted a formal assessment of treatment adherence; none addressed the issue of therapist competence.
For *JCCP*, 168 cognitive-behavioral intervention studies were identified. Of
these, 29.2% measured and reported adherence data; close to 10% included an
evaluation of therapist competence. As a follow-up, we subsequently focused on
the years 2001–2003 and added two additional journals that publish cognitive-
behavioral RCTs (*Behavior Research and Therapy, Cognitive Therapy and Research*; Nezu, Slome, Wilkins, & Nezu, 2004). Across these four journals, we
identified 114 such outcome investigations. Of these reports, although potentially denoting an increase in awareness, still less than half (approximately 43%)
included a formal method to assess the degree to which providers adhered to a

treatment manual. In addition, only 10.5% of the 114 RCTs included a formal procedure to assess provider competence.

2. *Think of treatment integrity as an integral part of the study.* Treatment integrity should not be an afterthought. In actuality, it should be considered as one of several interacting phases during the development and implementation of an outcome study. The first phase can be considered the hypothesis generation stage (i.e., concretizing the eventual specific set of questions that a study will be addressing). The second involves the development of a treatment manual (or manuals) that represents the operational definition of treatment(s) under investigation. A third phase in this endeavor involves training therapists or intervention providers. This should entail both the development of standardized training protocols in order to ensure that all therapists are trained in a similar manner, as well as the training itself. A fourth phase involves the development of a treatment integrity protocol, which should include a measure of therapist adherence and competence, and a means by which treatments can be differentiated if more than one intervention is being assessed.

Each phase should provide corrective feedback to the other stages in this process. For example, when training providers, it is possible that trainees may not understand what they should do in a given situation (e.g., what to do if a study participant does not complete a homework assignment for the second time) because the therapy manual does not provide such information. Such concerns should lead the investigators to revise the manual accordingly. Another example involves a situation when training integrity raters to assess for adherence. If an item is initially ambiguous regarding what should be rated (e.g., is the therapist providing empathy?), this should lead to revisions in either the treatment manual or the manner in which therapists are trained. In this way, investigators should view all such phases of developing and implementing a research study as having reciprocal influences.

3. *Develop the treatment manual with integrity issues in mind.* Given the notion of reciprocal relationships among the various development phases as noted earlier, investigators should keep the following in mind when developing treatment manuals: (a) Be certain to operationalize all treatment ingredients in concrete, understandable terms; (b) specify the structure of the intervention at all phases (e.g., group vs. individual, minutes per sessions, sequence of events); (c) specify provider *behaviors* (what to do and how to do it) when describing therapy components (e.g., therapist should explain the treatment rationale in detail, providing examples that are specific to the participant at hand); (d) provide relevant examples of "competent" versus "incompetent" behaviors; (e) differentiate provider behaviors by context if relevant (i.e., same behavior might be enacted differently at different times throughout the treatment); (f) build in flexibility (i.e., specifically state what to do if a study participant comes into a session with a new crisis when a new concept is slated to be taught that session); and (g) continuously revise until treatment integrity and treatment manuals are in sync.

4. *Develop training protocol with integrity issues in mind.* In a similar vein with regard to the reciprocal relationship between training therapists and treatment integrity, investigators should keep the following in mind when developing a training program for the providers: (a) Specify "job requirements" (i.e., define what previous training and practical experiences one needs in order to qualify for training); (b) develop a structured training protocol in order to standardize training; (c) specify training goals; (d) train providers in a consistent manner (across treatment sites and across time); (e) specify ongoing provider behaviors (e.g., the types of session notes that foster adherence and competence regarding the therapy under investigation); and (f) revise as part of the feedback loop among all development phases.

5. *Identify and appropriately operationally define those aspects of treatment that are considered crucial for integrity measurement.* Waltz et al. (1993) has identified four types of therapist behaviors that address treatment integrity: (a) those behaviors that are unique to a given intervention and essential to it (e.g., conducting relaxation induction for stress management training); (b) those behaviors that are essential to a treatment but not unique to it (e.g., establishing a positive therapeutic alliance); (c) behaviors that are compatible with the intervention under investigation but neither necessary nor unique (e.g., providing a treatment rationale); and (d) behaviors that are proscribed (e.g., assigning homework).

Another means of categorizing therapist behaviors involves the following (Nezu & Nezu, 2004): (a) *relationship-building behaviors* (those behaviors geared to foster a positive therapist-patient relationship, such as offering an empathetic response when the patient describes distressing experiences); (b) *protocol implementation behaviors* (those activities concerned with the mechanics of conducting treatment, such as describing the structure of future sessions); (c) *protocol-specific behaviors* (those behaviors that are unique to a given protocol but unrelated to specific hypothesized mechanisms of action, such as fostering group cohesion when the use of a group is not considered the essential means of achieving behavior change); and (d) *treatment-specific behaviors* (those activities that are unique and essential to a given intervention, such as identifying one's negative thinking that serves as a trigger for depression).

Using these types of classification approaches not only can provide for a comprehensive assessment of treatment adherence and therapist competence but also can help to discriminate among various treatments under investigation, as well as provide for useful process-outcome assessments. For example, one can determine the amount of variance accounted for in predicting outcome related to different types of therapist behaviors (e.g., relationship-building versus treatment-specific behaviors). In this way, a finer analysis of treatment outcome and those factors responsible for the outcome can be attained.

6. *Match the method by which integrity will be assessed with the question being asked.* The actual method of assessing fidelity often depends on the types of integrity issues a study raises, or which types of process-outcome questions are

being hypothesized. For example, adherence can be measured in terms of occurrence versus nonoccurrence, frequency, and or consistency. Competence can be measured along the dimensions of skill level, comprehensiveness of behavior, appropriateness of behavior, adeptness of behavior, and/or timing of behavior. Definitions of competence are closely tied to the operational definitions of an investigator's hypotheses regarding essential treatment components. The concern here is to ensure that all concepts are adequately and overtly defined.

An example of a therapist behavior that might be conceptually important in a particular group therapy protocol is "facilitates positive group interaction." Consider using a scale of 1 to 5, where 1 = not at all competent and 5 = very competent. A possible operational definition of a "1"-rated behavior is as follows:

> Provider never mentions idea of group interaction, does not ask follow-up questions of other group members based on what another participant stated, does not attend to issue of ensuring all group members have a chance to speak.

A rating of 5 (highly competent) behavior might be defined as follows:

> Provider mentions idea of positive group interaction and does engage in behaviors conducive to this, for example, asks follow-up questions of other group members based on what another participant stated, attends to issue of ensuring all group members have a chance to speak; in addition, engages in such behaviors in a therapeutic manner and repeatedly highlights the importance of positive group interaction throughout the session; provides continuous feedback to group members about this issue.

7. *Develop measures of behavior change principles.* In addition to focusing on specific therapist behaviors that occur in any given session, it may also be important to include "summary measures" that assess more global use of behavior change principles (Nezu & Nezu, 2004). For example, rather than only evaluating the competent frequency of teaching a patient to think in terms of "stimulus-behavior-response" within a cognitive-behavioral approach to treatment, a summary measure might also be included that asks raters to determine the degree to which such a principle was "taught, fostered, elicited, and reinforced" *throughout* a given session (or across sessions).

8. *Develop or use measures that provide for independent sources of fidelity.* During the earlier stages of assessing adherence in the literature, investigators relied on the therapists themselves to report the degree to which they adhered to a treatment manual. Just as an investigator would not rely on a therapist's judgment as the sole dependent variable regarding patient improvement, so should he or she not use providers as the primary source of integrity. Moreover, due to potential bias, neither should they be the judge of their own competence levels.

9. *Develop a protocol that provides for an adequate basis to assess fidelity.* Rating all sessions for integrity issues can be costly. However, this cost needs to be balanced against the concern for adequately evaluating fidelity. One issue concerns the difference between videotape and audiotape. Videotape is generally preferred but is more expensive and can potentially influence patient behaviors because it can be intrusive. It also can become more complicated from an ethics perspective (i.e., easier to identify a patient). However, if this leads one to choose audiotaping to obtain data for integrity analysis, it is important to remember to develop fidelity items in such a manner that precludes raters from having to "see" the behavior in order to rate it (e.g., do not define establishing a positive therapeutic relationship by having the therapist "maintain good eye contact" if audiotaping).

This issue also suggests that when developing treatment integrity measures, one needs to identify which sessions are essentially different from each other. For example, interventions are usually characterized by a first session in which therapists introduce themselves, provide for a treatment rationale, attempt to establish an initial positive relationship with a patient, describe the future structure, and so forth. This is usually vastly differently than the third session, for example, that is likely to be more treatment intensive. Evaluating all sessions for integrity is also likely to be costly, so when one randomly selects sessions to be reviewed, such differences among sessions should be taken into consideration (e.g., randomly select from blocks of sessions to identify ones to be rated for integrity). As an example, with regard to a protocol that involves 10 sessions of weekly individual therapy provided by four different therapists, the following approach can be applied: Randomly select 30% of all first sessions by therapist, randomly select 30% from all sessions numbered 2 through 9 by therapist, and randomly select from all last sessions by therapist. In this manner, one can obtain a more representative group of sessions.

10. *Develop standardized protocol for integrity raters.* Especially if fidelity raters are not seasoned experts, it is important to develop an integrity protocol that is standardized for all raters. This suggests that any training for such raters also be standardized. It is important to train raters to a predefined minimum level of competency to rate fidelity. As in other assessment situations that involve ratings, one should also check for interrater reliability.

11. *Assess the relationship between treatment integrity and patient outcome directly.* Perepletchikova and Kazdin (2005) provide excellent recommendations regarding this type of research, including controlling for various confounding factors (e.g., therapist characteristics), experimentally manipulating treatment integrity itself (e.g., vary the extent to which integrity procedures are implemented among conditions), and using various novel assessment and evaluation strategies (e.g., indirect assessment methods, such as written homework assignments).

■ Summary

This chapter focused on the issue of treatment integrity (also referred to as treatment fidelity), which is concerned with answering two basic questions with regard to treatment outcome studies: Did therapists adhere to treatment manuals, and did they do so in a competent manner? Although the basic assumption underlying the need for treatment integrity assessment suggests that the better the integrity, the better the outcome, the extant literature offers conflicting data. However, especially with the increased consensus across scientific disciplines regarding what constitutes the proper conduct of RCTs (e.g., CONSORT guidelines; see Chapter 2 of this volume), it is considered essential that all outcome investigations pay close attention to this issue. Last, various guidelines were offered to investigators interested in developing integrity measures as part of their outcome studies.

■ References

Armstrong, K. J., Ehrhardt, K. E., Cool, R. T., & Poling, A. (1997). Social validity and treatment integrity data: Reporting in articles published in the *Journal of Developmental and Physical Disabilities*, 1991–1995. *Journal of Developmental and Physical Disabilities, 9*, 359–376.

Barber, J. P., Crits-Christoph, P., & Luborsky, L. (1996). Effects of therapist adherence and competence on patient outcome in brief dynamic therapy. *Journal of Consulting and Clinical Psychology, 64*, 619–622.

Barber, J. P., Foltz, C., Crits-Christoph, P., & Chittams, J. (2004). Therapists' adherence and competence and treatment discrimination in the NIDA Collaborative Cocaine Treatment Study. *Journal of Clinical Psychology, 60*, 29–41.

Barber, J. P., Gallop, R., Crits-Christoph, P., Frank, A., Thase, M. E., Weiss, R. D., et al. (2006). The role of therapist adherence, therapist competence, and alliance in predicting outcome of individual drug counseling: Results from the National Institute on Drug Abuse Collaborative Cocaine Treatment Study. *Psychotherapy Research, 16*, 229–240.

Barber, J. P., Krakauer, I., Calvo, N., Badgio, P. C., & Faude, J. (1997). Measuring adherence and competence of dynamic therapists in the treatment of cocaine dependence. *Journal of Psychotherapy, Practice and Research, 6*, 12–14.

Barber, J. P., Liese, B. S., & Abrams, M. J. (2003). Development of the Cognitive Therapy Adherence and Competence Scale. *Psychotherapy Research, 13*, 205–221.

Barber, J. P., Mercer, D., Krakauer, I., & Calvo, N. (1996). Development of an adherence/competence rating scale for individual drug counseling. *Drug and Alcohol Dependence, 43*, 125–132.

Barsky, A., & Coleman, H. (2001). Evaluating skill acquisition in motivational interviewing: The development of an instrument to measure practice skills. *Journal of Drug Education, 31*, 69–82.

Billingsley, F., White, O. R., & Munson, R. (1980). Procedural reliability: A rationale and an example. *Behavioral Assessment, 2,* 229–241.

Borduin, C. M. (1999). Multisystemic treatment of criminality and violence in adolescents. *Journal of the American Academy of Child and Adolescent Psychiatry, 38,* 242–249.

Bright, J. I., Baker, K. D., & Neimeyer, R. A. (1999). Professional and paraprofessional group treatments for depression: A comparison of cognitive-behavioral and mutual support interventions. *Journal of Consulting and Clinical Psychology, 67,* 491–501.

Burke, B. L., Arkowitz, H., & Menchola, M. (2003). The efficacy of motivational interviewing: A meta-analysis of controlled clinical trials. *Journal of Consulting and Clinical Psychology, 71,* 843–861.

Carroll, K. M., Nich, C., Sifry, R. L., Nuro, K. F., Frankfurter, T. L., Ball, S. A., et al. (2000). A general system for evaluating therapist adherence and competence in psychotherapy research in the addictions. *Drug and Alcohol Dependence, 57,* 225–238.

Castonguay, L. G., Goldfried, M. R., Wiser, S., Raue, P. J., & Hayes, A. (1996). Predicting the effect of cognitive therapy for depression: A study of unique and common factors. *Journal of Consulting and Clinical Psychology, 64,* 497–504.

Crits-Christoph, P., Siqueland, S., Blaine, J., Frank, A., Luborsky, L., Onken, L. S., et al. (1999). The NIDA Collaborative Cocaine Treatment Study: Rationale and methods. *Archives of General Psychiatry, 54,* 721–726.

Crits-Christoph, P., Siqueland, S., Chittams, J., Barber, J. P., Beck, A. T., Frank, A., et al. (1998). Training in cognitive, supportive-expressive, and drug counseling therapies for cocaine dependence. *Journal of Consulting and Clinical Psychology, 66,* 484–492.

Davidson, K. W., Scott, J., Schmidt, U., Tata, P., Thorton, S., & Tyrer, P. (2004). Therapist competence and clinical outcome in the prevention of parasuicide by manual assisted cognitive behaviour therapy trial: The POPMACT study. *Psychological Medicine, 34,* 855–863.

DeRubeis, R. J., & Feeley, M. (1990). Determinants of change in cognitive therapy for depression. *Cognitive Therapy and Research, 14,* 469–482.

Dobson, K. S., Shaw, B. F., & Vallis, T. M. (1985). Reliability of a measure of the quality of cognitive therapy. *British Journal of Clinical Psychology, 24,* 295–300.

Elkin, I. (1999). A major dilemma in psychotherapy outcome research: Disentangling therapists from therapies. *Clinical Psychology: Science and Practice, 6,* 10–32.

Elkin, I., Parloff, M. B., Hadley, S. W., & Autry, J. H. (1985). NIMH Treatment of Depression Collaborative Research Program. *Archives of General Psychiatry, 42,* 305–316.

Gresham, F. M., MacMillan, D. L., Beebe-Frankenberger, M. E., & Bocian, K. M. (2000). Treatment integrity in learning disabilities intervention research: Do we really know how treatments are implemented? *Learning Disabilities Research and Practice, 15,* 198–205.

Haddock, G., Devane, S. Bradshaw, T., McGovern, J., Tarrier, N., Kinderman, P., et al. (2001). An investigation into the psychometric properties of the Cognitive Therapy Scale for Psychosis (CTR-Psy). *Behavioural and Cognitive Psychotherapy, 29,* 221–233.

Henggeler, S. W., & Borduin, C. M. (1992). *Multisystemic Therapy Adherence Scales.* Unpublished manuscript. Medical University of South Carolina.

Henggeler, S. W., Melton, G. B., Brodino, M. J., Scherer, D. G., & Hanley, J. H. (1997). Multisystemic therapy with violent and chronic juvenile offenders and their families: The role of treatment fidelity in successful dissemination. *Journal of Consulting and Clinical Psychology, 65,* 821–833.

Henggeler, S. W., Pickrel, S. G., & Brondino, M. J. (1999). Multisystemic treatment of substance abusing and dependent delinquents: Outcomes, treatment fidelity, and transportability. *Mental Health Services Research, 1,* 171–184.

Hill, C. E., O'Grady, K. E., & Elkin, I. (1992). Applying the Collaborative Study Psychotherapy Rating Scale to rate therapist adherence in cognitive-behavior therapy, interpersonal therapy, and clinical management. *Journal of Consulting and Clinical Psychology, 60,* 73–79.

Hoffart, A., Sexton, H., Nordahl, H. M., & Stiles, T. C. (2005). Connection between patient and therapist and therapist's competence in schema-focused therapy of personality problems. *Psychotherapy Research, 15,* 409–415.

Hollon, S. D., Evans, M. D., Auerbach, A., DeRubeis, R. J., Elkin, I., Lowery, A., et al. (1988). *Development of a system for rating therapists for depression: Differentiating cognitive therapy, interpersonal therapy and clinical management pharmacotherapy.* Unpublished manuscript, Vanderbilt University.

Huey, S. J., Henggeler, S. W., Brondino, M. J., & Pickrel, S. G. (2000). Mechanisms of change in multisystemic therapy: Reducing delinquent behavior through therapist adherence and improved family and peer functioning. *Journal of Consulting and Clinical Psychology, 68,* 451–467.

Jacobson, N. S., Dobson, K. S., Truax, P. A., Addis, M. E., Koerner, K., Gollan, J. K., et al. (1996). A component analysis of cognitive-behavioral treatment for depression. *Journal of Consulting and Clinical Psychology, 64,* 295–304.

Kazdin, A. E. (1986). Comparative outcome studies of psychotherapy: Methodological issues and strategies. *Journal of Consulting and Clinical Psychology, 54,* 95–105.

Liese, B. S., Barber, J. P., & Beck, A. T. (1995). *The Cognitive Therapy Adherence and Competence Scale.* Unpublished manuscript, University of Kansas Medical Center.

Madson, M. B., & Campbell, T. C. (2006). Measures of fidelity in motivational interviewing: A systematic review. *Journal of Substance Abuse Treatment, 31,* 67–73.

Madson, M. B., Campbell, T. C., Barrett, D. E., Brondino, M. J., & Melchert, T. P. (2005). Development of the Motivational Interviewing Supervision and Training Scale. *Psychology of Addictive Behaviors, 19,* 303–310.

Markowitz, J. C., Spielman, L. A., Scarvalone, P. A., & Perry, S. W. (2000). Psychotherapy adherence of therapists treating HIV-positive patients with depressive symptoms. *Journal of Psychotherapy Practice and Research, 9,* 75–80.

Miller, W. R. (2000). *Motivational Interviewing Skill Code (MISC): Coder's manual.* Unpublished manuscript, University of New Mexico.

Miller, W. R., & Rollnick, S. (2002). *Motivational interviewing: Preparing people to change* (2nd ed.). New York: Guilford.

Milne, D., Claydon, T., Blackburn, I.-M., James, I., & Sheikh, A. (2001). Rationale for a new measure of competence in therapy. *Behavioural and Cognitive Psychotherapy, 29,* 21–33.

Moncher, F. J., & Prinz, R. J. (1991). Treatment fidelity in outcome studies. *Clinical Psychology Review, 11,* 247–266.

Moyers, T., Martin, T., Manual, J. K., Hendrickson, S. M. L., & Miller, W. R. (2005). Assessing competence in the use of motivational interviewing. *Journal of Substance Abuse Treatment, 28,* 19–26.

Nezu, A. M. (2001, July). *Are we doing what we say we are doing? The importance of assessing treatment integrity.* Invited address presented to the World Congress of Behavioural and Cognitive Therapies, Vancouver, Canada.

Nezu, A. M., & Nezu, C. M. (2004, November). *Developing treatment integrity protocols for CBT outcome research: Ensuring manual adherence and therapist competence.* Advanced Methodology and Statistics Seminar presented to the Association for Advancement of Behavior Therapy, New Orleans.

Nezu, A. M., & Nezu, C. M. (2005). Comments on "Evidence-based behavioral medicine: What is it and how do we achieve it?": The interventionist does not always equal the intervention—The role of therapist competence. *Annals of Behavioral Medicine, 29,* 80.

Nezu, A. M., & Nezu, C. M. (in press). Treatment adherence and therapist competence. In D. McKay (Ed.), *Handbook of research methods in abnormal and clinical psychology.* Thousand Oaks, CA: Sage.

Nezu, A. M., Nezu, C. M., & Lombardo, E. R. (2004). *Cognitive-behavioral case formulation and treatment design: A problem-solving approach.* New York: Springer.

Nezu, A. M., Slome, B., Wilkins, V. M., & Nezu, C. M. (2004, November). *Assessment of treatment integrity in randomized clinical trials evaluating CBT interventions: An update.* Paper presented to the Association for Advancement of Behavior Therapy, New Orleans.

Perepletchikova, F., & Kazdin, A. E. (2005). Treatment integrity and therapeutic change: Issues and research recommendations. *Clinical Psychology: Science and Practice, 12,* 365–383.

Shaw, B. F., Elkin, I., Yamaguchi, J., Olmstad, M., Vallid, T. M., Dobson, K. S., et al. (1999). Therapist competence ratings in relation to clinical outcome in cognitive therapy of depression. *Journal of Consulting and Clinical Psychology, 67,* 837–846.

Startup, M., Jackson, M., & Pearce, E. (2002). Assessing therapist adherence to cognitive-behavior therapy for psychosis. *Behavioural and Cognitive Psychotherapy, 30,* 329–339.

Trepka, C., Rees, A., Shapiro, D. A., Hardy, G. E., & Barkham, M. (2004). Therapist competence and outcome of cognitive therapy for depression. *Cognitive Therapy and Research, 28,* 143–157.

Vermilyea, B. B., Barlow, D. H., & O'Brien, G. T. (1984). The importance of assessing treatment integrity: An example in the anxiety disorders. *Journal of Behavioral Assessment, 6,* 1–11.

Waltz, J., Addis, M. E., Koerner, K., & Jacobson, N. (1993). Testing the integrity of a psychotherapy protocol: Assessment of adherence and competence. *Journal of Consulting and Clinical Psychology, 61,* 620–630.

Weisman, A., Tompson, M. C., Okasaki, S., Gregory, M. J., Goldstein, M. J., Rea, M., et al. (2002). Clinicians' fidelity to a manual-based family treatment as a predictor of the one-year course of bipolar disorder. *Family Process, 41,* 123–131.

Wilkins, V. M., Nezu, A. M., & Nezu, C. M. (2001, November). *Treatment integrity in CBT: A 10-year "report card."* Paper presented to the Association for Advancement of Behavior Therapy, Philadelphia.

Yeaton, W., & Sechrest, L. (1981). Critical dimensions in the choice and maintenance of successful treatments: Strength, integrity, and effectiveness. *Journal of Consulting and Clinical Psychology, 49,* 156–167.

Young, J., & Beck, A. T. (1980). *The development of the Cognitive Therapy Scale.* Unpublished manuscript, Center for Cognitive Therapy, Philadelphia.

SECTION IV

DATA ANALYSIS ISSUES

14. DATA ANALYTIC FRAMEWORKS: ANALYSIS OF VARIANCE, LATENT GROWTH, AND HIERARCHICAL MODELS

C. Hendricks Brown, Tracy E. Costigan,
and Kimberly T. Kendziora

Many psychosocial investigations are concerned not only with outcome at one point in time but also with the pathway toward clinical improvement or prevention of poor outcomes over an extended period, such as across multiple treatment sessions, generalization to other contexts or follow-up periods, or across stages of life. The analysis of data from longitudinal research designs requires special treatment of repeated measures or developmentally related measures to arrive at accurate interpretations of results. This chapter addresses three major statistical approaches to longitudinal data analysis relevant to randomized controlled trials (RCTs): *analysis of variance models* (ANOVAs), *latent growth models* (LGMs), and *hierarchical linear models* (HLMs), or their generalization, *hierarchical models* (HMs). We also describe some use of nonlinear *generalized additive models* (GAMs).

■ Case Example: Baltimore Prevention Program

Throughout this chapter, the Baltimore Prevention Program's first RCT (Dolan et al., 1993; Kellam et al., in press) will serve as a case example to illustrate the various data analytic strategies. The Baltimore Prevention Program is conceptually grounded in *life course/social field theory* (Kellam, Branch, Agrawal, & Ensminger, 1975), which views behavior in the context of the social field (e.g., family of origin, classroom, or peer) in which it occurs. As the salience of these social fields varies throughout development, each has its own specific task demands to which all individuals respond. Each social field has natural raters, such as the teacher in the classroom, who rates the child's behavior either using formal measures, such as grades, or through informal means. Ratings of the process of demand and response are called *social adaptational status* (SAS). The theory holds that earlier SAS dimensions predict later SAS, such as school suspension. SAS is also reciprocally related to internal feelings about oneself, or psychological well-being. Thus, life course/social field theory emphasizes both the contextual and individual influences that enhance or inhibit the risk of mental health, behavioral, or social outcomes (Kellam, 1990; Kellam et al., 1975; Kellam & Ensminger, 1980; Kellam & Rebok, 1992).

Using this theory as a guide, the Baltimore Prevention Program applied a *prevention science* strategy, directing interventions at known early risk factors (disruptive classroom behavior and poor achievement); determining whether the risk factors improved; and then following participants to see if the distal outcomes of concern (e.g., youth violent behavior, drug use, school failure) were affected. To target the risk factor of poor achievement, the Mastery Learning (ML) program was administered (Dolan et al., 1993). To target disruptive classroom behavior, the Good Behavior Game (GBG) was implemented (Barrish, Saunders, & Wolf, 1969; Dolan et al., 1993).

Study Design

Three or four schools were selected in each of five sociodemographically distinct areas in eastern Baltimore, Maryland. Within these clusters, schools were randomly assigned to one of three conditions: ML, GBG, or no intervention control. Within each school, children were assigned to first-grade classrooms so as to be balanced within schools, and then classrooms within each school were randomly assigned to either that school's intervention condition or control. Teachers were randomly assigned to intervention conditions and implemented the classroom interventions following intensive training. Intervention and control teachers received equal attention and incentives. Design details are available in Kellam et al. (in press), and the statistical merits of this classroom randomized trial are described in Brown and Liao (1999).

Study Participants

Beginning in 1985, two successive cohorts ($N_1 = 1,196$; $N_2 = 1,115$) of urban first graders were recruited from 43 classrooms in 19 elementary schools and followed up yearly into middle school. Of the 2,311 children originally enrolled in Cohorts 1 and 2, 62% remained enrolled in the Baltimore City Public School System (BCPSS) at the end of the 1993–1994 year. Departure from BCPSS or transfer from a project to nonproject school was unrelated to assigned condition. During a 1998–2001 follow-up, when these former first graders were 19 to 21 years old, 1,648 (71%) of the members of Cohorts 1 and 2 were interviewed.

Measures

Extensive multimethod measurement of participants in the trials was carried out over a 15-year period, until study children were young adults. In addition to student self-report, investigators used teacher, parent, and peer report measures of social adaptational status and self-reports of psychological well-being, as well as direct observation of behavior and collection of school records. Most measures were administered during the fall and spring of each cohort's first-grade year, then each spring thereafter through seventh grade. As each cohort reached 19 to 21 years of age, researchers conducted comprehensive, standardized telephone interviews. Further information about measures may be obtained on the Johns Hopkins Center for Prevention and Early Intervention Web site (http://www.jhsph.edu/prevention/).

■ Analytic Frameworks for Evaluating Intervention Impact

Statistical modeling in randomized trials aims to explain intervention impact in terms of the patterns of variation within subjects over time, between subjects, and within different contexts. Intervention impact requires examination of changes in variance within and across subjects, and examination of the relationships among variables across time and dimension. The goal is to find the best fitting, most parsimonious model of intervention impact for the data from which inferences can be reasonably drawn. In RCTs, there are two particular emphases to statistical analysis: (a) modeling within-subject change across time, and (b) investigating the factors of greatest influence on subject change, including treatment effects on an entire group of individuals (e.g., students), on a particular subset (e.g., low achievers), or across a continuous baseline risk status measure (e.g., reading achievement; Brown, 1993b; Brown & Liao, 1999). Statistical tools for examining these questions are presented in this chapter; a glossary is included to help navigate the terms used to describe these models.

Historically, analysis of variance (ANOVA) and regression were used as the primary analytic procedures to investigate models involving repeated measures data. These techniques, though quite flexible in their ability to deal with a range of data issues (i.e., numbers of independent and dependent variables, categorical or continuous predictors, repeated observations, and fixed and random factors), have a limited ability to handle (a) nonindependence of observations, (b) complex growth trajectories, and (c) complex causal processes (i.e., path analysis). With advancements in methodologies and programming during the last decade, more complex techniques have been developed that are more readily accessible to the clinical or prevention researcher. These procedures include *hierarchical modeling* (HM)—often called multilevel modeling, random effect, or mixed modeling (Laird & Ware, 1982)—and *latent growth modeling* (LGM), which is linked closely to a *structural equation modeling* (SEM) framework. Though handled separately in many introductory texts, models in one framework can often be expressed in terms of another. In fact, many ANOVA models can be thought of as special cases of the more complex HM and LGM procedures, and either LGM or HM models can be expressed in terms of the other (Wang, Brown, & Bandeen-Roche, 2005).

■ Analysis of Variance Models

ANOVA and its closely related extensions test the effects of one or more independent variables on one or more dependent variables. As the simplest type, a one-way ANOVA examines the relationship of a single independent categorical variable, or factor, on the mean of a single continuous dependent variable. For example, in the Baltimore Prevention Program, one might examine differences between intervention type (i.e., GBG, ML, or control) on the outcome of teacher ratings of student aggressive behavior (the Baltimore team used the Authority Acceptance Subscale of the Teacher Observations of Classroom Adaptation—Revised [TOCA-R]; Werthamer-Larsson, Kellam, & Wheeler, 1991) using a one-way ANOVA model. Moreover, a second factor such as gender might be added to the model to account for differences between girls and boys in terms of the outcome. This factorial ANOVA not only would be used to investigate differences in TOCA-R between intervention types and difference in ratings as a function of gender but also could test how the effect of intervention on TOCA-R ratings may vary differentially by gender (i.e., the interaction between treatment type and gender). Multifactor ANOVA can also be used to test combined interventions, for example, varying the combination of reading and behavioral interventions in a single classroom.

Various ANOVA Designs

More complex extensions of ANOVA include repeated measures ANOVA, mixed ANOVA models, analysis of covariance (ANCOVA), and multivariate analysis of variance-covariance (MANOVA) models (Draper & Smith, 1998; Fisher, 1925; Scheffé, 1999; Morrison 2002). This class of analytical models is purposely broad; more than one categorical or continuous independent variable (IV) can be used, and one or more continuous dependent variable (DV) can be included. Repeated measures ANOVA and mixed ANOVA models also allow for the inclusion of random effects that can account for variation of results attributable to the person or at the level of classrooms, schools, and neighborhoods.

The specification of the particular ANOVA model used in an RCT varies greatly as a function of the number and types of data to be included in the study, the design conditions involving the level of random assignment, and the specific research questions that are being tested. Nonetheless, the same underlying principles apply to this family of analytic techniques. Table 14.1 summarizes common alternatives in ANOVA modeling techniques. In an RCT, data are usually collected at a minimum of two time periods—pretreatment and posttreatment—and preferably at one or more follow-up time periods. To test for changes in TOCA-R scores from pretest to posttest, the most common method is to use ANCOVA. This method computes means that are adjusted for pretest measures identical to that used in multiple regression, where the effect of one variable is measured as net of the other variables. Another approach is to use the difference score between posttest and pretest as an outcome variable, predicted by intervention status alone. This difference score method is generally inferior to that of ANCOVA—it routinely provides a poorer fit, for example—and is not recommended. For more than two time points (pre-, post-, follow-up, etc.), a repeated measures (RM) ANOVA would be used. Individuals' scores are compared across time points to determine whether there are systematic changes in score as a function of time. To build in the treatment effect, the RM ANOVA model may be factorial. In the preceding example, we might use a 2 (GBG vs. control) $\times$ 3 (time) to test for differences between intervention conditions across the three time points. Such models may still be inadequate because school and classroom factors are ignored.

A researcher may include more than one dependent variable in an RCT. A MANOVA tests for these differences on a set of outcomes, such as TOCA-R ratings and academic achievement scores. MANOVA examines all possible linear combinations of the DVs and can specify with high precision which linear combinations of the DVs are most strongly influenced by the factors (e.g., interventions). Also, because these take into account correlation among the DVs, the MANOVA can sometimes provide increased power over that of any single outcome. Several elements in the ANOVA models can be combined to examine more complex relationships among variables. For example, baseline continuous and discrete covariate measures can be used in combination with intervention factors to assess impact on multiple DV outcomes. This multivariate analysis of covariance (MANCOVA) could compensate for baseline TOCA-R scores and achievement, as well as poverty level and gender when examining the effect of an intervention TOCA-R and achievement scores. Specific MANOVA designs can also be used in the case of multiple repeated measures; in the Baltimore Prevention Program trial, for example, teacher ratings of aggressive behavior were collected annually from first through seventh grades. In this way, the investigator can test for linear or nonlinear growth with MANCOVA (Morrison, 2002). Most likely, researchers will need to incorporate many of these elements—multiple factors (IVs), multiple outcomes (DVs), repeated measures and covariates—into the model to test for effects in RCT.

Mixed ANOVA models provide a useful extension of these methods, combining both fixed and random predictors in the model. A fixed factor is a categorical

TABLE 14.1
ANOVA Models

Model	Research goal	Independent variables	Dependent variables	Common uses in RCTs
One-way	Tests for differences in the outcome between IV groups	1 IV, 2+ levels	1 DV	Compare intervention differences on means
Multifactor ANOVA	Tests for variations in the outcome as a function of main effects of factors and interactions between them	2+ IVs 2+ levels, each	1 DV	Compare impact of intervention on different subgroups or compare combined effects of different interventions
Analysis of covariance (ANCOVA)	Tests for variation in DV as a function of group differences, after controlling for covariate effects	1+ continuous IV (covariate) 1+ categorical IV	1 DV	Easily extended to examine interactions
Repeated measures ANOVA	Tests for variation in DV as a function of the repeated measure (e.g., time)	1 IV 3+ levels	1 DV	Examine impact of interventions on changes in individual scores over time
Mixed model ANOVA	Tests for variation in DV as a function of fixed factors and random factors	1+ fixed IV 1+ random IV	1 DV	Examine impact when intervention is applied at classroom or school level
Multivariate analysis of variance-covariance (MANOVA)	Tests for differences between groups on a linear combination of DVs	1 IV 2+ levels	2+ DVs	Examine impact on multiple, correlated outcomes
Multivariate analysis of covariance (MANCOVA)	Variation in multiple DVs as a function of group differences, after controlling for covariate effects	1+ continuous IV (covariate) 1+ categorical IV	2+ DVs	Easily extended to examine interactions

or nominal variable, such as intervention condition or gender, that is assumed to be measured without error (zero measurement variance), and for which the desired generalization is to the same values as those used in the study. A random factor indexes units, such as teachers or schools that would vary if the experiment were repeated; random factors are used when one intends to generalize beyond the individual units to a broader population (Searle, 1987). Thus, a random factor is one that is measured with sampling error because the categories of a given factor are sampled from a larger universe of categories. Models involving random factors are subsumed by the more general class of random effect or random regression modeling, whose varying coefficients can also assess change with continuous IVs (random slopes) and levels of nesting. The term *random effect modeling* is also used extensively in LGM and HM.

ANOVAs are generally robust and flexible, though as factors and variables are added, of course, more participants are required. Moreover, the inferential value of these models depends on whether assumptions about each model are met. These are addressed next.

Assumptions Involved in ANOVA Designs

All ANOVA-type models are conducted under certain assumptions, defined and summarized in Table 14.2. When certain assumptions are violated, the inferential qualities of the resulting statistics (point estimates, confidence intervals, and conclusions from testing) may be adversely affected. Table 14.2 orders assumptions by how severely each might affect the inferences. The first three, assignment bias, participation bias, and attrition bias (Brown & Liao, 1999), are often critical because these often reflect program design flaws that analytical methods may not be able to rectify. Although some corrections can be made in the analysis phase of a study; for example, inclusion of observed baseline covariates can correct for assignment bias, and participant selection problems may be addressed with complier-average causal effects (CACE) type models (Little & Yau, 1998; Jo & Muthén, 2001; Jo, 2002; Muthén, Jo, & Brown, 2003). However, if self-selection of the intervention does occur, the critical dimensions that distinguish those who choose different interventions may be missing entirely. In this case, unobserved characteristics may be too strong to overcome even with covariate adjustment.

The assumption of independence of observations—that inclusion of one subject does not influence the selection or inclusion of any other subject—is often not valid in educational or health settings where classrooms, schools, or provider effects are present. We know that nonindependence affects tests and confidence intervals more than point estimates. If children from the same classrooms are included but only individual outcomes are modeled, then the point estimates, such as means and regression coefficients, may be subjected to little bias and therefore are generally appropriate to report. However, nonindependence caused by clustering (i.e., the aggregation of correlated observations into units, such as similar students into a classroom) generally leads to variance estimates that are biased downward, thereby making p values appear more significant than they should be and confidence intervals shorter than they should be. Both of these can lead to seriously overestimating the importance of an intervention, particularly when it is randomly assigned at the group level (e.g., classroom or school; Murray, 1998). A

TABLE 14.2
Assumptions Used in ANOVA-Type Models

Severity	Assumption	Definition	Assumption is likely to be violated when	Alternative modeling approaches
High	No assignment bias	Subjects in each of the intervention conditions are equivalent to one another.	Nonrandomized and noncontrolled designs; subjects select their own interventions; failed random assignment.	Adjust for intervention selection factors with measured covariate, or adjust for selection with propensity scores.
High	No participation bias	Subjects receive the intervention they are assigned.	Contamination of interventions, intervention drift, low implementation, subjects fail to show up for intervention.	Perform CACE modeling.
High	No differential attrition bias	No differences in those who drop out before follow-up by intervention condition.	Side effects from intervention, inadequate randomized design.	Adjust for data that may or may not be missing at random.
High	Independence of observations	Response of one individual provides no information on that of any other individual.	Individuals are nested in classrooms, or repeated measures on same individuals.	Introduce random factor to account for clustering of classes or correlation of repeated measures for an individual.
High	Homogeneity of slopes (ANCOVA)	Mean difference in response between intervention conditions does not vary by baseline covariate.	Intervention impact varies by baseline risk.	Include interaction of intervention by baseline covariate.
High	Measurement error	Covariate's measurement error correlated with intervention condition or outcome.	Randomized design is corrupted, randomization occurs before consent.	Model measurement error explicitly or use an instrumental variable that is correlated with the true covariate, not its measurement error.

(*continued*)

TABLE 14.2 (*continued*)

Severity	Assumption	Definition	Assumption is likely to be violated when	Alternative modeling approaches
Medium	Linearity	The mean response is linearly related to a covariate.	Intervention only affects those at high or low risk.	Transform IV or DV nonlinearly (e.g., logarithm); use additive models.
Low	Homogeneity of variance	Variability around the mean predicted response is the same across all values of IVs.	DV has a skewed distribution, or censoring occurs.	Transform DV to reduce variance heterogeneity; model censoring directly; model variance directly as a function of mean.
Low	Normality	Univariate or multivariate distribution of the error terms in the model are normal.	Scales of the DV are ordinal or coarse, or DV is skewed or has heavy or light tails.	Transform DV toward normality; remove outliers or use robust methods; model as ordinal variable.
Low	Sphericity (RM ANOVA)	Covariances between repeated measures are the same for each pair.	Measures closer in time are more correlated.	Use MANOVA rather than univariate repeated measures.

number of methods can be used to overcome nonindependence, including multilevel modeling, discussed later, and adjustments of the variances themselves in generalized estimating equations (Zeger, Liang, & Albert, 1988).

Of high concern in cases of ANCOVA is whether slopes are homogeneous, that is, whether the intervention impact varies as a function of baseline characteristics. Such an interaction between baseline and intervention can lead to serious misspecification of impact if ignored.

Of just slightly less concern, the assumption of linearity implies that the mean response changes linearly with the continuous measures. That is, a one-unit change on a baseline risk factor at the low end of the scale produces the same amount of change in response as does a one-unit change at the high end of the risk scale. If the assumption of linearity cannot be met, then the traditional ANOVA-type models may misspecify the intervention's impact. Often adding quadratic and higher order polynomials can provide better fits than those of the standard linear models. However, including polynomials does not adequately represent intervention effects that are negligible below a certain risk score and exist only above a cutoff. A method of nonparametric regression called *additive models* (Hastie & Tibshirani, 1990; Brown, 1993a) provides a much richer class of intervention evaluations; examples of their use are found in Ialongo et al. (1999) and Kellam et al. (in press).

Measurement errors in the covariates can also cause bias in estimating the intervention effect, although well-conducted randomized trials protect against many of these problems far better than nonexperimental studies. A type of design that is particularly susceptible to these effects is one where random assignment takes place first, then individuals consent or not depending on their known assigned intervention condition. In this case, regressing on baseline covariates whose measurement errors are related to consent would introduce bias.

The remaining assumptions are important as well, but modest departures most often provide relatively slight changes in the adequacy of the inferential statements, at least with large sample sizes.

Although ANOVA-type models are often employed to analyze longitudinal or repeated measures data and may be sufficient in certain study designs, this approach is not sufficient to address design and research goals of RCTs with more complex designs (Willett, Ayoub, & Robinson, 1991). Thus, other techniques are needed to further the researcher's understanding of the complexity and variation in outcome in longitudinal models. The next sections turn to this topic by introducing LGM and HM. Because both of these methods have expanded their classes of analytic models and now overlap considerably, they share many analytic methods. Because of space limitations and without any intent to diminish the HM approach, we begin with LGM techniques and then describe additional hierarchical modeling techniques that are not easily run using LGM. We conclude with a comparison of their strengths.

■ Latent Growth Models

Many of the previously described ANOVA-type models can be used to assess impact of the intervention at a single follow-up point with data collected in a panel study. With repeated waves of data collected at distinct follow-up points, it is possible to evaluate impact separately at each time point. Alternatively, RM ANOVA allows for examination of any number of changes that may occur across measurement time. Both of these approaches have limitations, however. By analyzing data at each measurement occasion, one can introduce spurious results, or, if one wants to take into account the responses at previous time points, the models become exceedingly complex. RM ANOVA does not by itself provide an easy way to summarize impact—the degrees of freedom used to explain the intervention effect go up with the number of time points, for example. An alternative strategy is to summarize changes over time into a few parameters; this is the objective of growth modeling.

When there is particular interest in understanding how interventions affect development or change over the time, LGM can be used to examine a wide range of intervention hypotheses. Based in SEM, these models allow for the construction, estimation, and testing of complexities in developmental models. Growth modeling methods for analyzing impact of interventions are quite extensive, and these models can be carried out using Mplus (Muthén & Muthén, 2006), as well as other computer programs. Several of these statistical programs can now handle a wide range of outcome measures: continuous, discrete, ordinal, time to event, or nominal, as well as censoring and missing data. Mplus can handle both fixed observation times as in panel studies and time-varying observation times as one would find in clinic studies. Covariates can also be fixed (such as intervention condition) and time varying (such as current level of depressive symptoms). These models can also include cohort effects, the use of constant or time-dependent effects, and multidimensional repeated measures.

The graphs in Figure 14.1 show how to reduce the observed data to make inferences about patterns of growth for intervention and control conditions. Panel A shows, for a typical participant, scores on standardized achievement tests from grades 1 through 6, in which a 50-point gain is expected each year. Also shown are both a linear fit and a quadratic fit to these individual points; the latter suggests that achievement change is nearly linear. Panel B hides the individual-level observations but shows straight-line fits for multiple individuals in intervention and control conditions. Note that the solid lines, representing those receiving the active intervention, typically have higher slopes than do those for the dashed lines representing controls. These individual intercepts and slopes are latent, or unobserved; they can also be called *random effects*. LGM allows for modeling of these individual-level growth trajectories over time and examines how these growth patterns depend on covariates such as intervention condition. A powerful feature of LGM is its ability to examine individual means, variances, regression coefficients, and covariances for the random effects corresponding to, for example, an intercept, slope, and quadratic curve that characterize each individual's growth pattern. Within the same overall model, these means, variances, regression coefficients, and covariances can then be related to fixed discrete covariates, such as intervention condition, as well as continuous measured covariates and unmeasured or latent variables. Parameters involved with these effects can be allowed to vary freely, to be fixed to specified values, to be equal to one another, or to be constrained in a linear or nonlinear fashion. Models are generally fit using the marginal maximum likelihood technique. This general framework for LGM provides a very powerful means of testing intervention effects, some of which are presented in Table 14.3 and represented in Figures 14.1, Panels C through F. For example, growth models can examine intervention impact on the mean of the slope for intervention versus controls. Panel C replaces the lines in Panel B with points representing the intercept and slope for all intervention and control subjects. It is apparent from this plot that the intervention mean on the slope is higher than that for the controls. Also, there appears to be no difference in intercept means by intervention condition; this would be expected from an RCT that successfully balanced individuals at baseline. Growth modeling provides a direct test of the difference between the mean intervention and mean control slopes by adding intervention status as a predictor of the slope. This coefficient estimates the difference in slope means, and formal tests can be made either by comparing this coefficient to its standard error (a Wald test) or by assessing the improvement in model fit (a likelihood ratio test).

Other effects on the slope can be tested just as easily. For example, Panel D of Figure 14.1 uses box plots to show the distribution of slopes in intervention and control groups. Not only is there an increase in the mean, but also the intervention decreases the variance as well. A curriculum that has this effect would improve the class's overall achievement and also would lower the gap between low- and high-performing students. The Mastery Learning (ML) program is one such curriculum that claims to improve the mean and also reduce variance, but this second conclusion was not supported in the first Baltimore Prevention Program (Dolan et al., 1993; Brown, 1993a). To test whether the intervention has an effect on the variance of the slope, one can fit a model in Mplus separately to the intervention and control groups, then check how the model fit is affected when the variance of the slopes for intervention and control are set equal to one another.

A third example involves examining the differential effect of the intervention on the slope as a function of participants' initial levels at baseline. This relationship is called a baseline by intervention interaction on the slope trajectory. Panel E of Figure 14.1 indicates that the slope of intervention students is larger for initially low-achieving youth compared with the slope of control students who were similarly low achieving at baseline. At the right side of the figure, representing initially high-achieving youth, there is a much more modest gain. The impact of this baseline by slope interaction can be seen in Panel F, which examines the predicted achievement level across all grades for children who start with low achievement, those with medium levels of achievement, and those with high levels of achievement. In the intervention condition, represented by solid lines, all three groups have similar achievement by sixth grade. In the controls, their respective differences widen by sixth grade, and lower and medium level achievement at baseline remains well below all those in the intervention.

This interesting interaction between intervention status and the baseline level on growth patterns has been used to assess the impact of the Good Behavior Game (GBG) on aggression in the first Baltimore Prevention Program (Muthén & Curran, 1997). Such analyses have provided clear evidence that the universal GBG intervention had differential impact as a function of baseline aggressive behavior. Those males who had initially high TOCA-R scores in first grade benefited from the GBG intervention through elementary and middle school. Those with lower

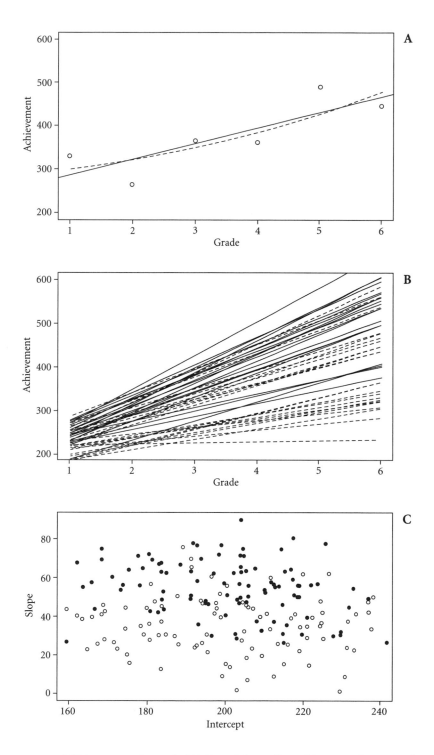

FIGURE 14.1. LGM patterns of growth. (A) Growth in reading achievement for one student; linear and quadratic fits; (B) linear growth curves for intervention and control students; (C) comparison of intercepts and slopes for intervention (solid) and control (open) subjects; (D) box plots of slopes for controls and intervention students; (E) relation between intercepts and slopes for intervention (solid) and control (open) subjects; (F) predicted growth in achievement for low, medium, and high achievers in first grade.

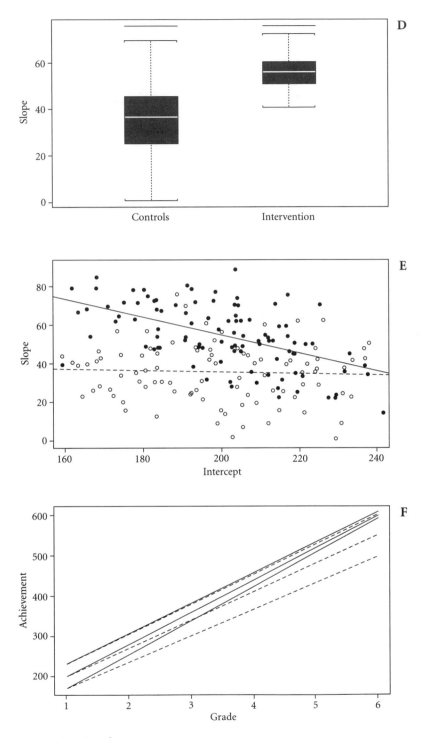

FIGURE 14.1. (*continued*)

TABLE 14.3
Types of Latent Growth Modeling Used to Examine Intervention Impact Across Time

Type of modeling	Application	Common ways to measure intervention effect	Other potential intervention effects
Latent growth modeling with a single class	Linear growth modeling	Change in mean of slope (Figure 14.1, Panels B, C)	Change in variance of slope (Figure 1D); correlation between slope and intercept (Figure 1E)
	Intercept by intervention interaction on growth trajectory	Slope affected by intervention (Figure 14.1, Panel E)	
	Piecewise and parametric latent growth modeling	Change in mean during or after intervention	Nonlinear change in growth; correlation between early change and later change
	Multivariate growth modeling	Change in mean slope of each developmental outcome (Figure 14.1, Panel F)	Change in the relationship between the slope and intercept as a function of intervention (Muthén & Curran, 1997)
Latent growth modeling with multiple classes	Growth mixture modeling	Multiple classes of growth trajectories (Muthén et al., 2002; Figure 14.3)	Simultaneous modeling of prevalence and quantity (Olsen & Schafer, 2001)
Generalized growth modeling	Proximal distal modeling	Intervention had different long-term effect across growth (Muthén et al., 2002)	
	Multilevel growth mixture modeling	Group-based intervention affects individual level trajectory classes differently (Asparouhov & Muthén, in press)	Discrete classes that exist at both the individual level and at the cluster level can interact (Asparouhov & Muthén, in press)

TOCA-R scores in first grade generally continued to have low levels of aggressive behavior over time and were not impacted by the intervention. Thus GBG's impact succeeded in reaching those who were most at risk without the need for separating and labeling those at the greatest risk of continued aggressive behavior.

Additional growth models are mentioned in Table 14.3, and the interested reader is referred to references by Muthén and colleagues (Muthén, 1991, 1997, 2002, in press; Muthén & Curran 1997; Muthén et al., 2002; Muthén et al., 2003; Muthén & Muthén, 2006), as well as by Nagin and colleagues (Nagin & Land, 1993; Nagin, 1999, 2005).

■ Growth Mixture Models

Despite the wide range of methods available in traditional latent growth modeling, there are interesting classes of intervention impact that cannot be assessed adequately with the methods just described. By introducing mixtures, or unobserved latent discrete classes, the growth mixture model (GMM) allows a broader flexibility in assessing impact. In statistical terms, a discrete mixture of two distributions occurs when participants come from two populations that are indistinguished, such as examining a histogram of aggression scores when gender is ignored. Empirical data consistently indicate that males overall have higher aggressive behavior scores than females. We may note from a histogram that ignores gender that some subjects are very high and others very low on aggressive behavior, but this separation is generally not sufficiently wide to classify individuals very well by gender based on this single outcome. Figure 14.2 provides some examples; Panel A shows two separate normal distributions with different mixing distributions than fifty-fifty, and Panel B shows the mixture itself. In this example, there is bimodality as well as skewness; if the two population means were closer together, one would see only skewness, not bimodality.

Besides this statistical view of mixtures, there is a conceptual one as well. Often mixtures occur because we know there is a missing attribute, such as gender in the last example. Examples of mixtures abound in medicine; for example, an abnormal response to a blood glucose test could be caused by one of two common types of diabetes. But often we may not have a clearly defined attribute in mind. Instead, mixtures may represent population subgroups that are thought to be present. Developmental psychology, for example, distinguishes normal development from abnormal development; in a population we can have a mixture of those who follow each growth trajectory, although heterogeneity of symptoms within each group may make it difficult to classify individual subjects. Because intervention impact may vary as a function of these trajectory classes, growth mixture models have been developed to examine how interventions can vary as a function of such trajectory classes.

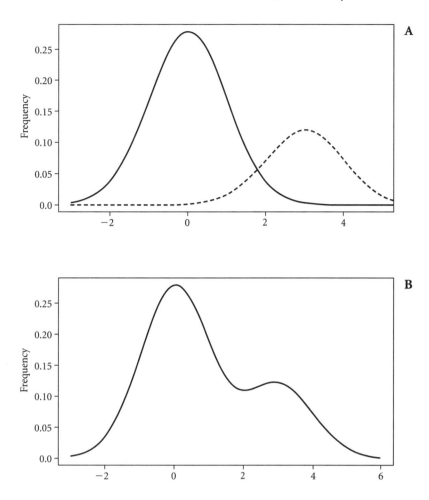

FIGURE 14.2. Histograms of population distribution for aggression, illustrating the results of mixing two discrete classes (males and females). (A) Two normal distributions; (B) mixture distribution from two normals.

An example of GMM is given in Figure 14.3. Along the x-axis is the grade level where aggressive behavior ratings are measured, with the letters F and S indicating fall and spring, respectively. A mixture of three distinct classes is identified, with one class of 14.5% of the sample beginning very high on aggressive behavior in first grade and remaining high through elementary to middle school. A second class of 49% starts moderately low and increases slightly throughout this period. The third class of 35.5% begins and remains low throughout. These data are for males, with solid lines representing growth curves for those given the GBG and dashed lines for no-intervention controls. Note that the intervention is effective in reducing aggressive behavior among the high-starters, or the most aggressive, but has no impact on the other two groups.

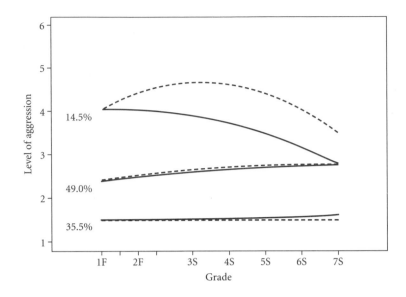

FIGURE 14.3. Growth mixture modeling with three trajectory classes for males' aggressive behavior from first grade to seventh grade in GBG and control classes.

The models we have just described can also be expanded to examine how disparate growth trajectories affect distal outcomes. Called *proximal-distal modeling,* these extensions relate how changes in growth patterns lead developmentally to outcomes that are later in time or farther removed in a theoretical mediating chain of developmental outcomes. For example, Muthén et al. (2002) examined how a distal outcome of juvenile delinquency through age 18 was related to the separate trajectory curves and interventions. This general growth mixture model (GGMM) allows for the growth trajectory classes to play a role of either a mediating or moderating effect on a distal outcome, which can be discrete, continuous, or time-to-event. In this case, GGMM results indicated that the GBG continued to have beneficial effects in reducing juvenile delinquency for the high aggressive trajectory class.

GMM and GGMM allow great flexibility in examining impact. But they must be specified accurately—with a myriad of mean, variance, covariance, regression, and loading parameters—or they will lose their inferential ability to examine intervention effects. Model inadequacy can be examined with statistical tests for each individual model constraint (Muthén & Muthén, 2006) or formal comparisons of two nested models using likelihood ratio tests or other fit statistics (Carlin, Wolfe, Brown, & Gelman, 2001). Perhaps the best way is to use graphic diagnostics to detect model misspecifications (Wang et al., 2005).

■ Missing Data

The handling of missing data is also crucial in analyzing data with growth modeling. Most often it is not appropriate to delete cases with any missing data because even a small proportion of missing data at each follow-up time will lead to a sizable proportion of the cases having some missing data. Instead, two general approaches are used, both of which are more intensive computationally, but they generally provide good estimates, confidence intervals, and tests. The first is full information maximum likelihood, which is an option available in Mplus, AMOS, and other such programs. This procedure fits the model to all the data that are observed for each subject. The second approach is to use multiple imputation (Schafer, 1997), which creates a set of complete data matrices by imputing each missing datum. A useful set of programs for generating imputed data sets can be found on the Penn State Methodology Center Web site (http://methodology.psu.edu/). Each of these data matrices is then used to fit the same growth curve; because the imputed values vary between data sets, the coefficients from these models are different. Standard procedures are available for combining the results of these separate fits to correctly account for the missing data; these are now handled directly in Mplus 4.2, for example.

There are some important points to note about these approaches. First, they both are excellent procedures when the data are "missing at random," a technical term that means whether a datum is missing is either unrelated to the data or related only to the variables that are observed. Although there are some specialized procedures for handling data that are not missing at random (Brown, 1990), it is virtually impossible to know when data are not missing at random, and even then the two procedures just mentioned generally produce reasonably good estimates. Second, if multiple imputation is used, care must be taken that the model used for imputation is more general than the model used for analysis. Otherwise, the imputed data would introduce unknown errors into the analysis. Generally, however, one set of multiple imputations is computed so that they can be used for all potential growth models that are fit.

■ Multilevel Models

Multilevel models provide a wide array of methods to evaluate intervention impact, and many of the growth models that we have just described can be fit using a wide assortment of multilevel software such as HLM (Raudenbush & Bryk, 2002), MLwiN (Goldstein, 2003), SAS's Proc MIXED (Littell, Milliken, Stroup, & Wolfinger, 1996; Singer, 1998), Supermix, and related earlier programs (Hedeker, Gibbons, & Flay, 1994; Hedeker & Gibbons, 1996; Gibbons & Hedeker, 1997), as well as similar programs in other packages such as SPSS,

STATA, Splus, and R. These approaches all have their roots in unbalanced ANOVA (Scheffé, 1959, republished 1999; Searle, 1987; Bryk & Raudenbush, 1987; Bock, 1988) and specification of one or more levels through random effects modeling (Laird & Ware, 1982; Aitkin & Longford, 1986; De Leeuw & Kreft, 1986; Goldstein, 1987).

There are a number of approaches to developing these multilevel models. As a consequence, these models are often described with different names: multilevel models, mixed effect models, hierarchical models, random effect models, or random slope or coefficient models. Despite these different names, they can all be approached in a similar way, and in this section we make no distinctions among these broad categories of HMs. All deal directly with correlated data, whether the correlation is based on repeated measures of the same subject over time (thus extending RM ANOVA) or is due to subjects being in one or more nested clusters, such as classrooms, schools, or neighborhoods. Growth curve modeling can be done within a two-level HM framework by specifying the distribution of individual-level scores at each time in the first level, then the subject-level parameters, say of intercept and slope, are involved in second-level modeling. Many (but not all) of the same types of models that are fit with LGM can be fit with two-level HM methods as well. Another common two-level HM involves nesting of individuals within clusters, such as schools. Correlation of subjects within schools is achieved by having all subjects share a common school-level random factor. A three-level HM is also common: the first level corresponds to individual-level measures at each time for each subject, the second is the person-level parameters that specify individual growth, and the third level corresponds to clusters of individuals. These three-level HMs are analogous to two-level LGMs already discussed. The number of "levels" in hierarchical and growth model frameworks only differs because time is considered another level in the hierarchical framework, whereas it is treated explicitly in the name latent growth model.

We provide one illustration of the use of HM for examining the impact of GBG. Figure 14.4 displays the fit of a general additive mixed model (GAMM) that simultaneously fits both individual-level and classroom-level first-grade measures to a distal outcome of diagnosis of illicit drug abuse/dependence disorder in young adulthood. The individual-level predictors include baseline TOCA-R scores in first grade and gender, while classroom is treated as a random effect whose mean is allowed to vary by intervention status. A significant interaction term between intervention and baseline TOCA-R is also included. The two fitted curves in Figure 14.4 show this interaction through nonparametric or nonlinear smooth curves (the "additive" part of GAMM). In the GBG group the chance of a diagnosis for those with low first-grade ratings is similar to control at the low end but rises much less steeply with GBG. Both of these curves were fit using nonlinear modeling so that we could examine whether there were change points or other nonlinearities that modified risk. In this instance there was no evidence of change points, but rather increasing benefit

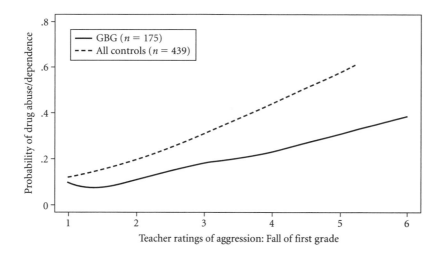

FIGURE 14.4. GBG impact on the risk of drug abuse/dependence on males and females as an adult through young adulthood evaluated using GAMM.

from GBG with increasing baseline level of risk. Formal testing of this model took into account the clustering effect of classrooms and showed there was a significant interactive relationship with baseline. Further details on the analytic method and results are provided in Kellam et al. (in press).

The analogies between the hierarchical and growth models go beyond the surface. Often, a model can be completely specified in one framework and then translated directly into the other, as shown with GGMM in Wang et al. (2005). Various limitations in today's computer programs still make it difficult, if not impossible, to specify one particular model in the LGM setting compared with the HM setting, or vice versa. However, advances in all these programs are closing gaps so that there is much more overlap between these two approaches. Indeed, a recent example was the modification of a small amount of Mplus code that permitted a rich class of traditionally considered two-level HMs to be fit (Dagne, Howe, Brown, & Muthén, 2002). In this era where programs are being quickly revised, then, it is useful to describe the general strengths and weaknesses inherent in the two approaches rather than make statements about what each model cannot now do.

When there are multiple nested levels of clustering, such as students within classes within schools, HMs excel, since it is easily represented in these models. Indeed, for mixed models or HLM, there is no inherent limit to the number of nestings, other than the number of units at each level and the respective precision that is affected by these respective sample sizes (Raudenbush, 1997; Murray, 1998; Brown & Liao, 1999; Raudenbush & Liu, 2000). For LGM, true multilevel capabilities are somewhat more awkward to represent, although substantial progress has been made in understanding and using these models.

A second situation where HMs have more inherent strength is with designs where observation times differ from individual to individual rather than coming at fixed times as in a panel study. The reason that HMs have an edge is that the correlations between observations on the same subject can be modeled explicitly as a function of time, something that is difficult to do in the latent variable approach. Another advantage related to this is that the observation times can differ dramatically from subject to subject without having to treat individuals as having any missing data.

Third, HMs can be represented in a Bayesian framework, thereby allowing fully Bayesian models to be specified with ease and opening up analyses to use fully Bayesian methods such as WinBUGS (Gilks, Thomas, & Spiegelhalter, 1994; Spiegelhalter, Thomas, & Best, 1999). Bayesian methods, although they often require lengthy computations, have advantages in producing inferences for small sample sizes, for fitting nonstandard random effect distributions, and for high dimensionality (Dagne et al., 2002).

Hierarchical models often have the edge when clusters are small, as, for example, when comparing outcomes for children within families. Recent work with multilevel growth models suggests that this gap is closing (Muthén, in press).

There are other areas where HMs are not inherently strong compared with LGMs. In particular, HMs traditionally do not provide extensive flexibility in analyzing multivariate measures that differ from one another as does the LGM approach. For example, analyzing the relationship between two growth patterns, one for a dichotomous variable and one for a continuous variable in a hierarchical analysis, presents real challenges but is much easier to express in the latent variable framework. Reported HMs do not often explicitly examine the multivariate structure of the data, so that the underlying correlation structure due to having measures taken on the same individuals over time may be misspecified. Sensitivity analysis and diagnostics (Seltzer, Novak, Choi, & Lim, 2002, Seltzer & Choi, 2002, Seltzer, Choi, & Thum, in press; Seltzer, in press), as well as model checking methods (Carlin et al., 2001), can be used for examining adequacy of fit.

HMs also have limited ability for modeling mediation, where one or more variables serve as both antecedents and consequences to other variables. They are not as well equipped to handle proximal-distal modeling as are those based on latent growth modeling and structural equation modeling frameworks.

Also, discrete mixtures are more challenging to fit in HMs than in LGMs. In the latter case, the mixtures that are represented by unobserved categorical variables can be related to observed items with latent class analysis, and their cross-classification probabilities can be examined with latent transition analysis (Muthén, in press).

■ Summary

This tour of analytic frameworks for examining intervention effect covers simple models involving comparisons of overall mean changes to more complex models of growth, change, and development in individuals and nested groups. We presented overviews of three broad classes of analysis, which are interrelated in many ways. As described in the preceding sections, many ANOVA-type models can be thought of as special cases of HM and LGM procedures. LGM and HM procedures themselves provide a great deal of overlap, as software program development is making it easier to translate one set of model specifications to another.

Our goal for this chapter was to leave the researcher with a basic understanding of analytic frameworks that are most effective in evaluating intervention impact. Further reading or training is required, of course, to implement some of these modeling techniques. However, with this introduction, we hope that readers will be enabled to expand their analysis plans in an RCT in order to ask more dynamic research questions about individual and group outcomes, developmental trajectories, and factors of influence.

■ Glossary

BAYESIAN ESTIMATION: Bayesian estimation provides an alternative to classical sampling theory. Instead of treating population parameters as fixed, Bayesian inference involves assigning probabilities or distribution to the possible values of a population parameter, and updating these probabilities based on the data obtained from the sample.

CENSORING: Observations are censored when the dependent variable of interest represents the time to a terminal event, and the duration of the study is limited.

CLUSTERING: The systematic aggregation of units, such as students into classrooms, classrooms into schools, or schools into districts. When clustering is present, subjects in the same cluster typically have more similar outcomes than do subjects in different clusters. Without adjusting for this, the usual estimates of precision for intervention effects are generally too small, resulting in erroneous inferences.

COMPLIER-AVERAGE CAUSAL EFFECT (CACE) MODELING: Assessing treatment effects among those who participate in or are exposed to the intervention. This requires modeling or adjusting for self-selection factors in the control group that is not offered the intervention.

GENERAL ADDITIVE MIXED MODEL: GAMM is a hierarchical model that simultaneously fits models of impact at the individual and clustered (e.g., school) levels. This analysis models nonparametric, nonlinear outcomes and interactions. See generalized linear models.

GENERAL GROWTH MIXTURE MODELING:　GGMM advances prior techniques by analyzing the effects of intervention on an entire trajectory at once, and not just a single end point. GGMM extends the use of random effects to test unobserved heterogeneity (individual differences) in the population and fixed effects to test interventions to include categorical latent variables (unobserved classes) to additionally detect effects on subgroups. GGMM extends growth mixture modeling (see below) by examining whether and how an intervention's impact on growth trajectories continues to influence one or more distal outcomes, such as psychiatric diagnoses, graduation, or drug use.

GENERAL LINEAR MODEL:　GLM is an extension of the basic regression model, in which a dependent variable may be estimated as an intercept plus a slope (or regression coefficient) times an independent variable. In matrix notation, the GLM can be described as

$$Y = XB + U$$

where Y is a matrix with series of multivariate measurements, X is a design matrix, B is a matrix containing parameters to be estimated, and U is a matrix containing residuals (i.e., errors). Residuals are assumed to follow a multivariate normal distribution.

The general linear model underlies ANOVA-type models, ordinary linear regression.

GENERALIZED LINEAR MODEL:　Although this shares a name similar to the general linear model, it is not the same; it includes linear multiple regression models but also includes Poisson models for count data, logistic regression, polytomous regression and log linear models for categorical data, and exponential modeling for time to event data. The generalized additive model allows modeling of nonlinear methods using this same broad class of outcomes.

GROWTH MIXTURE MODELING:　GMM allows treatment effects to vary across latent trajectory classes and among individuals within classes.

HIERARCHICAL MODELING:　HM is a generalization of hierarchical linear modeling (see below) that allows the measured variables to have binary, categorical, or other nonnormal distributions.

HIERARCHICAL LINEAR MODELING:　HLM relates the mean of an observed, normally distributed variable to fixed and random factors and covariates that operate at different levels of nesting, such as students within classrooms within schools, measured longitudinally over time. At each level beyond the first, the distribution of the random effects, or parameters governing growth or nesting effects, is related to relevant covariates.

MARGINAL MAXIMUM LIKELIHOOD:　MML estimation is a type of maximum likelihood (ML) estimation that averages over latent variables, representing random effects or discrete mixtures.

MAXIMUM LIKELIHOOD:　ML estimation identifies population parameters (e.g., mean, variance) that are most strongly supported by the sample data. Most often MLs are obtained through iterative computational procedures available in statistical packages.

STRUCTURAL EQUATION MODELING: In its broadest form, SEM examines the relationships between underlying latent continuous variables, as well as observed covariates, mediators, and outcomes. The structural part of the model examines how the latent variables relate to one another, and the measurement part of the model examines how the observed measures are related to hypothesized latent variables. It is a general technique that encompasses aspects of confirmatory factor analysis, path analysis, and growth modeling.

■ Acknowledgments

We are grateful for many discussions with our colleagues in the Prevention Science and Methodology Group, and especially to George Bohrnstedt, Bengt Muthén, Linda Muthén, Getachew Dagne, George Howe, Tihomir Asparouhov, Wei Wang, Peter Toyinbo, and Hanno Petras for their many insights. Special thanks are due to discussions with Drs. Sheppard Kellam, Jeanne Poduska, Nicholas Ialongo, and James Anthony for their leadership in developing the theoretical models and carrying out the randomized trials that have inspired and influenced many of the methods for evaluating intervention impact that are described here. The Baltimore Prevention Program has been supported by the National Institute of Mental Health and the National Institute on Drug Abuse through grants MH40859, MH38725, MH42968, MH42968–06A2, and DA09592. The principal collaborators have included Drs. Lisa Werthamer, C. Hendricks Brown, Sheppard G. Kellam, James C. Anthony, Lawrence Dolan, Jeanne Poduska, and Nicholas S. Ialongo. This work would not have been possible without the support and collaboration of the Baltimore City Public Schools and the parents, children, teachers, principals and school psychologists, and social workers who participated.

■ References

Aitkin, M. A., & Longford, N. (1986). Statistical modeling issues in school effectiveness studies. *Journal of the Royal Statistical Society, 149A,* 1–43.

Asparouhov, T., & Muthén, B. (in press). Multilevel mixture models. In G. R. Hancock, & K. M. Samuelsen (Eds.), *Advances in latent variable mixture models.* Charlotte, NC: Information Age.

Barrish, H. H., Saunders, M., & Wolf, M. M. (1969). Good behavior game: Effects of individual contingencies for group consequences on disruptive behavior in a classroom. *Journal of Applied Behavior Analysis, 2,* 119–124.

Bock, D. (Ed.). (1988). *Multilevel analysis of educational data.* San Diego, CA: Academic Press.

Brown, C. H. (1993a). Analyzing preventive trials with generalized additive models. *American Journal of Community Psychology, 21,* 635–664.

Brown, C. H. (1993b). Statistical methods for preventive trials in mental health. *Statistical Medicine, 12,* 289–300.

Brown, C. H., & Liao, J. (1999). Principles for designing randomized preventive trials in mental health: An emerging developmental epidemiology paradigm. *American Journal of Community Psychology, 27,* 673–710.

Bryk, A. S., & Raudenbush, S. W. (1987). Application of hierarchical linear models to assessing change. *Psychological Bulletin, 101,* 147–158.

Carlin, J. B., Wolfe, R., Brown, C. H., & Gelman, A. (2001). A case study on the choice, interpretation, and checking of multilevel models for longitudinal, binary outcomes. *Biostatistics, 2,* 397–416.

Dagne, G., Howe, G., Brown, C. H., & Muthén, B. (2002). Hierarchical modeling of sequential behavioral data: An empirical Bayesian approach. *Psychological Methods, 7,* 262–280.

De Leeuw, J., & Kreft, I. (1986). Random coefficient models for multilevel analysis. *Journal of Educational Statistics, 11,* 57–85.

Dolan, L. J., Kellam, S. G., Brown, C. H., Werthamer-Larsson, L., Rebok, G. W., Mayer, L. S., et al. (1993). The short-term impact of two classroom-based preventive interventions on aggressive and shy behaviors and poor achievement. *Journal of Applied Developmental Psychology, 14,* 317–345.

Draper, N. R., & Smith, H. (1998). *Applied regression analysis* (3rd ed.). New York: Wiley.

Fisher, R. A. (1925). *Statistical methods for research workers.* New York: Hafner.

Gibbons, R. D., & Hedeker, D. (1997). Random-effects probit and logistic regression models for three-level data. *Biometrics, 53,* 1527–1537.

Gilks, W. R., Thomas, A., & Spiegelhalter, D. J. (1994). A language and program for complex Bayesian modeling. *Statistician, 43,* 169–178.

Goldstein, H. I. (1987). *Multilevel models in education and social research.* London: Charles Griffin.

Goldstein, H. I. (2003). *Multilevel statistical models* (3rd ed.). London: Edward Arnold.

Hastie, T., & Tibshirani, R. (1990). *Generalized additive models.* London: Chapman & Hall.

Hedeker, D., & Gibbons, R. D. (1994). A random-effects ordinal regression model for multilevel analysis. *Biometrics, 50,* 933–944.

Hedeker, D., Gibbons, R. D., & Flay, B. R (1994). Random regression models for clustered data: With an example from smoking prevention research. *Journal of Clinical and Consulting Psychology, 62,* 757–765.

Ialongo, N. S., Werthamer, L., Kellam, S. G., Brown, C. H., Wang, S., & Lin, Y. (1999). Proximal impact of two first-grade preventive interventions on the early risk behaviors for later substance abuse, depression, and antisocial behavior. *American Journal of Community Psychology, 27,* 599–641.

Jo, B. (2002). Estimation of intervention effects with noncompliance: Alternative model specifications. *Journal of Educational and Behavioral Statistics, 27,* 385–409.

Jo, B., & Muthén, B. (2001). Modeling of intervention effects with noncompliance: A latent variable approach for randomized trials. In G. A. Marcoulides & R. E. Schumacker (Eds.), *New developments and techniques in structural equation modeling* (pp. 57–87). Hillsdale, NJ: Erlbaum.

Kellam, S. G. (1990). Developmental epidemiological framework for family research on depression and aggression. In G. R. Patterson (Ed.), *Depression and aggression in family interaction* (pp. 11–48). Hillsdale, NJ: Erlbaum.

Kellam, S. G., Branch, J. D., Agrawal, K. C., & Ensminger, M. E. (1975). *Mental health and going to school: The Woodlawn program of assessment, early intervention, and evaluation.* Chicago: University of Chicago Press.

Kellam, S. G., Brown, C. H., Poduska, J., Ialongo, N., Wang, W., Toyinbo, P., et al. (in press). Effects of a universal classroom behavior management program in first and second grades on young adult behavioral, psychiatric, and social outcomes. *Drug and Alcohol Dependence.*

Kellam, S. G., & Ensminger, M. E. (1980). Theory and method in child psychiatric epidemiology. In F. Earls (Ed.), *International monograph series in psychosocial epidemiology: Vol. 1. Studying children epidemiologically* (pp. 145–180). New York: Neale Watson Academic Publishers.

Kellam, S. G., & Rebok, G. W. (1992). Building developmental and etiological theory through epidemiologically based preventive intervention trials. In J. McCord & R. E. Tremblay (Eds.), *Preventing antisocial behavior: Interventions from birth through adolescence* (pp. 162–195). New York: Guilford.

Laird, N. M., & Ware, J. H. (1982). Random-effects models for longitudinal data. *Biometrics, 38,* 963–974.

Littell, R. C., Milliken, G. A., Stroup, W. W., & Wolfinger, R. D. (1996). *SAS system for mixed models.* Cary, NC: SAS Institute.

Little, R. J., & Yau, L. H. Y. (1998). Statistical techniques for analyzing data from prevention trials: Treatment of no-shows using Rubin's causal model. *Psychological Methods 3,* 147–159.

Morrison, D. F. (2002). *Multivariate statistical methods* (4th ed.). Pacific Grove, CA: Duxbury.

Murray, D. M. (1998). *Design and analysis of group-randomized trials.* New York: Oxford University Press.

Muthén, B. (1991). Analysis of longitudinal data using latent variable models with varying parameters. In L. Collins & J. Horn (Eds.), *Best methods for the analysis of change: Recent advances, unanswered questions, future directions* (pp. 1–17). Washington, DC: American Psychological Association.

Muthén, B. O. (1997). Latent variable modeling with longitudinal and multilevel data. In A. Raftery (Ed.), *Sociological methodology* (pp. 453–480). Boston: Blackwell.

Muthén, B. (2002). Statistical and substantive checking in growth mixture modeling. *Psychological Methods, 8,* 369–377.

Muthén, B. (in press). Latent variable hybrids: Overview of old and new models. In G. R. Hancock & K. M. Samuelsen. (Eds.), *Advances in latent variable mixture models*. Charlotte, NC: Information Age.

Muthén, B., Brown, C. H., Masyn, K., Jo, B., Khoo, S. T., Yang, C. C., et al. (2002). General growth mixture modeling for randomized preventive interventions. *Biostatistics, 3,* 459–475.

Muthén, B. O., & Curran, P. (1997). General longitudinal modeling of individual differences in experimental designs: A latent variable framework for analysis and power estimation. *Psychological Methods, 2,* 371–402.

Muthén, B., Jo, B., & Brown, C. H. (2003). Assessment of treatment effects using latent variable modeling: Comment on the Barnard, Frangakis, Hill & Rubin article: Principal stratification approach to broken randomized experiments: A case study of school choice vouchers in New York City. *Journal of the American Statistical Association, 98,* 311–314.

Muthén, B., & Shedden, K. (1999). Finite mixture modeling with mixture outcomes using the EM algorithm. *Biometrics, 55,* 463–469.

Muthén, L., & Muthén B. (2006). *Mplus user's manual, version 4.2.* Los Angeles: Muthén & Muthén.

Nagin, D. S. (1999). Analyzing developmental trajectories: A semi-parametric, group-based approach. *Psychological Methods, 4,* 139–157.

Nagin, D. S. (2005). *Group-based modeling of development.* Cambridge, MA: Harvard University Press.

Nagin, D. S., & Land, K. C. (1993). Age, criminal careers, and population heterogeneity: Specification and estimation of a nonparametric, mixed Poisson model. *Criminology, 31,* 327–362.

Olsen, M. K., & Schafer, J., L. (2001). A two-part random effects model for semi-continuous longitudinal data. *Journal of the American Statistical Association, 96,* 730–745.

Raudenbush, S. W. (1997). Statistical analysis and optimal design for cluster randomized trials. *Psychological Methods, 2,* 173–185.

Raudenbush, S. W., & Bryk, A. S. (2002). *Hierarchical linear models: Applications and data analysis methods* (2nd ed.). Newbury Park, CA: Sage.

Raudenbush, S. W., & Liu, X. (2000). Statistical power and optimal design for multisite randomized trials. *Psychological Methods, 5,* 199–213.

Schafer, J. L. (1997). *Analysis of incomplete multivariate data.* London: Chapman & Hall.

Scheffé, H. (1959). *The analysis of variance.* New York: Wiley.

Scheffé, H. (1999). *The analysis of variance.* Wiley Classics Library. New York: Wiley.

Searle, S. R. (1987). *Linear models for unbalanced data.* New York: Wiley

Seltzer, M. (in press). The use of hierarchical models in analyzing data from field experiments and quasi-experiments. In D. Kaplan (Ed.), *The handbook of statistical methods for the social sciences.* Thousand Oaks, CA: Sage.

Seltzer, M., & Choi, K. (2002). Model checking and sensitivity analysis for multilevel models. In N. Duan & S. Reise (Eds.), *Multilevel modeling: Methodological advances, issues, and applications* (pp. 29–52). Hillsdale, NJ: Erlbaum.

Seltzer, M., Choi, K., & Thum, Y. M. (in press). Examining relationships between where students start and how rapidly they progress: Using new developments in growth modeling to gain insight into the distribution of achievement within schools. *Educational Evaluation and Policy Analysis.*

Seltzer, M., Novak, J., Choi, K., & Lim, N. (2002). Sensitivity analysis for hierarchical models employing t level-1 assumptions. *Journal of Educational and Behavioral Statistics, 27,* 181–222.

Singer, J. D. (1998). Using SAS PROC MIXED to fit multilevel models, hierarchical models, and individual growth models. *Journal of Educational and Behavioral Statistics, 24,* 323–355.

Spiegelhalter, D. J., Thomas, A., & Best, N. G. (1999). *WinBUGS Version 1.2 user manual* (2nd ed.). Cambridge, England: Medical Research Council Biostatistics Unit.

Wang, C. P., Brown, C. H., & Bandeen-Roche, K. (2005). Residual diagnostics for growth mixture models: Examining the impact of a preventive intervention on multiple trajectories of aggressive behavior. *Journal of the American Statistical Association, 100,* 1054–1076.

Werthamer-Larsson, L., Kellam, S. G., & Wheeler, L. (1991). Effect of first-grade classroom environment on child shy behavior, aggressive behavior, and concentration problems. *American Journal of Community Psychology, 19,* 585–602.

Willett, J. B., Ayoub, C. C., & Robinson, D. (1991). Using growth modeling to examine systematic differences in growth: An example of change in the functioning of families at risk of maladaptive parenting, child abuse, or neglect. *Journal of Consulting and Clinical Psychology, 59,* 38–47.

Zeger, S. L., Liang, K. Y., & Albert, P. S. (1988). Models for longitudinal data: A generalized estimating equation approach. *Biometrics, 44,* 1049–1060. [Erratum appears in (1989) *Biometrics, 45 (1),* 347.]

15. ANALYZING AND PRESENTING OUTCOMES

Fiona Fidler, Cathy Faulkner, and Geoff Cumming

In this chapter we provide a model for analyzing and presenting data from RCTs. The worked example here is taken from a real study comparing a face-to-face therapy, an Internet intervention and a wait-list condition for treating body dissatisfaction and disordered eating in adults.

There are two main differences between the procedure we outline here and what might otherwise be found in textbooks or expository articles. First, we distinguish between "intention to treat" (ITT) analysis and "per protocol" (PP) analysis. Including PP analysis is essential if we want to answer the question: "*If a patient were to complete a course of therapy, what would the effects probably be?*" (Thomason & Gogos, 2007).

Second, we present effect size estimates and confidence intervals (CIs) as the primary outcomes of analysis, rather than statistical significance (i.e., null hypothesis significance tests [NHSTs] and associated p values). Our approach addresses the question, "How much of a difference does the therapy (or intervention) make?" rather than the more typical but less informative question "Does the therapy (or intervention) make a difference?"

Effect size estimates and CIs have been recommended by the American Psychological Association's *Publication Manual* (2001), the APA Task Force on Statistical Inference (Wilkinson & Task Force on Statistical Inference, 1999), and by scores of independent authors, including us (e.g., Cumming & Finch, 2005; Fidler, Thomason, Cumming, Finch, & Leeman, 2004). Consolidated Standards of Reporting Trials (CONSORT) also advocate this approach:

> Almost all methods of analysis yield an estimate of the treatment effect, which is a contrast between the outcomes in the comparison groups. In addition, authors should present a confidence interval for the estimated effect, which indicates a range of uncertainty for the true treatment effect." (CONSORT, n.d., checklist section)

We refer to this approach throughout this paper as an *estimation approach* and contrast it with the more traditional *statistical significance testing* approach.

■ Intention to Treat Versus Per Protocol

ITT analyses include all participants, regardless of whether they actually participated in the treatment. The Cochrane Collaboration describes the principle of
ITT in the following way: "The basic intention-to-treat principle is that participants in trials should be analysed in the groups to which they were randomized,
regardless of whether they received or adhered to the allocated intervention"
(module 14, http://www.cochrane-net.org/openlearning/HTML/mod14–4.htm).

In contrast, PP analyses exclude noncompleters. Criteria for "completion"
are, of course, context dependent. For example, completion may be attending
half or two thirds of therapy sessions, or a specified amount of some exercise or
intervention task. Criteria for completion should reflect the minimum amount
of intervention that might be capable of bringing about the hypothesized effect.
In addition, only participants who provided posttreatment data can legitimately be considered "completers."

The two analyses are not mutually exclusive—indeed, reporting both PP
and ITT analyses should perhaps be considered best practice. This is easily justified because the two analyses address substantially different questions.
Thomason and Gogos (2007) explain:

> A crucial goal of a medical Randomized Control Trial (RCT) should be to
> help answer the question: "*If* a patient were to take their medicine, what
> would the effects probably be?" Of course, there are other important
> questions as well, e.g., "What percent of the patients would actually com-
> ply with the regimen? To what degree?"(p. 1)

The first question is addressed by PP, the others by ITT. In the worked example presented in this chapter, we report PP analyses only. However, the estimation approach, and procedures we outline, can be easily applied to both PP
and ITT. We illustrate the approach only for PP to avoid repetition and because
PP is likely to be less familiar. We include some guidelines along the way for
how to adapt this for ITT.

■ Estimation Versus Statistical Significance Testing

There are many advantages of an estimation approach and, in particular, a
number of reasons why CIs are superior to sole reliance on p values. First, CIs
by definition contain point estimates of effect size—in readily interpretable
units of the original measurement scale. A CI around a mean difference will include a best estimate of mean difference, which is the raw effect size of the
study. Therefore when CIs are used to report results, effect size cannot be overlooked. By contrast, when reporting p values, it is common for researchers to
neglect effect size. Unfortunately, in psychological research effect sizes (includ-

ing the relevant mean differences) are all too often missing in articles reporting p values.

Second, CIs make uncertainty explicit. By this we mean that CIs offer immediate information about *precision*—again, in units of the original measurement scale. A wide interval indicates a lack of precision; a narrower interval, relatively better precision. A CI defines a set of plausible values for the population effect, so wider intervals rule out few values as not plausible. In other words, they give a less focused estimate of the effect. This means that studies with poor precision cannot be mistaken as evidence for nil effects, one of the major problems associated with p values.

Third, CIs do not preclude decisions. CIs can also be used to fail to reject or reject the null, when appropriate, by noting whether or not the null is captured. Though this is far from the most useful aspect of CIs, it is important to recognize that they are capable of fulfilling statistical decision needs when those needs exists. The links between CIs and p values may help ease the transition to estimation for the many researchers whose methodological and statistical training was dominated by a statistical significance testing view of research.

Finally, CIs may help facilitate meta-analytic thinking (Cumming & Finch, 2001, 2005). That is, they may assist thinking across the results of independent studies, acknowledging prior information with an emphasis on effect size, rather than making dichotomous "reject" or "fail-to-reject" decisions based on the outcome of single experiments. In an estimation approach, where the primary research outcome is an effect size, further research improves the precision of the effect size estimate, by narrowing the interval. Of course, decisions can still be made, but the illusion of objectivity provided by NHST is removed, and the uncertainty involved in any decision is made explicit. When authors fail to report effect sizes and estimates of their uncertainty, it is often not possible for their studies to be included in meta-analyses.

Results presented as merely "statistically significant" or "not significant" can create the illusion of inconsistency in the literature, particularly when review studies simply tally "significant" against "nonsignificant." CIs can help us identify patterns in data, and across studies, that statistical significance tests disguise. When presented visually, CIs may be even more effective in this role.

Lest the reader of this chapter think this approach is idiosyncratic, we emphasis that the APA Task Force on Statistical Inference made the same points. Its final report in *American Psychologist* (Wilkinson & Task Force on Statistical Inference, 1999) is a good starting point for guidance on statistical methodology. On effect sizes the task force wrote: "Reporting and interpreting effect sizes in the context of previously reported effects is essential to good research.... Reporting effect sizes also informs... meta analyses needed in future research." (p. 599). In support of CIs: "Comparing confidence intervals from a current study to intervals from previous, related studies helps focus attention on stability across studies.... Collecting intervals across studies also helps in constructing plausible regions for population parameters" (p. 599). Finally, on the general importance of cumulative research and meta-analysis: "Do not interpret a single study's results as having importance independent of the effects reported elsewhere in the relevant literature. . . . the results in a single study are important primarily as one contribution to a mosaic of study effects" (p. 602). The APA *Publication Manual* (2001) now also recommends effect sizes and calls CIs "the best reporting strategy" (p. 22).

■ The Data

The study we take as our example here assessed a manual-based 8-week group intervention for high body dissatisfaction and disordered eating in adults. The intervention sessions were facilitated by a therapist, delivered either face-to-face or in a synchronous Internet chat room. Women with high body dissatisfaction or bulimic symptoms were randomly allocated to either face-to-face delivery ($N = 42$), Internet delivery ($N = 38$), or delayed treatment control (DTC) or wait-list (N post $= 37$). (We use the terms *delayed treatment control* and *wait-list* interchangeably throughout this chapter, as is typical of this literature.)

Outcome measures can be divided into three main categories: (a) body image outcome measures, (b) eating and weight loss outcome measures, and (c) psychological outcome measures. Body image measures included the Body Shape Questionnaire (BSQ; Cooper, Taylor, Cooper, & Fairburn, 1987) and the Body Image Avoidance Questionnaire (Rosen, Srebnik, Saltzberg, & Wendt, 1991). In the following sections of this chapter we demonstrate, step by step, the analyses and presentation of results using the BSQ results only, the first measure listed in body image measures. The procedures followed here could of course be used with any of the outcome measures and/or repeated for all outcome measures.

■ A Model for Data Analysis and Presentation of Randomized Controlled Trials

Step 1. Inspect Rate of Completion

The first step in our analysis is defining what constitutes completion, so that we can then determine the completion rate and the effects of the treatment on those who received it. The criteria for what constitutes completion, or what it means to have completed the program, should be based on our judgment of the minimum number of sessions necessary to bring about the desired effect. This will be a value judgment and/or informed by past experience. Occasionally there may be guidance in the literature, but often there will not be. In this example case we decided that participants needed a minimum of four sessions. In addition, only participants who provided posttreatment data can legitimately be included in the analysis.

Once the criterion for completion has been established, we can calculate the completion rate of our study. This is simply the proportion of people, in each of the groups, who met the criterion for completion. In our case, this is the proportion of people in each group who attended four or more sessions and provided posttreatment data. We take the number of participants who attended four or more sessions and who also returned posttreatment data, divided by the total participants in that condition, multiplied by 100. For the face-to-face condition, $32/42 \times 100 = 76\%$ completion. In the Internet condition the completion rate was $24/38 \times 100 = 63\%$. For the waiting list it may be more meaningful to ignore the number of "sessions" attended and use all those returning "post" data.

As discussed previously, completion is one of the main outcomes of a study, and it is important to consider the implications of your completion rates: Was completion relatively high, or lower than expected? How did it compare with previous research? Was it substantially higher in one or more conditions? If so, what might have increased or decreased completion? Are there signs in the data, or given by participants, as to why noncompleters did not persist in the study? Are the reasons different for different conditions?

Step 2. Examine Overall Pattern of Results

Step 2 focuses on examining the effects of each condition, for those who received it (i.e. for the completers, since this is the PP analysis). Here we begin by examining histograms, to get a sense of the broad pattern of results. For this analysis, select completers only and exclude other participants. Our example histogram for pretreatment is shown in Figure 15.1.

Ideally, the distributions for each condition at pretreatment should have roughly similar means and spreads. This histogram provides the opportunity to detect any extreme outliers or any severe skewing. In making a visual assessment of the histograms, be sensitive to sample size. Small samples are likely to appear different simply because of sampling variability. For very large samples, marked differences in shape, or marked skewness, is more likely to indicate problems with the data that may need some action.

Figure 15.2 shows our posttreatment histogram. Questions to ask at this point include "Have the distributions shifted from the pretreatment data, hopefully in the predicted direction?," "Has one intervention had a larger effect than another?," and "How large are the effects, roughly speaking?"

In our example, the distributions for the face-to-face and Internet interventions have shifted considerably to the left from the pretreatment data and now appear to center on a score of around 100, whereas at pretreatment they were at around 130 or 140. Also, the wait-list condition is clearly to the right of the interventions at posttreatment, indicating improvement in both intervention

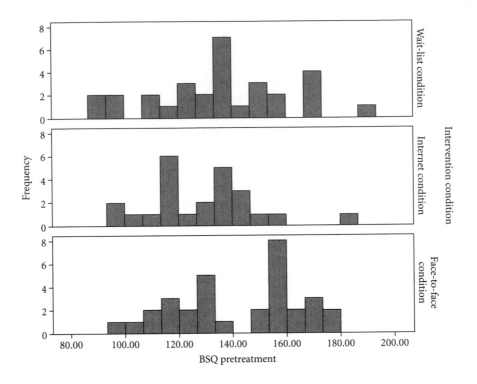

FIGURE 15.1. Histogram of pretreatment distribution of scores for one outcome variable (BSQ), for the three intervention conditions.

conditions relative to wait-list has been minimal. Note that figures produced in SPSS often have different scales, as in this example, which make shape comparisons between pre- and posthistograms slightly tricky. Check for extreme outliers or skewing, as with the pretreatment data.

Figure 15.3 shows our follow-up histogram. Here we include only participants who returned follow-up data and completed therapy. As in our case, there will probably be fewer participants at follow-up. Again, check for any extreme outliers and familiarize yourself with the pattern of follow-up data.

Once these distributions have been inspected, the next step is to calculate means and CIs. Figure 15.4 shows the list of values SPSS offers as default "descriptives." Unfortunately, n is not a default value in this list. In our case, n for face-to-face = 32, n for Internet = 24, and n for wait-list = 30. It is important to keep in mind that it is our choosing of completers that makes this a PP analysis, and therefore n in the pretest is determined by n at posttest. For an ITT analysis, we would follow the same steps but for *all* participants (i.e., not only those who attended four or more sessions). In ITT, cases where posttreatment data is not returned then become a missing data issue.

We recommend copying the output of Figure 15.4 into Microsoft Excel (see Figure 15.5) to create the graphical presentation shown in Figure 15.6. By formatting the data series and adding custom Y error bars, 95% CIs have been added to Figure 15.6. Clinically important cutoffs or other interpretative guidelines have been added with the drawing toolbar. In this figure the clinically significant criterion is taken to be 1 SD above the community mean in a previous study by Cooper et al. (1987).

We can now begin to interpret the pattern of our results. In our example, body image concerns have been reduced in both treatment conditions and have remained much the same in the wait-list condition. At pretreatment all three groups had similar BSQ scores. At posttreatment, the BSQ scores of the wait-list group are still above the clinically significant criterion for body dysphoria. In the Internet and face-to-face groups, BSQ scores have dropped below the clinical criterion.

We can make statistical inferences about the population BSQ scores based on the 95% CIs in Figure 15.6. Each CI gives information about the corresponding population mean; Cumming and Finch (2005) suggested several ways to interpret individual CIs and possible wording for discussing interpretations. Each 95% CI can be regarded as a set of plausible values for the true population mean. Values around the center of the CI are the best bet for the true value

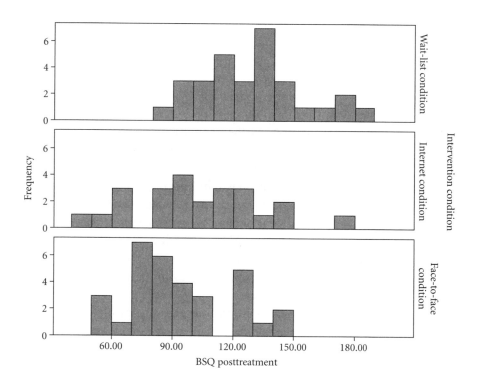

FIGURE 15.2. Histogram of posttreatment distribution of scores for one outcome variable (BSQ), for the three intervention conditions. Note that the *y*-axis scale in this figure is different from that in the pretreatment histogram in Figure 15.1. SPSS automatically produces different scales, which needs to be accounted for when comparing histograms from different time periods.

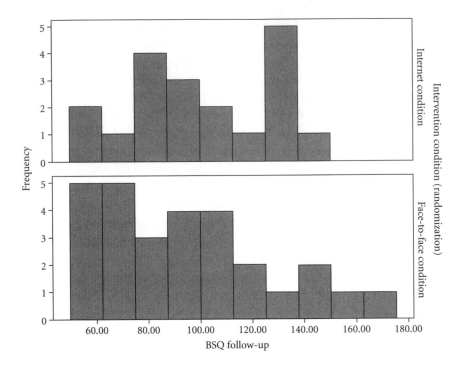

FIGURE 15.3. Histogram of follow-up distribution of scores for one outcome variable (BSQ), for the two intervention conditions assessed at this time period. Note again the difference in scale (as in Figure 15.2).

(Cumming, 2007), and values outside the CI are relatively implausible. The upper limit of the CI can be regarded as a likely upper bound for the true value, and the lower limit a likely lower bound.

Second, we can use the intervals shown in Figure 15.6 to compare any two means of different groups. If the 95% CIs of two independent groups overlap by no more than approximately one quarter of the total length, then the difference between the group means is statistically significant at $p < .05$, two-tailed (Cumming & Finch, 2005). Less overlap, or a gap between CIs, obviously indicates a greater difference; more overlap indicates that the difference fails to reach this statistical significance criterion.

In our example, there are statistically significant differences (at $p < .05$) between the waitlist condition and each of the treatment conditions at posttreatment and at follow-up, but there is no statistically significant difference between the Internet and face-to-face groups at any point.

Third, we can use the 95% CIs to assess which groups (if any) have improved to the extent that they are now distanced from the clinical range of body dysphoria (i.e., have moved convincingly below a BSQ score of 110). If the clinically significance criterion value is within a CI, this must be interpreted as a plausible value for the true mean. In our example in Figure 15.6, the 95% CIs for the Internet group at posttreatment and follow-up both include the clinical significance criterion. We interpret this as evidence that the population BSQ score for this group may be above, at, or below this criterion. For example, the Internet group may or may not have fallen below the clinical cutoff of 110 BSQ points. The CIs for the face-to-face group at posttreatment and at follow-up lie entirely below the clinical significance criterion, so at these time periods this group shows mean BSQ scores statistically significantly lower than the clinical cutoff of 110. Despite

Descriptives

Intervention Condition				Statistic	Std. Error
BSQ pretreatment	Face-to-face condition	Mean		142.4063	4.17362
		95% confidence Interval for mean	Lower Bound	133.8941	
			Upper Bound	150.9184	
		5% trimmed mean		142.8333	
		Median		147.5000	
		Variance		557.410	
		Std. deviation		23.60954	
		Minimum		97.00	
		Maximum		179.00	
		Range		82.00	
		Interquartile range		37.75	
		Skewness		−.241	.414
		Kurtosis		−1.061	.809
	Internet condition	Mean		128.9167	3.89859
		95% confidence Interval for mean	Lower Bound	120.8518	
			Upper Bound	136.9815	
		5% trimmed mean		127.9722	
		Median		130.5000	
		Variance		364.775	
		Std. deviation		19.09909	
		Minimum		97.00	
		Maximum		182.00	
		Range		85.00	
		Interquartile range		22.50	
		Skewness		.627	.472
		Kurtosis		1.334	.918
	Wait-list condition	Mean		136.3667	4.59872
		95% confidence Interval for mean	Lower bound	126.9612	
			Upper bound	145.7721	
		5% trimmed mean		136.2222	
		Median		138.0000	
		Variance		634.447	
		Std. deviation		25.18823	
		Minimum		89.00	
		Maximum		192.00	
		Range		103.00	
		Interquartile range		30.25	
		Skewness		−.008	.427
		Kurtosis		−.175	.833

FIGURE 15.4. Default output of the SPSS Explore procedure for pretreatment results for each of the three conditions (*n* for face-to-face = 32, *n* for Internet = 24, n for wait-list = 30). *Ns* given here are for completers at posttreatment in each intervention condition because we selected only these participants for the PP analysis. Note that *Ns* are not provided in the figure because they are not part of the SPSS "descriptives" default.

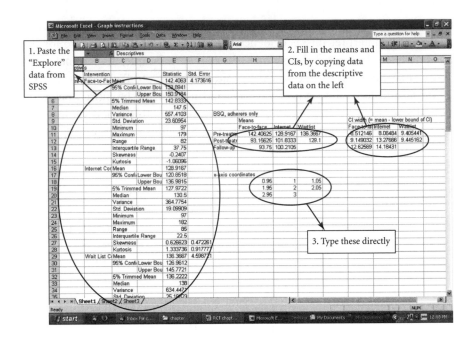

FIGURE 15.5. Steps to creating a graph of means and CIs in Microsoft Excel. Note that labels in Steps 2 and 3 (e.g., BSQ, completers only, *x*-axis coordinates) are typed directly into Excel.

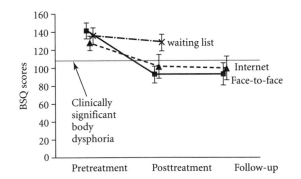

FIGURE 15.6. BSQ scores at pretreatment, posttreatment, and follow-up for the three intervention conditions. Pre- and posttreatment *N*s: face-to-face = 32, Internet = 24, waitlist = 30. Follow-up *N*s: face-to-face = 28, Internet = 19. Error bars are 95% CIs. Note that means have been slightly displaced horizontally so that CIs can be seen clearly. The clinically significant criterion of a BSQ score of 110 is provided by Cooper et al. (1987).

this difference in capture of the clinical cutoff between the Internet and face-to-face groups, the mean scores of these groups are in fact *not* statistically significantly different from each other. This is why it is essential to examine not only the statistical significance between intervention conditions but also each intervention condition individually against the clinical significance criterion.

Finally, note that although the intervals in Figure 15.6 are appropriate for assessing the difference between groups, and the inclusion or exclusion of the clinical significance criterion, they do *not* provide us with information about the statistical significance of change within groups. Just as the paired *t* test, unlike the independent-groups *t* test, is based on the SE of the paired *differences*, assessment of change within any group (i.e., a change involving a repeated measure) requires the CI on the differences, not the CIs on the individual means as shown in Figure 15.6 (Cumming & Finch, 2005). Step 3 explains how to assess change across time, within groups.

Step 3. Examine Change Across Time in Each Condition

First calculate differences scores for each participant, from pretreatment to posttreatment, for the outcome variable. Then select participants who returned posttreatment data and who completed therapy. Figure 15.7 shows the example histogram.

In our example, it appears that the face-to-face condition has had a larger change across time than the Internet condition. It is clear that participants in the Internet condition have also had a reduction in scores over time. At this stage we would also check for extreme outliers or a large amount of skewing. Using the same procedure, calculate difference scores for posttreatment to follow-up, and make histograms. After viewing the distributions in the histograms, mean differences and CIs can be calculated to analyze the change in each condition (see Figure 15.8).

Using Figure 15.8, we can examine change across time in each condition. In particular, we can investigate how precise the estimates are. For example, the improvement in BSQ score from pre- to posttreatment in the face-to-face group may be as little as about 40 points or as much as about 60 points. The width of the CI acts as a guide to precision (approximately corresponding to statistical power in an estimation approach). There can be no universal criteria for interpreting interval width, which needs to be assessed in the relevant clinical context, using clinical and research judgment.

Ideally, at follow-up, change will either be minimal, indicating maintenance of treatment gains, or will show further improvement. Figure 15.9 shows that in our example change from posttreatment to follow-up has been minimal, so treatment gains have been at least largely maintained.

Using Microsoft Excel, we can create a more sophisticated figure of the change from pre- to posttreatment (or from posttreatment to follow-up) using

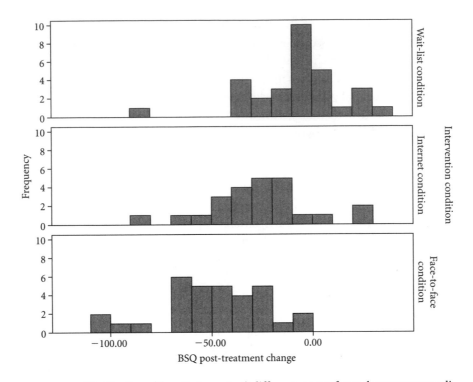

FIGURE 15.7. Distribution of (posttest – pretest) difference scores for each treatment condition.

the calculated means and 95% CIs. Figure 15.10 shows the Excel figure created for our example.

As shown in Figure 15.10, reference lines and labels can be added and used to guide interpretation of the results. If the outcome measure has clear interpretative guidelines, you can use those to indicate what would constitute a small, medium, large, or clinically important change. If no guidelines are available, you may choose to use Cohen's (1988) suggested benchmarks, which are that 0.2 SD is small, 0.5 SD is medium, and 0.8 is large. So, for example, for the reference line indicating a small effect, we calculated 0.2 × (pooled SD[1]) = 5.05 points on the BSQ (the primary outcome measure). Alternatively or in addition, Cohen's d may be calculated directly as the mean difference (post–pre BSQ) of a particular intervention group divided by the pooled standard deviation of that group, that is, the average of pre- and post-SD (see Cumming & Finch, 2001). A similar graph for the posttreatment to follow-up changes would assist interpretation of the maintenance of change caused by the interventions.

So far we have examined the distribution of raw scores for each condition across time, including the difference scores. We have then used means and CIs to examine and interpret group means at each time point, and then to estimate

1. Pooled SD is a weighted average of the pre- and post-SDs. One alternative is to use the pre-SD.

the size of the changes in each condition. Finally, we have made comparisons across conditions and relative to any important (e.g., clinically significant BSQ scores) reference points.

Step 4. Repeat Steps 2 and 3 for ITT and to Examine Outcomes of Other Variables

The procedures described here can be repeated for an ITT analysis simply by selecting *all* participants rather than only those who attended a select number of sessions such that face-to-face delivery $N = 42$, Internet delivery $N = 38$, and waitlist $N = 37$. Participants who do not return the posttreatment questionnaire then become a missing data issue.

The analysis, presentations, and interpretations can also be repeated for each variable of interest. Figures such as Figure 15.10 can easily be turned into panel graphs with the addition of more variables.

Step 5. Examine Moderating Effects

Paneled histograms and scatter graphs are useful for examining potential moderating effects. Figures 15.11 and 15.12 show some examples, with interpretations below. In these examples we have used fictional data because the sample

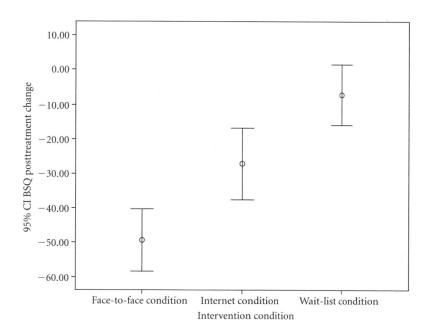

FIGURE 15.8. Simple graph of mean change scores, from pre- to posttreatment, with 95% CIs, as given by the SPSS "Simple" procedure. Pre- and posttreatment *Ns:* face-to-face = 32, Internet = 24, wait-list = 30.

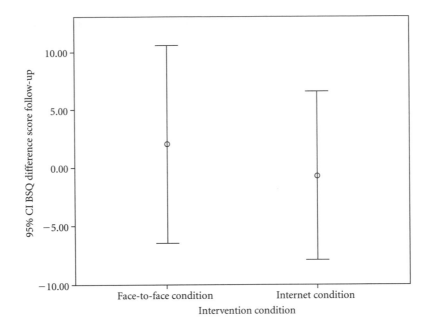

FIGURE 15.9. Example of mean difference scores with 95% CIs for the change from post-treatment to follow-up, for two treatment conditions. Follow-up *Ns:* face-to-face = 28, Internet = 19.

study we have described previously did not find any moderating effects. For this reason intervention conditions are now simply labeled Condition A, Condition B, and waitlist so as not to be confused with the real data we illustrate elsewhere in this chapter. Here we examine a participant's readiness for change (or "state of change") at pretreatment as a potential moderating variable on a fictional "outcome" variable.

Paneled histograms such as Figure 15.11 are useful for inspecting the impact of a categorical variable on a continuous variable. In our example, readiness to change (a categorical variable) has probably impacted on treatment effects. Particularly in Condition A, the participants who improved the most (i.e., decreased "outcome" scores of 50 to 100 points) are those who intended to change their behavior in the next 30 days. Similarly, those who were at a lower stage of readiness to change had generally smaller improvements (i.e., decreased "outcome" scores of between 0 to 50 points). If the histograms suggest important relationships between variables, relationships can be further examined by inspecting means and CIs. For the example shown in Figure 15.11, we would recommend calculating the means and CIs for participants in each condition, separating those who were ready to change in 30 days and those who were planning to change in 6 months.

If the potential moderating variable is continuous rather than categorical, use paneled scatter graphs (similarly generated in SPSS), as shown in Figure

15.12. The potential moderator under investigation in this figure is pretreatment severity. The question we ask is "Has pretreatment severity affected posttreatment improvement, such that participants with initially more severe scores improved more during treatment, regardless of the intervention condition?" Careful examination of the scatter plots in Figure 15.11 suggests that in this case we may have a floor effect, reflecting the fact that the pretreatment score sets an upper limit to the amount of improvement that is possible, because the dependent variable cannot take a negative value.

Step 6. Meta-analysis of Your Data Plus Data From Previous Studies

This final step involves comparing your results with those of previous studies. We mentioned earlier the importance of cumulative research and meta-analysis, and quoted from the APA Task Force on Statistical Inference, which strongly encouraged the use of meta-analysis. Some medical journals now require that any article presenting empirical results must either refer to a previous meta-analysis on the question or, if none exists, if possible conduct and report such a meta-analysis.

For this example, we illustrate a meta-analysis of one important outcome measure from the current study and three fictional previous studies addressing this question. The example meta-analysis estimates the effect of Internet therapy for body image concerns. The measure we focus on is once again BSQ score, in particular the change in BSQ score from pre- to posttreatment for the Internet condition. From Figure 15.8, we know that the change in BSQ for the Internet condition in our study was –27 points (post–pre BSQ) and that the half-width of the 95% CI for this change was 10.5. Imagine now that our care-

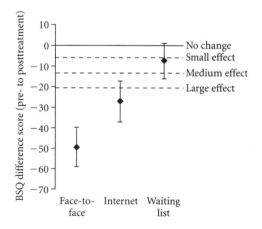

FIGURE 15.10. Pre- to posttreatment changes in each condition (face-to-face $n = 32$, Internet $n = 24$, wait-list $n = 30$), showing mean difference scores, 95% CIs, and reference lines and labels for selected effect sizes, to assist interpretation of clinical importance of the results.

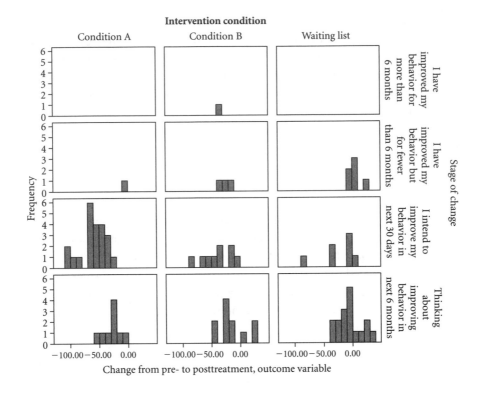

FIGURE 15.11. Paneled histogram of fictional data to examine a potential moderating variable. Participants' perceived "state of change" (on the second *y*-axis) is under investigation as a potential moderating variable on the "outcome" variable score from pre- to posttreatment (on the *x*-axis). Frequency of participants at each "state of change" and in each "outcome" variable score bracket is shown on the first *y*-axis.

ful literature search found three previous studies on this question that included a treatment we judged to be sufficiently similar to the Internet condition in our study. Figure 15.13 shows the three previous studies, each summarized as a mean decrease with its 95% CI, as P1, P2, and P3. Such a figure is known in medicine as a *forest plot*. Study size, and thus study weighting in the meta-analysis, is indicated approximately by the size of the mean circle and the thickness of the CI line. P1 was a small study, of low precision (wide CI), that found a large and statistically significant BSQ improvement. P2 and P3 were larger and more precise studies, each finding a small—or in the case of P3 very small—BSQ change, which was not statistically significantly different from zero. In Figure 15.13 the horizontal scale is the reverse of previous figures, that is, a decrease in BSQ is shown as a positive value. It is important to be aware that when using different pieces of software, defaults can give orderings that are inconsistent. Be alert to this, and before publication check that all such inconsistencies have been removed, by redefining variables or reversing the way an axis shows data in a figure.

M1 is the outcome of a simple meta-analysis of the three studies, and C the outcome of our study (from Figure 15.8). M2 is the best meta-analytic estimate of the effect of Internet therapy, based on all four studies. As we expect, its point estimate of 9 BSQ points improvement is the most precise estimate (shortest CI) shown.

Here we present only the simplest, first stage of a meta-analysis—the estimation of the effect of primary interest. A full meta-analysis would also assess other aspects, including consistency across studies and whether moderating variables might be playing a part.

■ Writing for Publication

In the final write-up, as in the analyses, we recommend a focus on estimation. The size of the effects and the uncertainty associated with those estimates (e.g., CIs) are the main outcomes of the study and should be discussed as such. Here we provide an example of how we would introduce and discuss results from the face-to-face condition. The following paragraphs are designed to give some guidance for the language that this new style of analyses and presentation might require.

Effects of the Face-to-Face Condition

The face-to-face condition had a 24% dropout rate; only 32 of the original 42 participants attended four or more sessions and returned posttreatment questionnaires. Participants who received the intervention had a pretreatment mean of 142 on the BSQ. This mean is typical of body image therapy patients and substantially above the criterion for clinical body dysphoria of 110 BSQ (Cooper, Taylor, Cooper, & Fairburn, 1987). Participants in this group had a

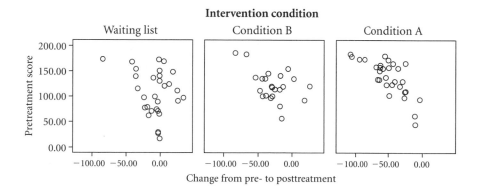

FIGURE 15.12. Example paneled scatter graph showing a fictional relationship between severity of symptoms at pretreatment and pre- to posttreatment change, for three hypothetical intervention conditions.

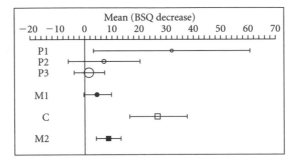

FIGURE 15.13. Meta-analysis for BSQ change (decrease) from pretreatment to posttreatment, for an Internet condition. Mean change is shown, with 95% CI. P1, P2, and P3 are fictional previously published studies, and C is the result from our current study, from Figure 15.8. M1 is the meta-analytic combination of the three previous studies, and M2 is the combination of all four studies. Our study has advanced the estimation of the true effect of an internet intervention from M1 to M2.

posttreatment mean of 96, well below the cutoff for clinically significant body dysphoria. Moreover, the 95% CI around the posttreatment mean BSQ lay entirely below the cutoff, so we conclude that the posttreatment population mean is not likely to be in the clinical range on this variable.

For those participants who were retained in therapy, the intervention had a very large (Cohen's $d = 1.9$) effect on improving body image, with the average effects in the population estimated to be an improvement of 48 points [95% CI: 26, 46] on the BSQ (see Figure 15.10). (The lower and upper limits of 95% confidence intervals are provided in square brackets following estimates mentioned in the text. This is the style we suggest should be used routinely for reporting CIs as numerical values.)

The face-to-face intervention had a distinctly greater effect than the Internet condition or waiting list. In Figure 15.10, the 95% confidence intervals overlap less than one quarter width, corresponding to a statistically significant effect at $p < .05$ (Cumming & Finch, 2005). The difference between face-to-face and other conditions was large (Cohen's $d = 1.0$ and 1.4 compared with the Internet and wait-list conditions, respectively). It is notable that these substantial improvements are very largely maintained at follow-up. Improvements of this size are clearly of considerable clinical value and would make a substantial improvement to the participants' quality of life.

■ Recommended Resources

Finally, we refer readers to the following sources for further guidance on using and interpreting the analyses described here. The APA Task Force on Statistical Inference report (Wilkinson, 1999) is a good starting point and includes many references. Kline (2004) provides excellent practical guidance on a wide range of statistical issues.

For further guidelines on CI interpretation, see Cumming and Finch (2001, 2005) and Cumming (in press). For an explanation of various types of effect sizes, see Kirk (1996), as well as Chapter 18 of this volume. A new statistical text for behavioral scientists, by Thompson (2006), outlines calculation procedures and interpretation for several types of effect sizes.

In 1999 the *Journal of Consulting and Clinical Psychology* ran a special section on clinical significance with articles that discussed methods, measures, and definitions of clinical significance. Kazdin (1999) provides an overview to the special section, and several practical "how-to" guides for clinical significance follow in the same section. See also Chapter 17 of this volume.

For a general background to statistical reform and surveys of changes to statistical practices in psychology journals, see Fidler et al. (2005) and, more recently, Cumming et al. (2007).

■ Acknowledgments

This research was supported by the Australian Research Council. We are extremely grateful to Susan Paxton, Sian McLean, and their coauthors for sharing their body image data with us for use in this chapter. Their manuscript presenting their study is currently under review: Paxton, S. J., McLean, S. A., Gollings, E. K., Faulkner, C., & Wertheim, E. (in press). Comparison of face-to-face and Internet interventions for body image and eating problems in adult women: An RCT. *International Journal of Eating Disorders*.

■ References

American Psychological Association. (2001). *Publication manual of the American Psychological Association* (5th ed.). Washington, DC: Author.

Cochrane Collaboration Opening Learning Material. *Module 14: Further issues in meta-analysis.* Retrieved September 15, 2006, from http://www.cochranenet.org/openlearning/HTML/mod14-4.htm

Cohen, J. (1988). *Statistical power analysis for the behavioral sciences* (2nd ed.). Hillsdale, NJ: Erlbaum.

Consolidated Standards of Reporting Trials (CONSORT). *12(a) Statistical methods used to compare groups for primary outcome(s).* Retrieved September 15, 2006, from http://www.consort statement.org/Downloads/checklist.pdf

Cooper, P. J., Taylor, M. J., Cooper, Z., & Fairburn, C. G. (1987). The development and validation of the Body Shape Questionnaire. *International Journal of Eating Disorders, 6,* 485–494.

Cumming, G. (2007). Inference by eye: Pictures of confidence intervals and thinking about levels of confidence. *Teaching Statistics, Teaching Statistics, 29,* 89–93.

Cumming, G., Fidler, F., Leonard, M., Kalinowski, P., Christiansen, A., Kleinig, A., et al. (2007). Statistical reform in psychology: Is anything changing? *Psychological Science, 18,* 230–232.

Cumming, G., & Finch, S. (2001). A primer on the understanding, use, and calculation of confidence intervals that are based on central and non-central distributions. *Educational and Psychological Measurement, 61,* 532–574.

Cumming, G., & Finch, S. (2005). Inference by eye: Confidence intervals, and how to read pictures of data. *American Psychologist, 60,* 170–180.

Fidler, F., Cumming, G., Thomason, N., Pannuzzo, D., Smith, J., Fyffe, P., et al. (2005). Toward improved statistical reporting in the *Journal of Consulting and Clinical Psychology. Journal of Consulting and Clinical Psychology, 73,* 136–143.

Fidler, F., Thomason, N., Cumming, G., Finch, S. & Leeman, J. (2004). Editors can lead researchers to confidence intervals but they can't make them think: Statistical reform lessons from medicine. *Psychological Science, 15,* 119–126.

Kazdin, A. E. (1999). The meanings and measurement of clinical significance. *Journal of Consulting and Clinical Psychology, 67,* 332–339.

Kirk, R. E. (1996). Practical significance: A concept whose time has come. *Educational and Psychological Measurement, 56,* 746–759.

Kline, R. B. (2004). *Beyond significance testing: Reforming data analysis methods in behavioral research.* Washington, DC: American Psychological Association.

Rosen, J. C., Srebnik, D., Saltzberg, E., & Wendt, W. (1991). Development of a body image avoidance questionnaire. *Psychological Assessment, 3,* 32–37.

Thomason, N., & Gogos, A. (2007). *Human randomized control trials don't give what we think they are giving us: The standard statistical test seriously misleads.* Manuscript in preparation.

Thompson, B. (2006). *Foundations of behavioral statistics: An insight-based approach.* New York: Guilford.

Wilkinson, L., & Task Force on Statistical Inference. (1999). Statistical methods in psychology journals: Guidelines and explanations. *American Psychologist, 54,* 594–604.

16. Methods for Capturing the Process of Change

Adele M. Hayes, Jean-Philippe Laurenceau, and LeeAnn Cardaciotto

The randomized clinical trial (RCT) has become the gold standard for determining whether treatments for specific clinical disorders meet the criteria for being empirically supported (Chambless et al., 1998; Chambless & Ollendick, 2001). Although there is considerable controversy over the specifics of this method of evaluation (e.g., Goldfried & Wolfe, 1996; Westen, Novotny, & Thompson-Brenner, 2004), there has been a proliferation of psychosocial interventions with data to support their efficacy and clinical utility (effectiveness). The field has reached a point at which there has been a resurgence of interest in understanding *how* treatments have their effects and for *whom* they work.

Process research has a long history but was overshadowed by the press to demonstrate the efficacy and effectiveness of psychotherapies (Pachankis & Goldfried, in press). The tide is changing, as researchers recognize the importance of process research in increasing our theoretical understanding of human change processes, improving the delivery of therapy, and maximizing treatment efficacy. A task force on psychotherapy research sponsored by Division 12 (Society for Clinical Psychology) of the American Psychological Association (APA) explicitly called for more research linking the process of change with treatment outcome (Weisz, Hawley, Pilkonis, Woody, & Follette, 2000). In line with this recommendation, Division 12 of the APA and the North American Society for Psychotherapy Research convened a group of leading psychotherapy researchers from a number of theoretical orientations to identify empirically supported principles of change that have emerged in the literature to date. In an edited volume, Castonguay and Beutler (2006) present principles that can be used to guide the treatment of four clusters of clinical problems: depression, anxiety disorders, personality disorders, and substance abuse. Kraemer and colleagues (Kraemer, Wilson, Fairburn, & Agras, 2002) urge researchers to routinely assess hypothesized moderators and mediators of change when designing an RCT. They view process research as vital to treatment development because such information can "guide the next generation of research and inform clinical applications" (p. 878).

The need is clear, but there are few guidelines on how to incorporate process research into the RCT design. Until recently, the traditional RCT design focused on the assessment of treatment outcome and was not designed to capture the process of change. We will describe how researchers can study the shape and process of change using both individual- and group-level data within the open trial and the full-scale RCT design. We will also illustrate how process research is an integral part of treatment development.

■ Questions That Process Research Can Address

We describe three central questions that process research can address within the RCT design: What is the *shape* of change?, What are the *moderators* of change?, and How does change occur (*predictors* of change, *mediators,* and *mechanisms*)? The methodological issues and statistical analyses will be organized around these questions. Process research is an integral part of psychotherapy development, refinement, and evaluation. It can be conducted during the open trial phase of development, using archived sessions from a completed trial, and it can also be incorporated into the newly designed RCT. We provide examples of each of these phases of process research. This chapter extends and elaborates on an earlier paper that provides a more general overview of process research methods (Laurenceau, Hayes, & Feldman, 2007).

The Shape of Change

In the traditional RCT design, symptoms are assessed at the beginning, middle, and end of treatment, and change is studied at the level of group averages. These snapshots of functioning do not capture the dynamic process of change over the course of therapy. For example, Figure 16.1 depicts three very different trajectories that cannot be distinguished by simple pre-mid-post change scores. In general, the traditional designs also do not allow for the study of discontinuities and nonlinear patterns of symptom change (Hayes, Laurenceau, Feldman, Strauss, & Cardaciotto, 2007).

With more frequent assessments, the shape of change can be studied over the course of therapy at the level of the individual and the group. An examination of the trajectories can reveal the rate of change and whether the rate is constant over the course of treatment. For example, change can occur smoothly and linearly over the course of therapy (as in Trajectory A in Figure 16.1), or most of the change can be concentrated at the beginning or end of therapy (as in Trajectory B), or change can take a cubic form of a decrease in symptoms, an increase, and then a decrease (as in Trajectory C). Pre- to posttreatment analyses of these data would suggest similar amounts of symptom change, but the *pattern* of change is not apparent unless trajectories are studied.

By studying trajectories of symptom change in cognitive-behavioral therapies for depression, researchers have identified three patterns of symptom

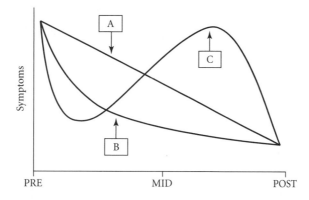

FIGURE 16.1. Examples of linear (A), quadradic (B), and cubic (C) trajectories of change over the course of therapy.

change that predict better treatment outcomes. The following examples illustrate the useful information that can be gleaned from an examination of weekly or biweekly data from individuals in clinical trials. Ilardi and Craighead (1994) identified an *early rapid response* pattern that is characterized by a rapid decrease in depression symptoms by session 4, after which change levels off (Trajectory B). The rapid response pattern even predicts symptom improvement in difficult-to-treat clinical disorders, such as bulimia (e.g., Grilo, Masheb, & Wilson, 2006; Wilson, Fairburn, Agras, Walsh, & Kraemer, 2002) and alcohol abuse (Breslin, Sobell, Sobell, Buchan, & Cunningham, 1997).

Tang and DeRubeis (1999) identified another pattern of change in the early sessions of cognitive therapy for depression that they call *sudden gains.* The sudden gain is a large improvement during a single between-session interval that does not reverse. Plots of averaged symptom change at pre-, mid-, and posttreatment suggest gradual and linear change, but Tang and colleagues (Tang & DeRubeis, 1999; Tang, DeRubeis, Beberman, & Pham, 2005) found that plots of *individual* symptom change over the course of therapy revealed that about 39 to 46% of patients experienced a sudden gain and that this nonlinear pattern predicted improvement in depression. Sudden gains also have been associated with better functioning at the end of treatment in supportive-expressive therapy (Tang, Luborsky, & Andrusyna, 2002), nonmanualized psychotherapies in routine clinical practices (Stiles et al., 2003), systematic behavioral family therapy (Gaynor et al., 2003), and cognitive-behavioral therapy (CBT) for recurrent and atypical depression (Vittengl, Clark, & Jarrett, 2005).

Our research group has identified a pattern of change that we call a *depression spike* in an exposure-based cognitive therapy for depression that we are developing. Hierarchical linear modeling (HLM) analyses revealed an overall S-shaped (cubic) trajectory of symptom change (Trajectory C). Individual trajectories revealed a rapid response pattern, as defined by Ilardi and Craighead

(1994), early in therapy. The phase of therapy that includes principles of exposure was characterized by depression spikes, which are large increases in depression during this phase, followed by a decrease in symptoms. The depression spike is the conceptual opposite of the sudden gain and is similar to the anxiety spike pattern described in exposure-based therapies for anxiety disorders (Heimberg & Becker, 2002). Patients were classified as having a rapid response and a depression spike or not. Both of these patterns of change predicted more improvement in depression at the end of treatment, after controlling statistically for previous levels of depression (Hayes, Feldman, Beevers, et al., 2007).

These three patterns of change (rapid response, sudden gain, depression spike) are discontinuous and nonlinear and therefore would not be apparent with pre-post analyses of group data, yet they mark important transition points that can reveal what therapists are doing to facilitate this transition and what is changing in patients during this time (Hayes, Laurenceau, Feldman, et al., 2007). Without such markers, the researcher is left to examine all the sessions and weeks of data to identify predictors of change, to randomly select sessions, or to select sessions from phases of therapy without regard to symptom change. Examining all the data is often too labor-intensive and inefficient. Random selection might miss the process variables of interest. Phase selection begins to isolate broad segments of therapy to study, but there is again the risk of missing the variables of interest if the selection method is too crude.

When significant transition points have been identified, they can guide further analyses to uncover the process of change. For example, Tang and DeRubeis (1999) found that there was more cognitive change in the session that immediately preceded the sudden gain (pregain session) than in the session that immediately preceded the pregain session (pre-pregain session). This suggests that cognitive shifts might be inducing the sudden gain in cognitive therapy. Similarly, Hayes and colleagues (Hayes, Beevers, Feldman, Laurenceau, & Perlman, 2005; Hayes, Feldman, Beevers, et al., 2007) studied patient narratives in the vicinity of the rapid response and depression spike patterns in a cognitive therapy that includes components of exposure. Consistent with Ilardi and Craighead's (1994) predictions, the narratives of rapid responders were associated with more hope than those of nonrapid responders. Narratives during the depression spike were characterized by more cognitive-emotional processing (a significant shift in perspective and emotional response) than those written by patients who did not experience this increase in affective arousal. This pattern and process of change is consistent with findings from exposure-based therapies for anxiety disorders (Foa & Kozak, 1986; Foa, Huppert, & Cahill, 2005). Identifying the shape of change can have important implications for testing theories of change, identifying predictors of symptom course, and treatment development.

An area that has received less emphasis in the process of change is what happens *after* the acute phase of therapy. This period traditionally has been viewed as relatively smooth, and researchers assess the maintenance of treatment outcomes at intervals of several months. Witkwiewitz and Marlatt (2007) propose that researchers and clinicians studying substance abuse could be more successful at predicting relapse if they were less dependent on linear, continuous models of relapse for a process that is more likely discontinuous. What seem to be minor changes in one risk factor (e.g., negative affect) can set off a rapid cascade of increased craving, positive outcome expectancies, and drug-seeking behavior that can quickly result in relapse. Hufford, Witkiewitz, Shields, Kodya, and Caruso (2003) applied catastrophe theory models of sudden and discontinuous change and demonstrated that the shift from recovery to relapse is indeed better predicted by nonlinear than linear models of change. Wikeiwitz and Marlatt (2007) replicated this finding with a larger sample size, a longer follow-up period, and a more sophisticated method of catastrophe cusp-fit modeling. After identifying the point of transition to relapse, distal and proximal risk factors of relapse can be identified. This method might be applied fruitfully to the study of relapse in other disorders.

Moderators of Change

Moderators clarify under what conditions and for whom an intervention works and does not work. These variables can help to explain individual differences in the effect of the treatment. A moderator has traditionally been defined as a variable that interacts with a predictor variable to influence the level of the dependent variable (Baron & Kenny, 1986; Holmbeck, 1997). When applied to psychotherapy trials, Kraemer et al. (2002) recommend two modifications. First, the moderator should precede treatment as a baseline or prerandomization characteristic. That is, a moderator should temporally precede the variable it is thought to modify, which distinguishes moderators from mediators and also makes more clear the temporal sequencing of variables. Second, a moderator is associated with outcome in either the treatment or control condition but not both. If the proposed moderator has a main effect only (i.e., associated with outcome regardless of treatment assignment), it is considered a nonspecific predictor of outcome rather than a moderator.

An increased understanding of moderators of change can improve treatment delivery and efficacy. For example, identifying moderators of change can allow for improved matching of patients with particular background characteristics to treatments with demonstrated efficacy. In an RCT of cognitive-behavioral therapy and interpersonal therapy (IPT) for bulimia, Constantino, Arnow, Blasey, and Agras (2005) identified moderators of therapeutic alliance quality, a well-established predictor of treatment outcome (Horvath & Bedi, 2002; Martin, Garske, & Davis, 2000). Patients with more interpersonal problems at baseline reported lower alliance quality at midtreatment in IPT, and those with more symptom severity at baseline reported lower alliance quality at midtreatment in CBT. Expectation for improvement predicted outcome in both therapies (main effect only, no interaction), and therefore is considered a non-specific predictor of outcome rather than a moderator.

Such research suggests avenues for treatment development to maximize treatment response for these difficult-to-treat patients. Identifying a moderator of change also can help to uncover potential mediators of change. Moderators can identify subgroups for whom a mediator of change contributes to improved outcomes and those for whom it does not (i.e., moderated mediation).

Predictors of Change, Mediators, and Mechanisms of Change (Why/How Is Change Occurring?)

Identifying mediators of treatment change can elucidate how psychotherapy has its effects on outcome. Mediators are the constructs or factors that an intervention program is designed to change and through which the therapy is thought to have its effects (Judd & Kenny, 1981). Researchers can identify predictors of therapeutic change in open trials and RCT designs, which can suggest possible mediators. Mediators, in turn, can suggest possible mechanisms of change, which are processes or events in psychotherapy that lead to and *cause* change in an outcome. A mediator that is a causal agent is a mechanism of change. As Kraemer et al. (2002) note, all mechanisms of change are mediators, but not all mediators will turn out to be mechanisms.

Kraemer et al.'s (2002) application of the original Baron and Kenny (1986) definitions of moderators and mediators to the RCT design include some important clarifications. In the study of change in the RCT, a putative mediator should precede change in outcome, occur during the course of treatment (between initiation of the treatment and the outcome), and have a main or interactive effect on outcome. A moderator is not correlated with treatment, whereas a mediator is. The proposed mediator should also be clearly distinguished from the therapy and from measures of outcome. For instance, if homework is assigned in one condition and not the other, homework is part of the therapy in one group and cannot be conceptualized as a mediator. In addition, if habituation is conceptualized as a mediator of change, it cannot be measured as both a mediator and an outcome. Kraemer et al. (2002) recommend a clear distinction between moderators and mediators in that the same variable cannot be both a moderator and a mediator. Directionality is also made clear by requiring temporal precedence of the mediator relative to the outcome, and the mediator is to follow treatment. In addition, these authors recommend using effect sizes to guide the evaluation of mediators rather than *p* values, which will change with sample size.

Understanding why therapies have their effects can lead to important advances in treatment development. If mediators of change can be identified, the potency and efficiency of treatments can be increased. For instance, Foa and Kozak (1986) proposed that emotional processing was a mediator of change in the efficacious therapies for anxiety disorders at the time. Emotional processing was defined as the modification of the pathological associations among stimuli, responses, and meaning (fear structure) with repeated exposure to feared stimuli, activation of the fear structure, and corrective information. Emotional processing has been examined as a mediator of exposure-based therapies in the context of the clinical trial, in naturalistic studies, and in laboratory studies that directly manipulate the proposed mediator. Exposure-based therapies have improved iteratively with this research. In a recent update of emotional processing theory, Foa et al. (2006) continue to clarify and refine the theory as new findings emerge from neurobiological and animal research. This updated theory can be tested in process research and perhaps further increase the potency of exposure-based therapies (McNally, 2007).

These innovations have implications for the theoretical understanding of change in anxiety disorders, for how therapy is delivered, and for the prevention of relapse. This is but one example of treatment development research that illustrates the interplay of theory, basic science research, process research, the evaluation of outcome, and further treatment development. It also illustrates how identifying a possible mediator across several treatments can facilitate consolidation and parsimony (Kazdin & Nock, 2003). Exposure-based therapies for anxiety disorders are among the most potent treatments available (Chambless & Ollindick, 2001).

A particularly interesting application of moderators and mediators is described by Collins, Murphy, and Bierman (2004). These authors explain how moderators and mediators of change that have been identified empirically can be used as "tailoring variables" for adaptive treatment strategies. Adaptive treatment approaches involve repeated adjustments of treatment level and type in response to individual patient needs over the course of therapy rather than the delivery of fixed treatment components to all participants. Adaptive treatment approaches represent a potentially powerful way to refine and optimize intervention packages.

Ultimately, clinical research that pursues these three types of process questions can contribute to advances in psychotherapy development. Some psychotherapy researchers (e.g., Kazdin & Nock, 2003) have argued that an increased focus on process-oriented questions will be the most rapid way that significant progress will be made in the study of psychotherapy. However, the traditional pre-post design of the randomized control trial that is typically used in most treatment outcome research can pose challenges for researchers interested in studying the process of change.

■ Design Considerations in Process Research

Whenever possible, it is wise to include measures that capture change over time because these measures describe the shape and timing of change, for whom and

under what circumstances the therapy works, how the therapy might be working, and also when and how the therapy does not work optimally. This information is useful in the early case series or open trial phase of new treatment development and also in the full-scale RCT. Clinical trial research takes many
years to complete, so incorporating measures of process can maximize the yield
of the research.

What to Measure: Selecting Assessments

Because neither researchers nor patients have unlimited resources investigators
must be judicious in their selection of measures and the frequency of assessments. It is most important to select measures that assess the primary constructs of interest. When possible, the measures should be based on a theory of
change and on previous research, but researchers in the exploration phase of
treatment development also can generate hypotheses from their data. As mentioned earlier, Ilardi and Craighead (1994) discovered the early rapid response
phenomenon and Tang and DeRubeis (1999) the sudden gain by plotting
symptom trajectories over the course of therapy and noticing a pattern of early
change that predicted better outcomes. Initially, these patterns were discovered
rather than predicted.

The process of change can be studied from the perspective of the patient
changes, therapist interventions, and the patient-therapist dyad such as the
therapeutic alliance. Researchers often focus on one of these perspectives, but
some measures allow for an assessment of multiple perspectives. For instance,
the first author has developed an observational coding system with which to
code the content of therapy sessions and patient narratives. The Change and
Growth Experiences Scale (CHANGE; Hayes, Feldman, & Goldfried, 2007) assesses patient variables (e.g., a focus on negative and positive view of self, hope,
avoidance, cognitive/emotional processing, and unproductive perseverative
processing), as well as therapist interventions (e.g., a focus on corrective information, supportive strategies, homework) and a focus on the therapeutic relationship. A measure that assesses multiple perspectives can be used to investigate models of change over time because patient, therapist, and the therapeutic
relationship variables are assessed at the same time points. Such a strategy is
more efficient than conducting separate studies focusing on one or the other of
the perspectives.

Another way to accomplish this is to include multiple measures of process
within the same study. In a study of experiential therapy for depression, Missirlian, Toukmanian, Warwar, and Greenberg (2005) included measures of emotional arousal and perceptual processing and also a measure of the working alliance between the patient and therapist. This allowed for a rich analysis of
change that was mapped onto a larger theory of emotional processing and
change (Greenberg, 2002). The study of change is not limited to the study of

individual therapy; it is also a vital part of treatment development for couples, families, and groups.

Where to Measure: Timing and Interval of Assessments

The goal of process research is to understand what happens between the beginning and end of treatment. It is therefore critical to obtain sufficient assessments of putative correlates of change, mediators, and symptoms to obtain an accurate and dynamic picture of how change unfolds over time. The temporal design (Collins, 2006; Collins & Graham, 2002) of a longitudinal study is an important but often underconsidered factor in RCT designs. Methodologists have long been aware of the issues related to the timing and spacing of assessments in longitudinal data and the potential effects of temporal design on findings (e.g., Windle & Davies, 1999), but these issues are less often discussed in guidelines for designs of psychotherapy trials. For instance, the Consolidated Standards of Reporting Trials (CONSORT; Begg et al., 1996) guidelines that outline consistent standards for the conduct and presentation of RCTs recommend assessments of outcome variables at pre- and posttreatment but do not provide guidelines on how researchers can use multiple assessments to enhance process research.

The temporal design of a psychotherapy trial can have important consequences for the evaluation of the three process questions discussed earlier—the shape of change, moderators of change, and mediators of change. If measurements are included only at pre- and posttreatment, curvilinear and cubic functions cannot be examined. Moreover, measurement error at the pre- and posttreatment assessments can make it difficult to precisely and reliably capture even linear change, unless more time points are obtained (Willett, 1988). It may also be difficult to evaluate pretreatment covariates as potential candidates for moderators of treatment, when the measure of change is a potentially unreliable pre-post difference. Measurement error in the pre-post difference score results in lower reliability of this measure of change, thus attenuating its associations with potential moderators or other covariates (Aguinis, 1995).

The temporal design of a clinical trial is particularly important for tests of mediation. Mediation cannot be tested in cross-sectional or two-wave pre-post designs (Singer & Willett, 2003). Three or more repeated measurements are necessary to adequately evaluate a mediation model, and the mediator must precede the measure of outcome (Kraemer et al., 2002). The putative mediator should show variability earlier in the treatment than the assessment of the outcome the mediator is purported to influence (Kraemer et al., 2002; Baron & Kenny, 1986). When the putative mediator is assessed at the same time as the outcome, the variable could be an epiphenomenon of symptom change or may no longer be relevant to change by the end of treatment. Another consideration is whether the mediator is assessed too far from the period at which the treatment effect on that mediator is strongest (too late) because this can lead researchers to the mistaken conclusion that there is no mediation. Even when symptoms are measured at multiple points between the beginning and end of treatment, few studies contain multiple measures of the correlates of change and putative mediators between pre- and posttreatment.

While adequate for establishing the efficacy of a treatment, two-wave pre-post designs for clinical trials do not provide psychotherapy researchers the opportunity to examine a range of process questions. Obtaining additional assessments of outcomes and putative mediators over the course of treatment allows for more complex shapes of change to be examined and increases the precision and reliability of change estimates (Willett, Singer, & Martin, 1998). A more appropriate temporal design can help researchers to identify when the greatest amount of change is taking place and when a potential mediator may be having an effect on outcome. We now turn to a discussion of ways to design clinical trials with more intensive temporal designs that can allow for more sophisticated process analyses. The literatures oriented toward methodologists who work with longitudinal data are invaluable resources for clinical research design (e.g., Collins, 2006; Collins & Graham, 2002; Singer & Willett, 2003; Willett et al., 1998; Windle & Davies, 1999).

SELECTING AN APPROPRIATE TIMING OF ASSESSMENTS

Psychotherapy researchers should carefully consider the timing of the effect of an intervention so that assessments are not taken too early or too late. Assessments can be distributed evenly across the course of therapy (e.g., weekly, bi-weekly) to increase the probability of capturing the phenomenon of interest, but at times such a strategy may not be efficient and may be too labor-intensive. In general, researchers should take more observations when change is occurring more quickly and fewer observations when change is more gradual (Collins & Sayer, 2000). Pilot work and initial open clinical trials of a treatment can provide useful information to guide temporal design decisions. Although these sources of information may not guarantee the optimal temporal design for a particular study, they are preferable to using an arbitrary, but typical, pre-mid-post design for studying all change processes or oversampling from every session.

The timing and spacing of repeated assessments can be based on a theoretically informed conceptualization of the treatment effect and theory of change for a particular psychotherapy (Collins & Graham, 2002). For example, given the consistent findings of a rapid response (Ilardi & Craighead, 1994) in CBT for depression, researchers planning an RCT of CBT versus some other intervention would be prudent to assess putative correlates of change, mediators, and outcomes multiple times and early in the treatment.

Some theories propose that a given process variable is most potent in a specific phase of therapy and that during that period it predicts treatment outcome. Two emotion-focused therapies for depression—experiential therapy (Greenberg & Watson, 2005) and exposure-based cognitive therapy (Hayes, Feldman, Beavers, et al. 2007)—are based on the assumption that cognitive/emotional processing occurs in the middle phase of therapy when affective arousal is highest. Indeed, in both therapies processing in the middle phase of therapy predicted more improvement in depression at the end of treatment than did processing in the early phase (Hayes et al., 2005; Hayes, Feldman, Beavers, et al., 2007; Missirlian et al., 2005). Studying process variables in phases of therapy sheds light on the temporal sequencing of variables. This sequencing is an important step in identifying possible mediators of change. These studies also make clear that the relationship between process and outcome can depend on when in therapy the process is measured (Missirlian et al., 2005).

Another way to pinpoint even more precisely where the action might be is to identify therapeutic events that are linked with theories of change and intensively study those events (Rice & Greenberg, 1984). In a clinical trial of experiential therapy for depression, Missirlian and colleagues (2005) used this method to identify emotion episodes, which are segments of therapy in which patients talk about having experienced an emotion. These episodes were then rated for affective arousal and extent of reflective processing. Emotional processing was operationalized as the combination of affective arousal and reflective processing. Emotional processing in the middle and late phases (and not the early phase) predicted more improvement in depression. This study illustrates how to use theory to guide the study of change, how to use a marker of therapeutic change to focus the process research, and how to use phases of therapy to clarify the temporal sequencing of process variables.

Researchers can also use periods of high risk to guide assessment. A number of disorders, such as personality disorders and substance abuse, are characterized by high rates of early dropout. In such cases, researchers can include baseline measures that might predict dropout and sample frequently during this period of increased risk.

The follow-up period after the acute phase of therapy is a time when the density of assessment of both outcome and process is very low, often separated by intervals of 3 to 6 months in the typical RCT design. Given the high rates of relapse in so many disorders, progress could be made in relapse prevention if researchers could understand better how relapse occurs. Witkiewitz and Marlatt (2007) describe some innovative attempts to remedy this problem and better capture the often nonlinear dynamics of relapse.

INCREASING THE DENSITY OF ASSESSMENT

One fairly direct approach to obtaining more frequent and closely spaced assessments is to use monitoring forms and worksheets that are used routinely in weekly psychotherapy sessions in many cognitive and behavioral therapies. For instance, clinicians routinely have patients monitor emotions, negative beliefs, and maladaptive urges and behaviors each week, and these ratings can be used as data. Researchers often do not take full advantage of the clinical monitoring that is part of therapy. The subjective units of distress (SUDS) ratings that are a routine part of exposure exercises are a good example of this. These ratings can be examined to study the peak levels of arousal and the shape of the anxiety response over the session and across sessions (e.g., Heimberg & Becker, 2002).

Another source for multiple assessments of putative change variables is the weekly narrative over the course of therapy. For instance, we have participants in an exposure-based cognitive therapy for depression write weekly narratives about their depression to facilitate processing and also to monitor change. These narratives take 20 minutes per week to complete and provide a window into the change process as the patient goes through the course of therapy. The content of these narratives is then coded and can reveal how the therapy might be having its effects and when the hypothesized change processes are activated (Hayes et al., 2005; Hayes, Feldman, Beevers, et al., 2007).

Diary methods are another way to increase the density of assessment. Experience sampling (Csikszentmihalyi, Larson, & Prescott, 1977), daily diaries (Eckenrode & Bolger, 1995), social interaction recording (Reis & Wheeler, 1991), and ecological momentary assessment (Stone, Shiffman, & DeVries, 1999) refer to a class of methodologies for examining everyday experience known broadly as diary methods (for a review, see Bolger, Davis, & Rafaeli, 2003). It may not be feasible to obtain daily assessments of putative mediators and outcomes across a whole course of therapy, but researchers can have a series of daily assessments in "bursts" at the beginning and at some other point in the course of therapy (e.g., Gunthert, Cohen, Butler, & Beck, 2004). These methods can be incorporated into psychotherapy process research to yield information on the links between events, emotion, cognition, and behavior in patients' day-to-day lives and to reduce retrospective bias by collecting information as it occurs. Researchers should also consider the potential costs of using narratives and diary methods, including increased costs, subject burden, and risk of dropout (Bolger et al., 2003).

Still another way to increase the density of assessment of variables is to create process data from an already conducted outcome trial. In a process study of an open trial of cognitive therapy for avoidant and obsessive-compulsive personality disorders (Strauss et al., 2006), the content of sessions was coded with the CHANGE observational coding system (Hayes, Feldman, & Goldfried, 2007) mentioned earlier. This system was used to code the first five sessions and then every fifth session thereafter. The focus of this study is to examine the roles of avoidance, ruminative thinking, and cognitive/emotional processing in personality symptom change. This design yielded up to 10 to 15 process data points for each participant rather than the pre-mid-post data available in the original outcome study. This density of assessment allows for the application of statistical methods, such as hierarchical linear modeling, to examine trajectories of variables over time. This is an example of the fruitful collaborations that outcome and process researchers can forge to identify important predictors of dropout and change. This research can guide future work, particularly in the early phases of treatment development. This also speaks to the importance of maintaining archived data of clinical trials so that attrition, outcome, relapse, and change can be studied from multiple perspectives, and researchers can make full use of the data collected in the labor-intensive RCT.

■ Statistical Innovations in the Study of Change

In this section, we focus on recent innovations in techniques for studying the process of change. We discuss individual growth curve modeling as a method for depicting change, as well as a more recent extension of growth curve modeling for capturing classes of individual growth trajectories called *growth mixture modeling*. Because the focus of this section is on statistical innovations that can be applied to process research, we provide only a brief overview of standard methods for testing moderators and mediators, as these have been reviewed comprehensively elsewhere.

The Shape of Change

INDIVIDUAL GROWTH CURVE MODELING

It is now well understood that to assess individual change appropriately over time, one needs repeatedly measured longitudinal data. With only two time points, change can only be viewed as an increment over time, and this measure of change can be unreliable due to difficulties separating the underlying true change score from measurement error (Rogosa, 1988; Singer & Willett, 2003). An alternative is to view change as a continuous process of learning over time and to collect more than two waves of assessment.

Work by methodologists has demonstrated that there are valid and reliable ways to measure change (and examine correlates of change) in the form of individual growth curve modeling (Rogosa 1988; Singer & Willett, 2003), hierarchical linear modeling (Raudenbush & Bryk, 2002), and random coefficient modeling (Hedeker, 2004). In order to take advantage of and apply appropriately these more modern methods for assessing change in psychotherapy, researchers need to have an appropriate temporal design.

In essence, individual growth modeling takes place at two levels. The first level consists of fitting a regression model (linear or nonlinear) to each participant's repeated measures data (capturing intraindividual change). The second level consists of estimating average parameters of change and the amount of individual variability around these average parameters (capturing interindividual variability in intraindividual change). It is this interindividual variability in change that is typically treated as error variance in traditional ANOVA-based approaches. Individual growth modeling allows researchers to model (i.e., explain) this individual variability in change with covariates of interest that may predict the shape and rate of change.

Researchers are using individual growth curve modeling to address the three process-oriented questions of the shape of change, moderators of change, and mediators of change. Individual growth curve modeling provides a way for researchers to directly examine the shape of change in an outcome over time. The term *growth curves* implies that the outcome needs to be smoothly increasing, but this does not need to be so. The trajectory describing the outcome can be increasing, decreasing, quadratic, or cubic. For example, Hayes, Feldman, Beevers, et al. (2007) reported a significant cubic pattern of change in depression in an exposure-based cognitive therapy for depression. This overall pattern could be used to then identify periods of early rapid response and other periods of depression spikes underlying this overall cubic pattern.

Willett and colleagues (1998) recommend a minimum of three time points to specify a linear model, four points for a quadratic model, and five points for a cubic model. When reaearchers use more than the minimum number of time points, they can increase the precision with which parameters of change are captured can be increased. Depending on the number of repeated measures taken, many growth curve models can provide more statistical power than ANOVA approaches (Muthén & Curran, 1997), with the important feature of revealing the shape of change. Moreover, Muthén and Curran (1997) suggest that treatment effect size can be obtained in growth curve models by comparing intercept differences when time is centered on the last time point.

A trajectory may also show some complex combination of these patterns over distinct pieces of the assessment period (Singer & Willett, 2003). This approach is an extension of growth curve modeling, known as *piecewise linear modeling* (Raudenbush & Bryk, 2002), that allows the model of intraindividual change to be different for different portions of therapy. An application of piecewise linear modeling to intervention data can be found in Svartberg, Stiles, and Seltzer (2004). In this study, the authors compared the rates of progress over the course of treatment and over a follow-up period in patients with Cluster C personality disorders. Patients were randomized to receive short-term dynamic psychotherapy or cognitive therapy. Symptom distress and interpersonal problems were assessed at pretreatment, midtreatment, and posttreatment, and then 6, 12, and 24 months after treatment. Piecewise growth analyses revealed that both treatment groups showed significant improvement over the course of treatment on distress and interpersonal problems, but the rate of improvement for interpersonal problems was greater after treatment in short-term dynamic psychotherapy than in cognitive therapy.

GROWTH MIXTURE MODELING

As discussed earlier, individual growth curve modeling focuses on capturing the typical trajectory for a sample, as well as the degree to which individuals differ in the parameters that define the typical trajectory. One assumption of this approach is that all individuals have been drawn from the same population, with common population parameters defining the typical trajectory. That is, the heterogeneity that may be observed in growth trajectories is captured by continuous individual differences in trajectory parameters. Growth mixture modeling (GMM; Muthén, 2004; Muthén, 2001) allows for parameter differences to come from subpopulations (i.e., discrete classes) that may be reflected in the sample. Thus, the GMM approach can allow for different classes of average growth trajectories, with individuals varying around these latent trajectory classes, as compared with assuming individual variability around a single average growth curve. Interestingly, class can be thought of as having a moderating effect, with the different classes of trajectory shapes indicating qualitative types of change. GMM represents a combination of continuous and categorical latent variables in a growth curve framework, where a latent categorical variable is used to estimate the probability of membership in a particular class.

Consistent with a GMM approach, some psychotherapy researchers have noted the importance of detecting and examining potential subgroups of trajectories beyond the average trajectory (e.g., Krause, Howard, & Lutz, 1998). When applied to data in a psychotherapy trial, GMM allows process researchers to ask intriguing questions about the number of discrete trajectory classes that best describe the ways in which participants change over the course of therapy, the parameters that best describe the shape of change for each class, and the antecedent variables and distal outcomes associated with participants belonging to particular classes. An interesting application of GMM to psychotherapy data can be found in Szapocznik et al. (2004). In this application, GMM was used to explore whether there were classes of trajectories that represented differential response to Structural Ecosystems Family Therapy in HIV-seropositive, inner-city, African American women. Three classes emerged: One trajectory class consisted of high baseline distress that decreased over time, one consisted of high baseline distress that increased over time, and one consisted of low baseline distress that decreased over time. Different change processes may be associated with each of these classes.

GMM is superior to a post-hoc clustering approach for determining the number of trajectory classes because the clusters from the latter assume error-free classification. GMM provides a probability of class membership that takes unreliable classification into account. However, at this point, we would recommend that clinical researchers conduct post-hoc exploration of trajectory clusters and explore potential correlates of these clusters. These analyses can form the basis for generating future tenable hypotheses for more stringent analyses.

An important potential limitation of the application of GMM to data from psychotherapy trials concerns sample size and power considerations. At this point, relatively little is known about power and sample size requirements for GMM. Based on some simulation data on an example growth mixture model, Muthén (2004) has used 300 participants to obtain reasonable power for analysis. GMM is probably best utilized with data sets from multisite collaborative studies (e.g., Keller et al., 2000), where sample sizes may be sufficient. However, if the differing classes of trajectories are very well defined and clearly separable, smaller sample sizes may still be useful. Another potential limitation of GMM is that clinical researchers need to learn specialized statistical software for this type of data analytic approach (see Muthén, 2004).

Moderators and Mediators

As we reviewed earlier, Kraemer et al. (2002) clarified the Baron and Kenny (1986) definitions of moderators and mediators and conditions for testing them in the context of the RCT and longitudinal data. A number of papers present the basics of how to conduct these analyses with standard regression analysis (Holmbeck, 1997; Kazdin & Nock, 2003; Rose, Holmbeck, Coakley, & Franks, 2004), structural equation modeling (SEM; Cole & Maxwell, 2003; Holmbeck, 1997), latent growth curve modeling (Cheong, McKinnon, & Khoo, 2003; Khoo, 2001), and survival analyses (Tein & MacKinnon, 2003), as well as more general overviews (MacKinnon, 2006).

The general strategy for testing moderation is to examine the treatment variable and moderator as predictors of outcome followed by the interaction term of the treatment variable and moderator. The variables should be centered before creating the interaction term (Aiken & West, 1991). Centering involves subtracting the mean from all individual scores, which produces a revised sample mean of zero. Regression strategies tend to underestimate the effect size of the interaction term, particularly as measurement error in the predictor and moderator variable increases, and SEM is preferred when there is more than one measure for a construct (Holmbeck, 1997). Researchers can also use individual growth curve modeling to examine moderators of change. A pretreatment between-subjects covariate can be used as a predictor of variability in intraindividual change. If this covariate interacts with a treatment factor in such a way as to have an impact on an outcome, the between-subject covariate may be considered a moderator of individual treatment change (Cheong et al., 2003).

A mediation analysis can identify a putative variable (or set of variables) that transmits the effect of treatment on an outcome. In a recent review of mediation in psychological theory and research, MacKinnon, Fairchild, and Fritz (2007) summarize the important reasons for using mediation analysis in intervention research. In addition to the reasons discussed in earlier sections of this chapter, MacKinnon et al. (2007) emphasize that mediation analysis in an intervention setting can also identify which part of the chain of transmission of treatment effect is *not* working. If the treatment was efficacious but did not affect the putative mediator, it is possible that the mediator was not effectively manipulated or that the mediator was not adequately measured. On the other hand, if the treatment is related to the mediator but the mediator is not related to the outcome, then the treatment effects might be attributed to a different mediator, or the expected effects on the mediator might be occurring at a different time than was measured.

Kazdin and Nock (2003) provide a clear outline of the conditions for testing statistical mediation in intervention contexts:

1. The intervention (A) must be related to therapeutic change or treatment outcome (C).
2. The intervention (A) is related to the proposed mediator (B).
3. The mediator (B) must precede and be related to therapeutic change (C); the mediator must be conceptually distinct from the measure of outcome.
4. The relation between the intervention (A) and therapeutic change (C) must be reduced after statistically controlling for the proposed mediator (B).

In regression-based analysis, these authors recommend simultaneous entry of the intervention and proposed mediator as predictors of outcome. In path analysis, all effects in the mediation model can be entered simultaneously with the potential benefit of testing the indirect effect (i.e., mediation pathway) directly rather than using the traditional Baron and Kenny (1986) mediation procedure, which has been demonstrated to have lower power (MacKinnon, Lockwood, Hoffman, West, & Sheets, 2002).

Individual growth curve modeling also can be used to examine links between a putative mediator as a time-varying covariate and an outcome (Cheong et al., 2003). A piecewise linear modeling approach can be used as a way to examine mediation, where the treatment factor influences the trajectory of a putative repeatedly measured mediator in the first piece of treatment, and the slope of the mediator trajectory influences the slope of the outcome in the second piece of treatment (Khoo, 2001). Methodologists are currently working on more formal ways of examining mediation in a growth curve modeling framework (e.g., Cheong et al., 2003). Although beyond the scope of this chapter, it should be noted that it is also possible to examine multiple mediators and also chains of mediators over time (Kraemer et al., 2002; MacKinnon, 2006).

To establish a mediator as a mechanism of change, it is essential to demonstrate a causal relation between the putative mechanism and treatment outcome. The putative mechanism can be examined in RCTs or laboratory-based studies that directly manipulate the putative mechanism (Kazdin & Nock, 2003). Establishing a variable as a mechanism is an iterative process that often proceeds from the identification of predictors of change and mediators to multiple tests and perspectives that together support that variable as a mechanism of change. This information then feeds back to treatment refinement, development, and new applications.

Conclusion

Process research is enjoying a renaissance as a method by which to understand how therapy has its effects and for whom or under what conditions the therapy is more and less effective. Understanding the processes of change in any psychotherapy is an iterative process that cannot be accomplished in a single study. For example, researchers can identify putative mediators in existing trials or data sets, manipulate these mediators in laboratory studies, and then follow up with RCTs that include a higher dose of the mediator of change to test the hypothesis that the enhanced treatment is associated with more change than the original treatment. The types of analyses that can be conducted and the quality of the findings are dependent on the research design. We described ways to enhance the temporal design and the spacing of assessments to maximize the ability to capture the shape of change, moderators of change, and mediators of change. The combination of a strong theory of the nature of change in psychotherapy, a well-conceived research design (including temporal design issues), and the application of modern methods for the analysis of change will be most likely to produce a fruitful line of psychotherapy process research.

Acknowledgment

Preparation of this chapter was supported by National Institute of Mental Health grants R21MH062662 awarded to the first author and K01MH64779 awarded to the second author.

References

Aguinis, H. (1995). Statistical power problems with moderated multiple regression in management research. *Journal of Management Research, 21,* 1141–1158.

Aiken, L. S., & West, S. G. (1991). *Multiple regression: Testing and interpreting interaction.* Newbury Park, CA: Sage.

Baron, R. M., & Kenny, D. A. (1986). The moderator-mediator variable distinction in social psychological research: Conceptual, strategic, and statistical considerations. *Journal of Personality and Social Psychology, 51,* 1173–1182.

Begg, C. B., Cho, M. K., Eastwood, S., Horton, R., Moher, D., Olkin, I., et al. (1996). Improving the quality of reporting of randomized controlled trials: The CONSORT statement. *Journal of the American Medical Association, 276,* 637–639.

Bolger, N., Davis, A., & Rafaeli, E. (2003). Diary methods: Capturing life as it is lived. *Annual Review of Psychology, 54,* 579–616.

Breslin, F. C., Sobell, M. B., Sobell, L. C., Buchan, G., & Cunningham, C. J. (1997). Toward a stepped care approach to treating problem drinkers: The predictive utility of within-treatment variables and therapist prognostic ratings. *Addiction, 92,* 1479–1489.

Castonguay, L. G., & Beutler, L. E. (Eds.). (2006). *Principles of therapeutic change that work.* New York: Oxford University Press.

Chambless, D. L., Baker, M. J., Baucom, D. H., Beutler, L. E., Calhoun, K. S., Crits-Christoph, P., et al. (1998). Update on empirically validated therapies, II. *Clinical Psychologist, 51,* 3–16.

Chambless, D. L., & Ollendick, T. H. (2001). Empirically supported psychological interventions: Controversies and evidence. *Annual Review of Psychology, 52,* 685–716.

Cheong, J., McKinnon, D., & Khoo, S. T. (2003). Investigation of mediational processes using parallel process latent growth curve modeling. *Structural Equation Modeling, 10,* 238–262.

Cole, D. A., & Maxwell, S. E. (2003). Testing mediational models with longitudinal data: Questions and tips in the use of structural equation modeling. *Journal of Abnormal Psychology, 112,* 558–577.

Collins, L. M. (2006). Analysis of longitudinal data: The integration of theoretical model, temporal design and statistical model. *Annual Review of Psychology, 57,* 505–528.

Collins, L. M., & Graham, J. W. (2002). The effect of the timing and temporal spacing of observations in longitudinal studies of tobacco and other drug use: Temporal design considerations. *Drug and Alcohol Dependence, 68,* S85–S96.

Collins, L. M., Murphy, S. A., & Bierman, K. (2004). A conceptual framework for adaptive preventive interventions. *Prevention Science, 5,* 185–196.

Collins, L. M., & Sayer, A. G. (2000). Growth and change in social psychology research: Design, measurement, and analysis. In H. Reis & C. Judd (Eds.), *Handbook of research in social psychology* (pp. 478–495). Cambridge, England: Cambridge University Press.

Constantino, M. J., Arnow, B. A., Blasey, C., & Agras, W. S. (2005). The association between patient characteristics and the therapeutic alliance in cognitive-behavioral and interpersonal therapy for bulimia nervosa. *Journal of Consulting and Clinical Psychology, 73,* 203–211.

Csikszentmihalyi, M., Larson, R., & Prescott, S. (1977). The ecology of adolescent activity and experience. *Journal of Youth and Adolescence, 6,* 281–294.

Eckenrode, J., & Bolger, N. (1995). Daily and within-day event measurement. In S. Cohen, R. C. Kessler, & L. U. Gordon (Eds.), *Measuring stress: A guide for health and social scientists* (pp. 80–101). New York: Oxford University Press.

Foa, E. B., Huppert, J. D., & Cahill, S. P. (2006). Emotional processing theory: An update. In B. O. Rothbaum (Ed.), *The nature and treatment of pathological anxiety* (pp. 3–24). New York: Guilford.

Foa, E. B., & Kozak, M. J. (1986). Emotional processing of fear: Exposure to corrective information. *Psychological Bulletin, 99,* 20–35.

Gaynor, S. T., Weersing, V. R., Kolko, D. J., Birmaher, B., Heo, J., & Brent, D. A. (2003). The prevalence and impact of large sudden improvements during adolescent therapy for depression: A comparison across cognitive-behavioral, family, and supportive therapy. *Journal of Consulting and Clinical Psychology, 71,* 386–393.

Goldfried, M. R., & Wolfe, B. E. (1996). Psychotherapy practice and research: Repairing a strained alliance. *American Psychologist, 51,* 1007–1016.

Greenberg, L. S. (2002). Integrating an emotion-focused approach to treatment in psychotherapy integration. *Journal of Psychotherapy Integration, 12,* 154–189.

Greenberg, L. S., & Watson, J. (2005). *Emotion-focused therapy of depression.* Washington, DC: American Psychological Association.

Grilo, C. M., Masheb, R. M., & Wilson, T. G. (2006). Rapid response to treatment for binge eating disorder. *Journal of Consulting and Clinical Psychology, 74,* 602–613.

Gunthert, K. C., Cohen, L. H., Butler, A. C., & Beck, J. S. (2004). Predictive role of daily coping and affective reactivity in cognitive therapy outcome: Application of a daily process design to psychotherapy research. *Behavior Therapy, 36,* 70–90.

Hayes, A. M., Beevers, C., Feldman, G., Laurenceau, J.-P., & Perlman, C. A. (2005). Avoidance and emotional processing as predictors of symptom change and positive growth in an integrative therapy for depression. *International Journal of Behavioral Medicine, 12,* 111–122.

Hayes, A. M., Feldman, G., Beevers, C., Laurenceau, J.-P., Cardaciotto, L. A., & Lewis-Smith, J. (2007). Discontinuities and cognitive change in an exposure-based cognitive therapy for depression. *Journal of Consulting and Clinical Psychology, 75,* 409–421.

Hayes, A. M., Feldman, G. C., & Goldfried, M. R. (2007). The Change and Growth Experiences Scale: A measure of insight and emotional processing. In L. G. Castonguay & C. Hill (Eds.), *Insight in psychotherapy* (pp. 441–454). Washington, DC: American Psychological Association.

Hayes, A. M., Laurenceau, J.-P., Feldman, G. C., Strauss, J. L., & Cardaciotto, L. A. (2007). Change is not always linear: The study of discontinuities and nonlinear patterns of change in psychotherapy. In D. Hope & A. M. Hayes (Eds.), New approaches to the study of change in cognitive behavioral therapies. *Clinical Psychology Review, 27,* 715–723.

Hedeker, D. (2004). An introduction to growth modeling. In D. Kaplan (Ed.), *The Sage handbook of quantitative methodology for the social sciences* (pp. 215–234). Thousand Oaks, CA: Sage.

Heimberg, R. G., & Becker, R. E. (2002). *Cognitive-behavioral group treatment for social phobia: Basic mechanisms and clinical applications.* New York: Guilford.

Holmbeck, G. N. (1997). Toward terminological, conceptual, and statistical clarity in the study of mediators and moderators: Examples from the child-clinical and pediatric psychology literatures. *Journal of Consulting and Clinical Psychology, 65,* 599–610.

Horvath, A. O., & Bedi, R. P. (2002). The alliance. In J. C. Norcross (Ed.), *Psychotherapy relationships that work: Therapist contributions and responsiveness to patients* (pp. 37–69). New York: Oxford University Press.

Hufford, M. H., Witkiewitz, K., Shields, A. L., Kodya, S., & Caruso, J. C. (2003). Applying nonlinear dynamics to the prediction of alcohol use disorder treatment outcomes. *Journal of Abnormal Psychology, 112,* 219–227.

Ilardi, S. S., & Craighead, W. E. (1994). The role of nonspecific factors in cognitive-behavior therapy for depression. *Clinical Psychology: Science and Practice, 1,* 138–156.

Judd, C. M., & Kenny, D. A. (1981). *Estimating the effects of social interventions.* New York: Cambridge University Press.

Kazdin, A. E., & Nock, M. K. (2003). Delineating mechanisms of change in child and adolescent therapy: Methodological issues and research recommendations. *Journal of Child Psychology and Psychiatry, 44,* 1116–1129.

Keller, M. B., McCullough, J. P., Klein, D. N., Arnow, B., Dunner, D. L., Gelenberg, A. J., et al. (2000). A comparison of Nefazodone, the cognitive-behavioral analysis system of psychotherapy, and their combination for the treatment of chronic depression. *New England Journal of Medicine, 342,* 1462–1470.

Khoo, S. T. (2001). Assessing program effects in the presence of treatment-baseline interactions: A latent curve approach. *Psychological Methods, 6,* 234–257.

Kraemer, H. C., Wilson, G. T., Fairburn, C. G., & Agras, W. S. (2002). Mediators and moderators of treatment effects in randomized clinical trials. *Archives of General Psychiatry, 59,* 877–883.

Krause, M. S., Howard, K. I., & Lutz, W. (1998). Exploring individual change. *Journal of Consulting and Clinical Psychology, 66,* 838–845.

Laurenceau, J.-P., Hayes, A. M., & Feldman, G. C. (2007). Statistical and methodological issues in the study of change in psychotherapy. In D. Hope & A. M. Hayes (Eds.), New approaches to the study of change in cognitive behavioral therapies. *Clinical Psychology Review 27,* 682–695.

MacKinnon, D. P. (2006). *Introduction to statistical mediation analysis.* Mahwah, NJ: Erlbaum.

MacKinnon, D. P., Fairchild, A. J., & Fritz, M. S. (2007). Mediation analysis. *Annual Review of Psychology, 58,* 593–614.

MacKinnon, D. P., Lockwood, C. M., Hoffman, J. M., West, S. G., & Sheets, V. (2002). A comparison of methods to test the significance of the mediated effect. *Psychological Methods, 7,* 83–104.

Martin, D. J., Garske, J. P., & Davis, M. K. (2000). Relation of the therapeutic alliance with outcome and other variables: A meta-analytic review. *Journal of Consulting and Clinical Psychology, 68,* 438–450.

McNally, R. J. (2007). Mechanisms of exposure therapy: How neuroscience can improve psychological treatments for anxiety disorders. In D. Hope & A. M. Hayes (Eds.), New approaches to the study of change in cognitive behavioral therapies. *Clinical Psychology Review, 27,* 750–759.

Missirlian, T. M., Toukmanian, S. G., Warwar, S. H., & Greenberg, L. S. (2005). Emotional arousal, client perceptual processing, and working alliance in experiential psychotherapy for depression. *Journal of Consulting and Clinical Psychology, 73,* 861–871.

Muthén, B. (2001). Second-generation structural equation modeling with a combination of categorical and continuous latent variables: New opportunities for latent class growth modeling. In L. Collins & A. Sayer (Eds.), *New methods for the analysis of change* (pp. 291–322). Washington, DC: American Psychological Association.

Muthén, B. (2004). Latent variable analysis: Growth mixture modeling and related techniques for longitudinal data. In D. Kaplan (Ed.), *Handbook of quantitative methodology for the social sciences* (pp. 345–368). Newbury Park, CA: Sage.

Muthén, B. O., & Curran, P. J. (1997).General longitudinal modeling of individual differences in experimental designs: A latent variable framework for analysis and power estimation. *Psychological Methods, 2,* 371–402.

Pachankis, J. E., & Goldfried, M. R. (in press). On the next generation of process research. In D. Hope & A. M. Hayes (Eds.), Towards the understanding of the mechanisms and process of change in cognitive-behavioral therapy: Linking innovative methodology with fundamental questions. *Clinical Psychology Review.*

Raudenbush, S. W., & Bryk, A. S. (2002). *Hierarchical linear models: Applications and data analysis methods* (2nd ed.). Thousand Oaks, CA: Sage.

Reis, H. T., & Wheeler, L. (1991). Studying social interaction with the Rochester Interaction Record. In M. P. Zanna (Ed.), *Advances in experimental social psychology* (Vol. 24, pp. 270–318). San Diego, CA: Academic Press.

Rice, L. N., & Greenberg, L. S. (Eds.). (1984). *Patterns of change.* New York: Guilford.

Rogosa, D. R. (1988). Myths about longitudinal research. In K. W. Schaie, R. T. Campbell, W. M. Meredith, & S. C. Rawlings (Eds.), *Methodological issues in aging research* (pp. 171–209). New York: Springer.

Rose, B., Holmbeck, G. N., Coakley, R. M., & Franks, L. (2004). Mediator and moderator effects in developmental and behavioral pediatric research. *Journal of Developmental and Behavioral Pediatrics, 25,* 1–10.

Singer, J. D., & Willett, J. B. (2003). *Applied longitudinal data analysis: Modeling change and event occurrence.* Oxford, England: Oxford University Press.

Stiles, W. B., Leach, C., Barkham, M., Lucock, M., Iveson, S., Shapiro, D. A., et al. (2003). Early sudden gains in psychotherapy under routine clinic conditions: Practice-based evidence. *Journal of Consulting and Clinical Psychology, 71,* 14–21.

Stone, A. A., Shiffman, S. S., & DeVries, M. (1999). Rethinking our self-report assessment methodologies: An argument for collecting ecologically valid, momentary measurements. In D. Kahneman, E. Diener, & N. Schwarz (Eds.), *Well-being: The foundations of hedonic psychology* (pp. 26–39). New York: Sage.

Strauss, J. L., Hayes, A. M., Johnson, S. L., Newman, C. F., Brown, G. K., Barber, J. P., et al. (2006). Early alliance, alliance ruptures, and symptom change in a nonrandomized trial of cognitive therapy for avoidant and obsessive-compulsive personality disorders. *Journal of Consulting and Clinical Psychology, 74,* 337–345.

Svartberg, M., Stiles, T., & Seltzer, M. (2004). Effectiveness of short-term dynamic psychotherapy and cognitive therapy for Cluster C personality disorders: A randomized controlled trial. *American Journal of Psychiatry, 161,* 810–817.

Szapocznik, J., Feaster, D. J., Mitrani, V. B., Prado, G., Smith, L., Robinson-Batista, C., et al. (2004). Structural ecosystems therapy for HIV-seropositive African American women: Effects on psychological distress, family hassles, and family support. *Journal of Consulting and Clinical Psychology, 72,* 288–303.

Tang, T. Z., & DeRubeis, R. J. (1999). Sudden gains and critical sessions in cognitive-behavioral therapy for depression. *Journal of Consulting and Clinical Psychology, 67,* 894–904.

Tang, T. Z., DeRubeis, R. J., Beberman, R., & Pham, T. (2005). Cognitive changes, critical sessions, and sudden gains in cognitive-behavioral therapy for depression. *Journal of Consulting and Clinical Psychology, 73,* 168–172.

Tang, T. Z., Luborsky, L., & Andrusyna, T. (2002). Sudden gains in recovering from depression: Are they also found in psychotherapies other than cognitive-behavioral therapy? *Journal of Consulting and Clinical Psychology, 70,* 444–447.

Tein, J.-Y., & MacKinnon, D. P. (2003). Estimating mediated effects with survival data. In H. Yanai, A. O. Rikkyo, K. Shigemasu, Y. Kano, & J. J. Meulman (Eds.), *New developments in psychometrics* (pp. 405–412). Tokyo: Springer-Verlag Tokyo.

Vittengl, J. R., Clark, L. A., & Jarrett, R. B. (2005). Validity of sudden gains in acute phase treatment of depression. *Journal of Consulting and Clinical Psychology, 73,* 173–182.

Weisz, J. R., Hawley, K. M., Pilkonis, P. A., Woody, S. R., & Follette, W. C. (2000). Stressing the (other) three Rs in the search for empirically supported treatments: Review procedures, research quality, and relevance to clinical practice. *Clinical Psychology: Science and Practice, 7,* 243–258.

Westen, D., Novotny, C. M., & Thompson-Brenner, H. (2004). The empirical status of empirically supported psychotherapies: Assumptions, findings, and reporting in controlled clinical trials, *Psychological Bulletin, 130,* 631–663.

Witkiewitz, K., & Marlatt, A. (2007). Modeling the complexity of post-treatment drinking: It's a rocky road to relapse. In D. Hope & A. M. Hayes (Eds.), New approaches to the study of change in cognitive behavioral therapies. *Clinical Psychology Review, 27,* 724–738.

Willett, J. B. (1988). Questions and answers in the measurement of change. In *Review of research in education* (Vol. 15, pp. 345–422). Washington DC: American Educational Research Association.

Willett, J. B., Singer, J. D., & Martin, N. C. (1998). The design and analysis of longitudinal studies of development and psychopathology in context: Statistical models and methodological recommendations. *Development and Psychopathology, 10,* 395–426.

Wilson, G. T., Fairburn, C. G., Agras, W. S., Walsh, B. T., & Kraemer, H. (2002). Cognitive-behavioral therapy for bulimia nervosa: Time course and mechanisms of change. *Journal of Consulting and Clinical Psychology, 70,* 267–274.

Windle, M., & Davies, P. (1999). Developmental theory and research. In K. E. Leonard & H. T. Blane (Eds.), *Psychological theories of drinking and alcoholism* (2nd ed.; pp. 164–202) New York: Guilford.

17. Assessing the Clinical Significance of Outcome Results

Michael J. Lambert, Nathan B. Hansen, and Stephanie Bauer

In general, three groups of statistics have been used to express the conse-quences of psychotherapy for patients: statistical significance of within-group and between-group differences, effect size, and clinical significance. This chapter provides an overview of the third method—clinical significance. First we put clinical significance in the context of other methods for evaluating treatment effects. We then define clinical significance, provide methods of calculation with illustrations, and end with a discussion of limitations.

The data produced by research projects designed to evaluate the efficacy or effectiveness of therapy is typically submitted to statistical tests of significance. Treatment means are compared, the within-group and between-group variability is considered, and the analysis produces a numerical figure, which is then checked against critical values. An outcome achieves *statistical* significance if the magnitude of the mean difference is beyond what could have resulted by chance alone. Statistical analyses and statistical significance are essential for therapy evaluation because they inform us that the degree of difference was not due to chance. However, sole reliance on statistical significance can lead to per-ceived differences (i.e., treatment gains) as potent, when in fact they may be clinically insignificant.

For example, consider a weight loss treatment group that is compared with a control group. Forty individuals who are at extreme risk for detrimen-tal physical consequences related to their obesity are selected to participate in the study. After 2 months the 20 individuals receiving treatment have lost an average of 8 pounds. The comparison group has lost no weight during the time that elapsed. The statistical test reveals a statistically significant finding for the treatment group as compared with the control group. These statistical effects suggest that the differences between the groups are important as op-posed to differences that are "illusory, questionable, or unreliable" (Jacobson & Truax, 1991, p. 12). However, the statistical test does not give information regarding the variety of responses to treatment within the treated group. With an average of 8 pounds weight loss, some individuals who received treatment may have lost 16 pounds, whereas others who received treatment lost no weight or even gained weight.

Similarly, significance testing gives us evidence that the performance of the treatment is unlikely to be the result of a chance finding, but it gives us no information regarding the size, importance, or clinical significance of the results. As a group, the participants in the study remain classified as extremely obese. Even though the 20 treated individuals lost an average of 8 pounds, many, if not all of them, remain extremely overweight and are likely to experience the physical consequences of extreme obesity despite treatment. In a pragmatic or clinical sense, the treatment and control groups may be considered identical (with regard to meaningful change) after 2 months of treatment.

The effect size (ES) statistics deal with one shortcoming of statistical significance by providing information about the degree or magnitude of the relationship between variables. These statistics have proved especially valuable for meta-analytic reviews of studies by allowing researchers to sum and average the size of treatment effects across different measures and studies, thereby estimating the percentage of patients who benefit from treatments. Smith, Glass, and Miller (1980) applied these methods to psychotherapy research in their extensive review of the literature. A small effect indicates a smaller difference in group means than does a large effect. Even ES numbers, however, do not give us information regarding within-group variation or the clinical relevance of group or individual change.

For literature reviews, the effect size is invaluable, but for consumers to evaluate the clinical relevance of our weight loss study, one must know how much weight each individual lost, and one must then make some value judgments as well as empirical observations concerning the importance of the weight loss for each individual (who began treatment as extremely obese). Is the quality of life for a person in the treated group improved? Does the person's weight loss make a difference in terms of the probability of negative physical consequences of obesity? Has the individual returned to a "normal" weight for his or her height and bone structure? These are the types of questions that are at the heart of clinical significance methods. What is the clinical importance of changes for each individual patient?

All three methods are useful in the assessment of treatment outcome. Given the complex nature of change, it is essential to evaluate treatment with consideration of all three approaches. Statistically significant improvements are not equivalent to "cures," and clinical significance is an additional, not a substitute, evaluative strategy. Statistical significance is required to document that changes were beyond those due to chance alone, and the effect size tells how large group differences were, yet it is useful to also consider if the changes returned dysfunctional clients to within normative limits on the measures of interest.

■ A Brief History

As early as the 1970s (Bergin, 1971; Kazdin, 1977; Lick, 1973), the examination of individual changes occurring during formal psychotherapy research projects was seen as important to examine as a needed supplement to statistical significance. However, psychotherapy studies that included clinical significance were relatively rare outside of behavior therapy. Early in the 1980s, Jacobson, Follette, and Revenstorf (1984) presented a statistical solution for systematically estimating the clinical significance of change based on self-report scales completed by distressed couples undergoing couple therapy by reanalyzing data from a clinical trial. Since this work was published, there has been a steady refinement of methods and statistical formulas, as well as increased applications in clinical trials. In fact, these methods form a core condition for the emerging line of psychotherapy research aimed at monitoring and improving individual patient treatment response—patient-focused research (Lambert, 2001; Lambert et al. 2003).

Historically, two rather independent bodies of literature evolved for designating the clinical significance of psychotherapy: social validity and clinical significance. Social validity (Kazdin, 1977; Wolf, 1978) emerged as a method of assessing the perspective of individuals *outside* the therapeutic relationship regarding the importance of psychosocial interventions and outcomes. Social validity provides a cohesive rationale and two specific methodologies (subjective evaluation and social comparison) for evaluating the relevance of client change. Subjective evaluation refers to gathering data about clients by individuals who are "likely to have contact with the client or are in a position of expertise" (Kazdin, 1998, p. 387). This allows the researcher to understand if the client has made qualitative changes that are in turn observable by others. The underlying premise is that socially valid changes due to the intervention in question will result in the client's postintervention behavior being indistinguishable from that of a normal reference group.

Although social validity emphasizes an examination of practical change from the perspective of societal members, clinical significance takes a slightly narrower view of meaningful change by identifying methods defined by clinician-researchers (Ogles, Lunnen, & Bonesteel, 2001). The two most prominent definitions of clinically significant change are (a) treated clients make statistically reliable improvements as a result of treatment (Jacobson, Roberts, Berns, & McGlinchey, 1999), and (b) treated clients are empirically indistinguishable from "normal" or nondeviant peers following treatment recovery (Kendall, Marrs-Garcia, Nath, & Sheldrick, 1999). Several statistical methods are used to evaluate these propositions. Before turning to these, it is important to note that the use of such methods broadens and modifies our views of the effects of psychotherapy. In general, the consequence of using clinical significance methods softens our claims for the effects of psychotherapy and makes it clear that a portion of patients who undergo treatment do not respond and that a small group of patients (perhaps 5 to 10%) actually worsen (Lambert & Ogles, 2004).

For example, Ogles, Lambert, and Sawyer (1995) examined the clinical significance of the Treatment of Depression Collaborative Research Program (TD-CRP) data. When combining estimates across three empirically supported treatments (interpersonal psychotherapy [IPT], cognitive-behavioral therapy [CBT], and imipramine plus clinical management) and three measures, they found that 69 (55%) of the 125 clients who participated in a minimum of 12 sessions and 15 weeks of treatment met the criteria for clinically meaningful change on all three measures. Many other studies provide similar analyses of clinical significance following the standard statistical comparison of group averages (e.g., Freestone et al., 1997). Hansen, Lambert, and Forman (2002) summarized across 28 clinical trials that studied a variety of disorders and treatment methods and found that on average 58% of patients met the criteria for clinically significant change following an average of 13 treatment sessions. We might summarize this clinical significance data by saying that if we give our best treatments, in high doses (relative to routine care), a patient has about a 50% chance of reliably changing and reentering the ranks of normal functioning.

We will return to this issue at the end of this chapter but for now turn our attention to calculations of clinically significant change.

■ Methods of Calculating Clinical Significance

The Jacobson-Truax Method

As mentioned earlier, Jacobson et al. (1984) introduced a first statistical method to assess clinically significant change. All methods outlined in this chapter suggest a two-step criterion for clinically significant change based on this original proposal and its minor modifications formulated by Jacobson and Truax (1991). The first step is to determine whether the observed change from pretest to posttest is *statistically reliable,* that is, whether the observed difference in scores can be attributed to real change rather than the measurement error of the outcome instrument. This reliable change index (RCI) is calculated by dividing the difference between the observed posttest (x_{post}) and pretest (x_{pre}) scores by the standard error of differences (Jacobson & Truax, 1991):

$$RCI = \frac{(x_{post} - x_{pre})}{\sqrt{2S_E^{\,2}}} \tag{1}$$

The size of the standard error of measurement (S_E) depends on the reliability (r) of the outcome measure:

$$S_E = SD\sqrt{1-r} \tag{2}$$

This means that the more reliable the instrument, the smaller the resulting standard error and thus the smaller the observed change between pre- and posttest score required to achieve a statistically reliable change. In the discussion of which reliability score is most accurate for the calculation of the RCI, Martinovich, Saunders, and Howard (1996), as well as Tingey, Lambert, Burlingame, and Hansen (1996), recommended the use of internal consistency rather than of test-retest reliability scores. If the RCI is smaller than -1.96, a person scored reliably lower on the posttest compared with the pretest assessment ($p < .05$) and thus has shown reliable improvement on the outcome measure.

The second step in the calculation of clinical significance is the estimation of a cutoff point between a patient (dysfunctional) and a nonpatient (functional) population. Jacobson et al. (1984) proposed "that a change in therapy is clinically significant when the client moves from the dysfunctional to the functional range during the course of therapy" (p. 340). They suggested three different cutoff scores, labeled A, B, and C, that should be calculated depending on the available patient and/or nonpatient data sets and the distribution characteristics (Jacobson et al., 1999).

Cutoff A is defined as the point two standard deviations below the pretreatment mean score of a patient population:

$$\text{Cutoff A} = M_{patient} - 2SD_{patient} \tag{3}$$

Cutoff B is defined as the point two standard deviations above the mean score of a nonpatient sample:

$$\text{Cutoff B} = M_{nonpatient} + 2SD_{nonpatient} \tag{4}$$

Finally, *Cutoff C* is a weighted midpoint between the means of a patient and a nonpatient population:

$$\text{Cutoff C} = \frac{(SD_{patient}M_{nonpatient}) + (SD_{nonpatient}M_{patient})}{(SD_{patient} + SD_{nonpatient})} \tag{5}$$

The use of Cutoff C is recommended when adequate normative data sets (patient and nonpatient) are available, and there is overlap between the two distributions. In contrast, when the distributions are nonoverlapping, Cutoff B should be used. When data from nonpatient samples are not available, Cutoff A is the only cutoff point that can be calculated.

In summary, according to Jacobson et al.'s (1984) two-step criterion, for a pre-posttest change to be considered a clinically significant change, (a) it must be proved to be statistically reliable, and (b) the score must pass from the dysfunctional to the functional distribution. Using these two steps, each individual can be classified as Recovered (passed both criteria), Improved (passed only the RCI criterion in the positive direction), Unchanged (did not pass the RCI criterion), or Deteriorated (passed the RCI criterion in the negative direction).

Illustrative Example

To illustrate the Jacobson-Truax method, we provide data from three patients who underwent psychotherapeutic treatment. Outcome was assessed with the Outcome Questionnaire (OQ-45; Lambert et al., 2004), a 45-item questionnaire widely used in psychotherapy outcome research that assesses psychological impairment via three subscales (symptom distress, interpersonal relations, and social role functioning) and a total score. The range of the total score is 0 to 180, with higher scores indicating more impairment. All relevant information for computing clinical significance for each patient, including normative data from functional and dysfunctional samples, is presented in Table 17.1.

CALCULATION OF CUTOFF SCORE

Because normative data are available from both functional and dysfunctional data sets for the OQ-45, the calculation of Cutoff C is recommended. However, for the purpose of illustration, we also provide scores for Cutoffs A and B.

$$\text{Cutoff A} = M_{patient} - 2SD_{patient} = 84.7 - 48.2 = 36.5$$

$$\text{Cutoff B} = M_{nonpatient} + 2SD_{nonpatient} = 45.2 + 37.2 = 82.4$$

$$\text{Cutoff C} = \frac{(SD_{patient} M_{nonpatient}) + (SD_{nonpatient} M_{patient})}{(SD_{patient} + SD_{nonpatient})}$$

$$= \frac{(24.1 * 45.2) + (18.6 * 84.7)}{(24.1 + 18.6)} = 62.4$$

The implications of choosing one of the cutoff scores as opposed to another are as follows: Whereas Cutoff A has high sensitivity (i.e., a posttreatment score below this cutoff score is very unlikely to belong to the dysfunctional population, and the risk of falsely classifying a score as functional is very small), Cutoff B has high specificity (i.e., a score above this cutoff score is very likely to belong to the dysfunctinal population, and the risk of falsely classifying a score as dysfunctional is small). In other words, Cutoff A is difficult to reach for many patients undergoing psychotherapeutic treatment, whereas a posttreatment score below Cutoff B will be observed in a high percentage of patients. These differences should be kept in mind when interpreting rates of clinically significant change. As mentioned before, Cutoff C is the cutoff of choice in our example. Cutoff C equals 62.4 for the OQ total score. Thus, in this illustration a score of 63 or higher is considered to belong to the dysfunctional range, and scores of 62 or lower are considered to belong to the functional range.

TABLE 17.1

Individual Patient and Normative Sample Pre- and Posttreatment OQ-45 Scores for Computing Clinical Significance Using Jacobson et al. (1984) Method

Individual patient information	Patient A	Patient B	Patient C
Pretreatment OQ total score	72	95	68
Posttreatment OQ total score	52	70	58

Normative sample information	Functional distribution		Dysfunctional distribution	
	Mean	SD	Mean	SD
Pretreatment OQ total score	45.2	18.6	84.7[a]	24.1[b]
Posttreatment OQ total score	n.a.	n.a.	67.2	27.1

[a]Internal consistency: Cronbach's alpha = .93.
[b]Standard error of measurement: $S_E = SD\sqrt{1-r} = 6.38$.

CALCULATION OF RELIABLE CHANGE INDEX (RCI)

The computation of RCI for each patient is demonstrated as follows:

Patient A:

$$RCI = \frac{(x_{post} - x_{pre})}{\sqrt{2S_E^2}} = \frac{(52 - 72)}{\sqrt{2*6.38^2}} = 2.21$$

Patient B:

$$RCI = \frac{(x_{post} - x_{pre})}{\sqrt{2S_E^2}} = \frac{(70 - 95)}{\sqrt{2*6.38^2}} = 2.77$$

Patient C:

$$RCI = \frac{(x_{post} - x_{pre})}{\sqrt{2S_E^2}} = \frac{(58 - 68)}{\sqrt{2*6.38^2}} = 1.11$$

These results indicate that Subjects A and B show reliable improvement in their OQ scores (RCI smaller than -1.96), whereas Subject C does not meet the criterion for reliable change (at the $p < .05$ level). Subject A additionally meets the Cutoff criterion, displaying a dysfunctional score ($x_{pre} > 63$) before treatment and a functional score ($x_{pre} < 63$) thereafter. Thus, Subject A can be classified as Recovered, Subject B as Improved (yet remaining within the dysfunctional range), and Subject C as Unchanged. In terms of clinical significance, Subject A is the only subject showing clinically significant change.

Other Formulas

To date, the Jacobson and Truax (JT) method has been the most frequently reported method for assessing clinically meaningful change in psychotherapy outcome studies (Ogles et al., 2001). Several authors have criticized the JT method on statistical grounds and suggested alternative methods that they believed would yield more accurate estimates of meaningful change than the original conceptualization. We want to briefly introduce the six alternative methods for the calculation of the RCI that have been used in comparative studies (see later discussion) investigating convergences and divergences in classification rates of different methods.

The main point of criticism addressed by newer approaches was that the JT approach did not take into account regression to the mean. Regression to the mean implies that in repeated assessments with the same (not perfectly reliable) outcome measure, more extreme scores naturally become less extreme over time. Criticizing the JT method for not accounting for this phenomenon, Hsu (1989, 1999) suggested the Gulliksen-Lord-Novick (GLN) method. The GLN formula for calculating the RCI includes estimates of the population mean and standard deviation toward which scores are assumed to regress. It is problematic, however, because these means and standard deviations are rarely known (Maassen, 2000). In this case, Hsu (1999) recommended using the pretreatment mean and standard deviation scores.

The problem of regression to the mean was also noted by Speer (1992), who suggested the Edwards-Nunnally (EN) method. The EN method uses an estimated true score based on the obtained pretest score to minimize the presumed effects of regression to the mean. The posttreatment score is then evaluated in relation to a confidence interval that was calculated around the pretreatment score ($\pm 2SD$). Similar to the EN method, in the Nunnally-Kotsch (NK) method, the pretreatment scores are adjusted for regression to the mean by replacing the raw pretreatment score by the estimated true pretreatment score. In contrast to the GLN, EN, and NK methods, the Hsu-Linn-Lord (HLL) formula uses deviation scores of the observed scores from the pretreatment as well as the posttreatment means (Hsu, 1989).

The most recent and most significant revision to calculate clinically significant change was formulated by Hageman and Arrindell (HA; 1999). Similar to the EN method, the HA approach includes the reliability of the outcome measure at pre- and posttreatment assessment. Hageman and Arrindell (1999) also suggested applying corrections for regression to the mean to the cutoff criterion and provided a modified formula for the calculation of the cutoff. Furthermore, they provided separate formulas for the calculation of group-based analyses (for details, see Hageman & Arrindell, 1999).

In another suggested procedure, Speer (1992) generally criticized the use of two-wave designs to assess change in psychotherapy research and recommended the use of growth curve modeling (e.g., hierarchical linear modeling [HLM]; Bryk & Raudenbush, 1992) for the study of clinically significant change. HLM is believed to estimate the RCI more accurately because it uses longitudinal data instead of only pre- and posttest scores. Further advantages are the possibility of handling missing data and the use of the empirical Bayes estimation (Bryk & Raudenbush, 1992).

The formulas of the six alternative methods to calculate reliable change mentioned here are displayed in Table 17.2.

Comparisons of Choice of Methods and Their Consequences

Although addressing methodological and statistical controversies on how to calculate clinical significance most accurately is important, of more pressing concern to psychotherapy researchers is the question of what are the practical consequences of using one method instead of another. Three empirical studies have addressed this question and investigated the convergences and divergences in classifications between different methods.

Speer and Greenbaum (1995) included in their study the JT approach and four alternative methods and compared the classification rates of 73 patients based on the RCI. In addition to the JT method, they included the EN, the HLL, the NK, and the HLM methods. The results showed relatively high rates of agreement (78% to 81%) between four (JT, EN, NK, HLM) of the methods. Compared with these, the HLL method led to higher rates of deterioration and lower rates of improvement, and showed only 51% agreement with the other methods. Based on their results, Speer and Greenbaum (1995) recommend the use of HLM when longitudinal data exist and identifying deteriorated patients is not of interest (due to HLM classifying none of the 73 patients in their sample as reliably deteriorated). Otherwise they recommend the use of the JT method.

McGlinchey, Atkins, and Jacobson (2002) compared five methods of estimating clinical significance rates in a sample of 128 patients with depression. Three of the methods (JT, EN, HLM), were identical to those used by Speer and Greenbaum (1995). In addition, McGlinchey et al. (2002) included the GLN and the HA approach. Instead of comparing rates of *statistically* significant client change as did Speer and Greenbaum (1995), McGlinchey et al. (2002) compared rates of *clinically* significant change, by including not only the RCI criterion but also the cutoff criterion. The HA method was found to provide the most conservative estimations, and to differ significantly from three of the other methods (JT, GLN, EN). Furthermore, the EN classifications differed from the JT and HLM results. All other paired comparisons were nonsignificant, that is, the methods produced similar change rates.

TABLE 17.2

Formulas for the Calculation of Individual Reliable Change

Method	Calculation of RCI	
Gulliksen-Lord-Novick (GLN)	$$\dfrac{(x_{post} - M) - r_{xx}(x_{pre} - M)}{SD_{pre}\sqrt{1 - r_{xx}{}^2}}$$	(6)
Edwards-Nunnally (EN)	$$[r_{xx}(x_{pre} - M_{pre}) + M_{pre}] \pm 2SD_{pre}\sqrt{1 - r_{xx}}$$	(7)
Nunnally-Kotsch (NK)	$$\dfrac{x_{post} - \left\lfloor r_{IC(pre)}(x_{pre} - M) + M \right\rfloor}{\sqrt{\left[r_{IC(pre)}{}^2 SD_{pre}{}^2\left(1 - r_{IC(pre)}\right)\right] + \left[SD_{pre}{}^2\left(1 - r_{IC(post)}\right)\right]}}$$	(8)
Hsu-Linn-Lord (HLL)	$$\dfrac{\left(x_{post} - M_{post}\right) - r_{xx}\left(x_{pre} - M_{pre}\right)}{SD_{pre}\sqrt{1 - r_{xx}{}^2}}$$	(9)
Hagemann-Arrindell (HA)	$$\dfrac{\left(x_{post} - x_{pre}\right)r_{dd} + \left(M_{post} - M_{pre}\right)\left(1 - r_{dd}\right)}{\sqrt{r_{dd}}\sqrt{2S_E{}^2}}$$	(10)
Hierarchical linear modeling (HLM)	$$\dfrac{B^*}{\sqrt{V^*}}$$	(11)

Note. x_{pre} = raw pretreatment score; x_{post} = raw posttreatment score; SD_{pre} = standard deviation of pretreatment scores; SD_{post} = standard deviation of posttreatment scores; S_E = standard error of measurement; r_{xx} = reliability of measure; M_{pre} = mean of pretreatment scores; M_{post} = mean of posttreatment scores; M = mean of a relevant group (e.g., the group from which participants were selected for treatment; Hsu, 1999). If not available, the use of the pretreatment mean score is recommended.; $r_{IC(pre)}$ = internal consistency reliability of pretreatment scores; $r_{IC(post)}$ = internal consistency reliability of posttreatment scores; r_{dd} = reliability of difference scores (see formula 12); r_{pre} = reliability of pretreatment scores (see formula 13); r_{post} = reliability of posttreatment scores (see formula 14); $r_{pre^* post}$ = correlation between pretreament and posttreatment scores; B^* = empirical Bayes estimate of linear slope; $V^{*1/2}$ = standard deviation of the empirical Bayes estimate.

$$r_{dd} = \frac{SD_{pre}{}^2 r_{pre} + SD_{post}{}^2 r_{post} - 2SD_{pre}SD_{post}r_{pre^* post}}{SD_{pre}{}^2 + SD_{post}{}^2 - 2SD_{pre}SD_{post}r_{pre^* post}} \tag{12}$$

$$r_{pre} = \frac{SD_{pre}{}^2 - S_E{}^2}{SD_{pre}{}^2} \tag{13}$$

$$r_{post} = \frac{SD_{post}{}^2 - S_E{}^2}{SD_{post}{}^2} \tag{14}$$

In addition to comparing concordance between the estimations, McGlinchey et al. (2002) went one step further and investigated the prognostic validity of the five methods by assessing relapse rates within 2 years after treatment. They found all methods to discriminate significantly between patients who relapsed and those who did not. The differences in classification did not lead to a significantly greater accuracy of one method over another in predicting relapse.

Bauer, Lambert, and Nielsen (2004) compared the classification rates of the same five methods (JT, EN, HLM, GLN, HA) as McGlinchey et al. (2002) in a sample of 386 patients who were treated in routine care at a university-based outpatient clinic. The average agreement of one method with the other four ranged from 71% (HA) to 85% (GLN). The highest paired agreement was found between the JT and the GLN method. The EN method provided the most liberal estimations of change, and the HA method the most conservative. This trend is in line with the findings reported by McGlinchey et al. (2002).

Instead of using empirical data, Atkins, Bedics, McGlinchey, and Beauchaine (2005) recently conducted a simulation study to systematically explore the performance of four methods (JT, GLN, EN, HA) by varying several relevant parameters (effect sizes, reliabilities, pre-post correlations). This allowed them to evaluate not only the question *if* the methods differ but also *under which conditions* they differ. Overall, the results showed considerable agreement between methods, especially in the case of high reliability in the outcome measure. The differences between methods identified by Atkins et al. (2005) confirm the empirical results of Bauer et al. (2004): The JT and GLN methods resulted in almost identical classifications, the EN method was the most liberal, and the HA approach the most conservative approach.

In contrast to comparing classification rates of different methods, several studies have investigated to what extent the use of different outcome measures and different perspectives (e.g., therapist, client, and spouse ratings) produces comparable estimations of clinically significant change. The results of these studies indicate that different measures produce largely varying rates of clinically significant change (e.g., Beckstead et al., 2003). Consequently, it is important to keep in mind that the rates of clinically significant change are dependent both on the specific outcome measures that are used and on the statistical methods used to estimate clinically significant change.

Recommendations

It is important to differentiate between the most accurate way to calculate rates of clinically significant change and the practical relevance of differences between methods for psychotherapy research. The results of the three comparative studies indicate that convergences and divergences between methods vary from study to study. We agree with other authors who suggested ceasing the formulation of new methods until we get a better understanding of the performance of current approaches (McGlinchey et al., 2002; Speer, 1999) and recommend the use of the JT method for routine use in outcome research. Several points lead to this recommendation: First and most important, it has yet to be demonstrated that any other approach is superior in terms of more accurate estimations of clinically significant change (McGlinchey et al., 2002). As noted by Hsu (1999), it is inappropriate to recommend a particular method based on its production of higher improvement rates. Due to the lack of validation studies (with the exception of McGlinchey et al., 2002, who did not find differences in the performance of the different methods), it remains an open question as to which method is most sensitive to detecting meaningful changes in patients undergoing psychotherapeutic treatment. Second, as noted by Maassen (2000), the newer methods require generally unknown population information to make more precise estimates than the JT method. Maassen (2000) as well as Atkins et al. (2005) conclude that the JT method has been undeservedly regarded as inferior, and also recommend the use of the JT approach. Finally, third, the JT method is relatively easy to compute and already the most popular approach (Ogles et al., 2001), which allows for comparisons of change rates across studies.

■ Limitations to Clinical Significance

Despite the potential advantages to using clinical significance methods in reporting outcome, there are numerous limitations to these methods. These include (a) the inability to adequately categorize change in the large number of patients who enter treatment already scoring in the functional range on outcome measures, (b) the lack of methodology to categorize change in chronically ill populations, (c) the lack of suitable norms for many potentially useful outcome measures and for many relevant clinical populations, and (d) the fact that clinical significance relies on categorization that is unreliable at the category edges.

Patients Entering Treatment in the Functional Range

The first limitation, the inability of clinical significance to adequately categorize change in patients entering treatment already in the functional range, is captured in the interchange between Gray (2003) and Hansen, Lambert, and Forman (2003). Depending on the clinical setting, a large number of patients may initiate treatment with low to mild levels of psychiatric symptoms, and have little room for improvement. If these patients score at or below the established cutoff score between the functional and dysfunctional normative distributions, it will be impossible for them to meet the criteria for *recovery* using clinical significance methodology. For this reason, Tingey et al. (1996) recommended viewing patient functioning as a continuum, rather than using a dichotomous functional/dysfunctional operationalization of patient functioning. Based on a continuum, appropriate cutoffs can be created between any two relevant populations, assuming they form distinct distributions by meeting specified criteria for nonoverlap. Tingey et al. (1996) demonstrated this procedure using the Symptom Checklist 90, Revised (Derogatis, 1983) by defining cutoffs between severe and moderate symptom ranges, moderate and mild symptom ranges, and mild and asymptomatic symptom ranges. Thus, for patients who enter treatment in a mildly distressed range, an appropriate asymptomatic range of functioning can be defined and relevant normative data can be collected to establish a cutoff point and an RCI. As demonstrated by Tingey et al. (1996) and others (Grundy, Lambert, & Grundy, 1996; Seggar, Lambert, & Hansen, 2002), identifying, recruiting, and assessing asymptomatic participants from the community that are comparable to mildly symptomatic patients to form a normative distribution for establishing clinical significance cutoffs and RCIs is a labor- and resource-intensive process.

Therefore, Tingey et al. (1996) suggested a more practical, if less elegant, approach for addressing low-scoring (or very high-scoring) patients, namely, relaxing the rather stringent clinical significance methodology to include a category for "improvement" based on meeting criteria for reliable change alone. Although this moves away from the intended rationale of clinical significance, that is, establishing *recovery* as a "gold standard" for treatment outcome, it greatly increases the applicability of clinical significance. First, it helps to address the problem of patients who begin treatment already within the functional distribution. Although these patients cannot cross the cutoff point defining normal functioning (clinically significant change), it is possible for them to achieve *reliable improvement*. As has been demonstrated (Ankuta & Ables, 1993; Lunnen & Ogles, 1998), *reliable improvement* is clinically meaningful and represents a positive treatment outcome short of *recovery*.

Second, the concept of *reliable improvement* is useful for patients who begin treatment with extremely elevated distress that is unlikely to remit to the stage of *recovery (normal functioning)* without extensive intervention over long periods of time. Indeed, for some patients with chronic physical and mental health needs, the concept of *recovery* is impractical, as will be discussed later. Finally, *reliable improvement* provides a positive intermediate outcome that is useful for brief interventions and for situations where *recovery* may be an overly stringent goal.

A potential problem with viewing functioning as a continuum rather than as discrete populations is the previously mentioned phenomenon of regression to the mean (Speer, 1992). For example, from the continuum perspective, the general population mean would be expected to be the functional mean, and dysfunctional groups would represent scores toward the tail of the distribution. Therefore, changes that bring extreme scores closer to the population mean could be expressions of regression to the mean rather than therapeutic change. In fact, this description fits the observed course of many psychiatric symptoms, because distress does tend to remit with time and, in many cases, with or without treatment (Lambert, 1976). Treatment, however, does appear to accelerate this process. For example, in an RCT with a sample of bereaved, HIV-positive men and women who lost loved ones to AIDS, the same disease that threatens their own lives, it was found that at immediate postassessment, participants in a group intervention had significantly greater reductions in grief, psychiatric distress, and depression (Sikkema, Hansen, Kochman, Tate, & DiFranceisco, 2004) and increases in health-related quality of life (Sikkema, Hansen, Meade, Kochman, & Lee, 2005). By the end of a 12-month follow-up period, however, participants in the treatment-upon-request comparison condition had matched the gains of the intervention group, although the intervention was more effective in resolving grief for participants with higher levels of psychiatric distress (Sikkema et al., in press). Despite the potential limitation of regression to the mean, however, this approach does offer great practical value and extends the use of clinical significance methodology across a much wider range of treatment outcome research.

Additional suggestions for addressing patients who score below a clinical significance cutoff point are to assess outcome using a different instrument that is more relevant to the patient's presenting problems—for instance, rather than measuring patient change in psychiatric distress, measure interpersonal problems, social role functioning, ability to cope, or life satisfaction. Whereas limitations related to low scores at intake are a critical problem in effectiveness research examining outcomes in routine care, they are generally of less concern in RCTs with inclusion criteria of clinically notable levels of psychopathology and distress at intake.

Chronically Ill Populations

As noted earlier, with many chronically ill populations (including both physical and mental illness), clinically significant change may be an impractical goal. Patients with severe and persistent mental illness may never approach a "normal" level of functioning, but that does not mean they are incapable of achieving significant and meaningful improvements through treatment. Additionally, for chronically physically ill patients, and even relatively healthy people living in chronically stressful situations (i.e., extreme poverty, areas of violence, and in the aftermath of natural disasters), "normal" and expected functioning may be outside the range of typically identified functional distributions.

This is another area where the approach of viewing functioning along a continuum suggested by Tingey et al. (1996) has merit. For example, with patients who have severe and persistent mental illnesses, the typical creation of discrete functional and dysfunctional distributions does not offer a realistic chance for clinically significant improvement (i.e., *recovery*) to occur. These patients may make great improvements without coming close to reaching the functional distribution. Using the relaxed criteria of reliable change, being considered *reliably improved* offers a partial solution to this problem. However, with the extensions proposed by Tingey et al. (1996), a dysfunctional distribution may be defined as an inpatient or partial hospital population, with a functional distribution defined as a partial hospital or an outpatient treatment sample. Within this procedure an inpatient might be considered "recovered" if his or her functioning changes over the course of treatment to be more characteristic of an outpatient population. In this sense the patient has moved from a population that could be described as fully affiliated with a "sick role" to one that is healthier. Such possible applications of clinical significance make clear another limitation to the standard methodology, however, namely, the lack of suitable measures, and a lack of norms for many potentially useful outcome measures and for many relevant clinical populations.

Lack of Suitable Measures and Norms

For a measure to be useful in the assessment of clinical significant change, it must be sensitive to change and have adequate reliability. Several measures of global functioning and psychiatric distress exist that are sensitive to change and have high reliabilities (<0.9), but there is a lack of normative data relevant to specialized populations (e.g., substance abuse, survivors of trauma, general health). Additionally, there is a lack of more specialized measures that have adequate reliability or have adequate norms for computation of clinical significance criteria.

An example will highlight this problem. A strength of clinical significance methodology is that it considers change on the individual patient level, which makes it useful for small-N studies where power to detect statistical differences may be lacking, and where individual changes may be masked by group variance. Therefore, in a recent report on a small-N pilot study of a new group treatment for HIV-positive adult survivors of childhood sexual abuse (Sikkema et al., 2004), clinical significance methodology was used to report patient outcome. The first problem encountered in this study was the lack of trauma-focused assessment tools for assessing outcome with adequate reliability for use with clinical significance methods and demonstrated sensitivity for assessing therapeutic change. The second problem was the selection of appropriate normative populations for a functional distribution. Because the patient sample was drawn from a low-income, mostly ethnic minority population, and all were living with HIV infection and had experienced sexual abuse as children, should a functional sample consist of similar patients living with HIV infection but who were not abused as children? Should it consist of non-treatment-seeking people who were abused as children but who are not HIV-infected? Is a general community sample adequate, or should it be a community sample composed mostly of low-income ethnic minorities? And because none of these samples actually exist in the literature on the outcome measure, are there resources available to collect a relevant sample?

As described earlier, Jacobson and Truax (1991) provide methods for computing clinical significance when relevant normative samples are not available, including ending treatment with posttreatment outcome scores within two standard deviations of the mean of a functional distribution (Cutoff A), or two standard deviations away from the mean of a dysfunctional distribution (Cutoff B). In the current example, the lack of a relevant functional distribution made Criterion A unavailable. Also, the only available dysfunctional sample of HIV-positive, sexually abused adults was the study sample. This makes Criterion B a poor choice because, by definition, a subset of the sample begins treatment above the mean and would therefore be required to experience change of more than two standard deviations to achieve clinically significant change. Therefore, in this example, although not an ideal solution, normative samples were selected from the literature such that a general community sample served as a functional sample (though it is unrealistic to expect the severely stressed and traumatized, chronically ill study sample to achieve a level of functioning consistent with a general community), and a sample of treatment-seeking adult survivors of childhood sexual abuse was used as a dysfunctional distribution (though the study sample scored, on average, much higher than the normative sample across all scales of traumatic stress). Despite this less than optimal application of clinical significance methodology, which essentially reduced the chance of patients achieving clinically significant change (*recovery*), more than 75% of the sample achieved *reliable improvement* on at least one scale of traumatic stress (Sikkema et al., 2004).

■ Summary

Although much more research is needed to fully evaluate the optimal application of clinical significance methodology, including establishing adequate measurement tools and normative data, sufficient evidence exists to guide routine use of clinical significance evaluation in research. We would advise that researchers be cognizant of the measurement of the clinical significance of change in study design, including establishing inclusion and exclusion conditions and the selection measures for assessment batteries, to avoid some of the pitfalls that limit the ability to assess clinical significance noted in this chapter. Researchers should maximize the use of measures with adequate psychometric properties and relevant norms for study populations when possible.

In short, three categories of statistical methods can be applied in clinical trials to evaluate the consequences of interventions, including statistical significance, effect size, and clinical significance. Each addresses an important component of change, including probability, magnitude, and meaningfulness, respectively. We recommend that all three statistical methods be routinely reported in reports of clinical trials research. Clinical significance methods have the advantage of categorizing the change reported by individual patients and estimating the degree to which normal functioning has been achieved. Failing to include these types of analytical tools in the evaluation of interventions can result in overstating the value of treatments and exaggerating the comparative effects of study treatments over competing interventions.

■ References

Ankuta, G. Y., & Ables, N. (1993). Client satisfaction, clinical significance, and meaningful change in psychotherapy. *Professional Psychology: Research and Practice, 24,* 70–74.

Atkins, D. C., Bedics, J. D., McGlinchey, J. B., & Beauchaine, T. P. (2005). Assessing clinical significance: Does it matter which method we use? *Journal of Consulting and Clinical Psychology, 73,* 982–989.

Bauer, S., Lambert, M. J., & Nielsen, S. L. (2004). Clinical significance methods: A comparison of statistical techniques. *Journal of Personality Assessment, 82,* 60–70.

Beckstead, D. J., Hatch, A. L., Lambert, M. J. Eggett, D. L., Vermeersch, D. A., & Goates, M. K. (2003). Clinical significance of the Outcome Questionnaire (OQ-45.2). *Behavioral Analyst Today, 4,* 74–90.

Bergin, A. E. (1971). The evaluation of therapeutic outcomes. In S. L. Garfield & A. E. Bergin (Eds.), *The handbook of psychotherapy and behavior change.* New York: Wiley.

Bryk, A. S., & Raudenbush, S. W. (1992). *Hierarchical linear models: Applications and data analysis methods.* Newbury Park, CA: Sage.

Derogatis, L. R. (1983). *SCL-90-R: Administration, scoring, and procedures manual* (2nd ed.). Towson, MD: Clinical Psychometric Research.

Freestone, M. H., Ladouceur, R., Gagnon, F., Thibodeau, N., Rheaume, J., Letarte, H., et al. (1997). Cognitive-behavioral treatment of obsessive thoughts: A controlled study. *Journal of Consulting and Clinical Psychology, 65,* 405–413.

Gray, G. V. (2003). Psychotherapy outcomes in naturalistic settings: A reply to Hansen, Lambert, and Forman. *Clinical Psychology: Science and Practice, 10,* 505–506.

Grundy, C. T., Lambert, M. J., & Grundy, E. M. (1996). Assessing clinical significance: Application to the Hamilton Rating Scale for Depression. *Journal of Mental Health, 5,* 25–33.

Hageman, W. J., & Arrindell, W. A. (1999). Establishing clinically significant change: Increment of precision between individual and group level of analysis. *Behavior Research and Therapy, 37,* 1169–1193.

Hansen, N. B., Lambert, M. J., & Forman, E. M. (2002). The psychotherapy dose-response effect and its implications for treatment delivery services. *Clinical Psychology: Science and Practice, 9,* 329–343.

Hansen, N. B., Lambert, M. J., & Forman, E. M. (2003). The psychotherapy dose-effect in naturalistic settings revisited: Response to Gray. *Clinical Psychology: Science and Practice, 10,* 507–508.

Hsu, L. M. (1989). Reliable changes in psychotherapy: Taking into account regression toward the mean. *Behavioral Assessment, 11,* 459–467.

Hsu L. M. (1999). Caveats concerning comparisons of change rates obtained with five methods of identifying significant client changes: Comment on Speer and Greenbaum (1995). *Journal of Consulting and Clinical Psychology, 67,* 594–598.

Jacobson, N. S., Follette, W. C., & Revenstorf, D. (1984). Psychotherapy outcome research: Methods for reporting variability and evaluating clinical significance. *Behavior Therapy, 15,* 336–352.

Jacobson, N. S., Roberts, L. J., Berns, S. B., & McGlinchey, J. B. (1999). Method for defining and determining the clinical significance of treatment effects: Description, application, and alternatives. *Journal of Consulting and Clinical Psychology, 67,* 300–307.

Jacobson, N. S., & Truax, P. (1991). Clinical significance: A statistical approach to defining meaningful change in psychotherapy research. *Journal of Consulting and Clinical Psychology, 59,* 12–19.

Kazdin, A. E. (1977). Assessing the clinical or applied importance of behavior change through social validation. *Behavior Modification, 1,* 427–452.

Kazdin, A. E. (1998). *Research design in clinical psychology* (3rd ed.). Boston: Allyn & Bacon.

Kendall, P. C., Marrs-Garcia, A., Nath, S. R., & Sheldrick, R. C. (1999). Normative comparisons for the evaluation of clinical significance. *Journal of Consulting and Clinical Psychology, 67,* 285–299.

Lambert, M. J. (1976). Spontaneous remission in adult neurotic disorders: A revision and summary. *Psychological Bulletin, 83,* 107–119.

Lambert, M. J. (2001). Psychotherapy outcome and quality improvement: Introduction to the special section on client-focused research. *Journal of Consulting and Clinical Psychology, 69,* 147–149.

Lambert, M. J., Morton, J. J., Hatfield, D., Harmon, C., Hamilton, S., Reid, R. C., et al. (2004). *Administration and scoring manual for the OQ-45.2.* Salt Lake City, UT: OQMeasures.

Lambert, M. J., & Ogles, B. M. (2004). The efficacy and effectiveness of psychotherapy. In M. J. Lambert (Ed.), *The handbook of psychotherapy and behavior change* (5th ed.). New York: Wiley.

Lambert, M. J., Whipple, J. L., Hawkins, E. J., Vermeersch, D. A., Nielsen, S. L., & Smart, D. W. (2003). Is it time for clinicians to routinely track patient outcome? A meta-analysis. *Clinical Psychology: Science and Practice, 10,* 288–301.

Lick, J. (1973). Statistical vs. clinical significance in research on the outcome of psychotherapy. *International Journal of Mental Health, 2,* 26–37.

Lunnen, K. M., & Ogles, B. A. (1998). A multiperspective, multivariable evaluation of reliable change. *Journal of Consulting and Clinical Psychology, 66,* 400–410.

Maassen, G. H. (2000). Principles of defining reliable change indices. *Journal of Clinical and Experimental Neuropsychology, 22,* 622–632.

Martinovich, Z., Saunders, S., & Howard, K. (1996). Some comments on "assessing clinical significance." *Psychotherapy Research, 6,* 124–132.

McGlinchey, J. B., Atkins, D. C., & Jacobson, N. S. (2002). Clinical significance methods: Which one to use and how useful are they? *Behavior Therapy, 33,* 529–550.

Ogles, B. M., Lambert, M. J., & Sawyer, J. D. (1995). Clinical significance of the National Institute of Mental Health Treatment of Depression Collaborative Research Program data. *Journal of Consulting and Clinical Psychology, 63,* 321–326.

Ogles, B. M., Lunnen, K. M., & Bonesteel, K. (2001). Clinical significance: History, application, and current practice. *Clinical Psychology Review, 21,* 421–446.

Seggar, L. B., Lambert, M. J., & Hansen, N. B. (2002). Assessing clinical significance: Application to the Beck Depression Inventory. *Behavior Therapy, 33,* 253–269.

Sikkema, K. J., Hansen, N. B., Ghebrenichael, M., Kochman, A., Tarakeshwar, N., Meade, C. S., et al. (in press). A randomized controlled trial of a coping group intervention for AIDS-bereaved HIV-positive adults: Longitudinal effects of grief. *Health Psychology.*

Sikkema, K. J., Hansen, N. B., Kochman, A., Tate, D. C., & DiFranceisco, W. (2004). Outcomes from a randomized controlled trial of a group intervention for HIV-positive men and women coping with AIDS-related loss and bereavement. *Death Studies, 28,* 187–209.

Sikkema, K. J., Hansen, N. B., Meade, C. S., Kochman, A., Lee, R. S. (2005). Improvements in health-related quality of life following a group intervention for coping with AIDS-bereavement among HIV-infected men and women. *Quality of Life Research, 14,* 991–1005.

Sikkema, K. J., Hansen, N., Tarakeshwar, N., Kochman, A., Tate, D., & Lee, R. S. (2004). The clinical significance of change in trauma-related symptoms following a pilot group intervention for coping with HIV-AIDS and childhood sexual trauma. *AIDS and Behavior, 8,* 277–291.

Smith, M. L., Glass, G. V., & Miller, T. I. (1980). *The benefits of psychotherapy.* Baltimore: Johns Hopkins University Press.

Speer, D. C. (1992). Clinically significant change: Jacobson & Truax (1991) revisited. *Journal of Consulting and Clinical Psychology, 60,* 402–408.

Speer, D.C. (1999). What is the role of two-wave designs in clinical research? Comment on Hagelman and Arindell. *Behavior Research and Therapy, 37,* 1203–1210.

Speer, D. C., & Greenbaum, P. E. (1995). Five methods for computing significant individual client change and improvement rates: Support for an individual growth curve approach. *Journal of Consulting and Clinical Psychology, 63,* 1044–1048.

Tingey, R. C., Lambert, M. J., Burlingame, G. M., & Hansen, N. B. (1996). Assessing clinical significance: Proposed extensions to method. *Psychotherapy Research, 6,* 109–123.

Wolf, M. M. (1978). Social validity: The case for subjective measurement or how applied behavior analysis is finding its heart. *Journal of Applied Behavior Analysis, 11,* 203–214.

18. Assessing the Effect Size of Outcome Research

Ralph L. Rosnow and Robert Rosenthal

The *effect size* (ES), a concept developed by Jacob Cohen (1969) in his seminal text on statistical power analysis, is generally used in behavioral and biomedical research to refer to the magnitude of an outcome result or to the strength of the relationship between two variables (e.g., an independent and a dependent variable). The ES does not tell us whether there was a causal relationship—which is a complex and philosophically controversial question (e.g., Pearl, 2000)—but gives us a sense of "the *degree* to which the phenomenon is present in the population" (Cohen, 1988, p. 9). In this chapter we provide a sampling of ES indices in three general classes: (a) the difference family (illustrated here by Cohen's *d*, Hedges's *g*, and the risk difference); (b) the correlation family (illustrated by the point-biserial *r*, the phi coefficient, r_{alerting}, $r_{\text{effect size}}$, r_{contrast}, and r_{BESD}); and (c) the ratio family (illustrated by the odds ratio and relative risk). When a decision needs to be made to convert effect sizes to a common index, we recommend the correlation (or *r*-type) family primarily because *r*-type indices can be used in all situations in which difference and ratio indices are used, and *r*-type indices associated with contrasts can be used in situations in which difference and ratio indices are not naturally applicable.

Among the reasons effect sizes should be of interest is that funding agencies often require that a power analysis be part of the grant application, and some expectation of the ES is an imperative of power analysis. A second reason is that effect sizes are the coin of the realm in meta-analysis, which has become an increasingly popular mode of research synthesis in the behavioral and biomedical sciences (e.g., Cooper & Hedges, 1994). A third reason is that recommended reforms for the treatment of statistical results in psychological research have emphasized the reporting of effect sizes and interval estimates for principal outcomes (Wilkinson & Task Force on Statistical Inference, 1999). Similar counsel can be found in the *Publication Manual of the American Psychological Association* (APA, 2001), which urges researchers to report "one-degree-of-freedom effects—particularly when these are the results that inform the discussion" (p. 26). (The expression *one-degree-of-freedom effects* refers to outcome indicators that are generally associated with focused statistical procedures, including all contrasts, all *t* tests, *F* tests with numerator $df = 1$, and 1-df χ^2 tests.)

However, the most fundamental reason that effect sizes should be of interest is implied in the following conceptual equation:

$$\text{Significance test} = \text{Size of effect} \times \text{Size of study} \qquad (1)$$

which indicates that all significance tests (t, F, χ^2, etc.) can be parsed into one or more definitions of ES multiplied by one or more definitions of study size (e.g., the total sample size, N, or the n per group). The larger the ES and the larger the study, the larger will be the value of the significance test, and, therefore, the smaller (and usually more coveted) will be the p value. (If the ES were exactly zero, increasing the N would not produce a result that is any more significant than a smaller N would produce.) Thus, reporting only that a statistical test was, or was not, *significant* reveals nothing specifically about the size of the effect in question. The test result might be statistically significant because the effect was large, or the total N was large, or both, or the test might fail to achieve a desired level of significance because there was not enough power to detect an effect that truly exists. In a classic case, Cohen (1962) found the median power to detect what he called "medium" effects at $p = .05$ in studies published in one APA journal was no better than the flip of a coin. Remarkably, two decades later, Sedlmeier and Gigerenzer (1989) reported that the median power of studies published in another incarnation of the journal was slightly worse than before!

Difference Indices for Means

COHEN's d

When practical implications of the dependent measure are transparent (e.g., the daily number of cigarettes smoked, employee absences from work, incidents of disruptive behavior), the raw mean or median may be pregnant with practical meaning. Cohen (1988) recognized, however, that a limitation of most raw unit measures has to do with the arbitrariness of the scalar units in behavioral research. For example, the practical meaning of the absolute size of scores on judgment scales is not obvious without detailed information about characteristics of the scale and the observed data. One useful option is to express effects in standard deviation units. This strategy enables us not only to compare transformed raw unit measures on a common metric but also to draw implications for the populations based on characteristics of the cumulative normal distribution (illustrated shortly). Cohen proposed that, when using the t test to compare two independent means, a useful "pure number" ES (i.e., free of the original measurement unit) is

$$d = \frac{M_1 - M_2}{\sigma_{\text{pooled}}} \qquad (2)$$

which is Cohen's d, where the numerator indicates the difference between two observed means, and the denominator is the common within-group σ. A caveat, particularly in small-sample studies, is that one or more outliers might inflate the denominator of Equation 2, causing d to be small even when there is a large difference between groups (Wilcox, 2005). An outlier that is an error can often be dealt with by equitable trimming, whereas a far-out score that is not an error cautions us to look deeper into the data (Rosenthal & Rosnow, 2008, pp. 309–311).

With Cohen's d the ES index, one way of thinking about the t test for independent means in the framework of Equation 1 is

$$t = d \times \left[\frac{\sqrt{n_1 n_2}}{n_1 + n_2} \times \sqrt{df} \right] \tag{3}$$

with the estimate of d given by Equation 2. When $n_1 = n_2$, the first term in the brackets of Equation 3 simplifies to 1/2, and we can write

$$t = d \times \frac{\sqrt{df}}{2} \tag{4}$$

Thus, given t and the two sample sizes ($n_1 = n_2$), we can estimate d from t by

$$d = \frac{2t}{\sqrt{df}} \tag{5}$$

Suppose 80 patients were randomly assigned in equal numbers ($n = 40$) to a therapy and a wait-listed control group, and $t(78) = 2.21$, $p = .03$ two-tailed. Equation 5 yields $d = .50$, or one half a standard deviation difference between the two means. Based on the cumulative normal distribution, $d = .50$ implies (a) 33% nonoverlap of normal population distributions (67% overlap); (b) that the highest 59.9% of one population will exceed the lowest 59.9% of the other population; and (c) the upper half of the latter population will exceed 69.1% of the former population (Cohen, 1988, p. 22). Whether this kind of information is useful in a practical sense, Cohen left to the reader's judgment. He noted that another way of thinking about d was in terms of r or r^2, in which case $d = .5$ corresponds to $r = .24$ and $r^2 = .06$ (we return to r^2 in the next section on correlation indices).

Equation 5 can also be useful when no formal ES is available. Suppose we had the Mann-Whitney U probability that patients in the experimental group ranked higher than the patients in the control group. The Mann-Whitney U test yields an exact p value, but no generally accepted ES estimate exists for this test. We simply find the value of t corresponding to the exact p and df and then substitute in Equation 5 to obtain what is denoted as $d_{\text{equivalent}}$, the value of d

analogous to the result for an exactly normally distributed outcome with $N/2$ units in each group and the obtained p (Rosenthal & Rubin, 2003). (The t value can be determined by computer programs and at reliable Web sites, such as http://calculators.stat.ucla.edu.)

The 95% confidence interval (CI) for Cohen's d on independent means is obtained by

$$95\%\text{CI} = d \pm t_{(.05)} \left(S_{\text{Cohen's } d} \right) \tag{6}$$

where $t_{(.05)}$ is the critical value of t at $p = .05$ two-tailed for $df = n_1 + n_2 - 2$, and $S_{\text{Cohen's } d}$ is the square root of the variance of Cohen's d from

$$S^2_{\text{Cohen's } d} = \left[\frac{n_1 + n_2}{n_1 n_2} + \frac{d^2}{2(df)} \right] \frac{n_1 + n_2}{df} \tag{7}$$

Substituting in Equation 7 the results of the illustration above—where $d = .50$, $n_1 = n_2 = 40$, and $df = n_1 + n_2 - 2 = 78$—we find

$$S^2_{\text{Cohen's } d} = \left[\frac{40 + 40}{(40)(40)} + \frac{.50^2}{2(78)} \right] \frac{40 + 40}{78} = .053$$

so $S_{\text{Cohen's } d}$ is $\sqrt{.053} = .230$. With $df = 78$, the critical value of $t_{(.05)}$ is 1.99, and substitution in Equation 6 yields $95\%\text{CI} = .50 \pm 1.99(.230) = .50 \pm .458$, which indicates that there is a 95% probability that the population value of d falls between .042 and .958.

UNEQUAL SAMPLE SIZES

In behavioral research of many different types it is common to have unequal sample sizes, for example, when the treatment is much more expensive to administer than is the control procedure. For any given study in which $n_1 + n_2 = N$ (the total sample size), we increasingly lose statistical power the more that n_1 and n_2 differ in size for any specific value of N. It will then often be useful to compare the power of our statistical tests for different degrees of heterogeneity of the sample sizes when we are planning the research.

We can calculate the retention of power in the unequal-n design from the ratio of the harmonic mean sample size (n_h) to the arithmetic mean sample size ($\bar{n}$). Subtracting that value from unity gives the proportional loss of relative efficiency (Rosenthal, Rosnow, & Rubin, 2000), that is,

$$\text{Loss} = 1 - \left(\frac{n_h}{\bar{n}} \right) \tag{8}$$

where the harmonic mean sample size in $k = 2$ samples of n_1 and n_2 size is

$$n_h = \frac{1}{\left(\frac{1}{2}\right)\left(\frac{1}{n_1 + n_2}\right)} = \frac{2(n_1 n_2)}{n_1 + n_2} \qquad (9)$$

Because the harmonic mean sample size equals the arithmetic mean sample size when $n_1 = n_2$, the ratio of n_h to $\bar{n}$ is always 1.0 in equal-n designs, and Equation 8 therefore yields a value of zero loss in such designs. In samples of unequal sizes, the harmonic mean is less than the arithmetic mean, and the value given by Equation 8 increases with corresponding increases in the inequality of the sample sizes.

In studies with unequal sample ns, the valid estimate of d is still given by Equation 2, but we modify the equal-n equation for estimating d from t (Eq. 5) as follows:

$$d = \left(\frac{2t}{\sqrt{df_{within}}}\right)\sqrt{\frac{\bar{n}}{n_h}} \qquad (10)$$

In studies with equal ns, it makes no difference whether we use the equal-n equation (Eq. 5) or the unequal-n equation (Eq. 10) to estimate d from t. However, the more unequal the ns, the more will Equation 5 underestimate d.

Cohen (1969, 1988) recognized that investigators might prefer to think of effect sizes for mean differences in terms of r rather than d. We can convert d into the point-biserial r in an unequal-n design by

$$r = \frac{d}{\sqrt{d^2 + 4\left(\frac{\bar{n}}{n_h}\right)}} \qquad (11)$$

Suppose group means of 6.0 and 4.8, σ of 2.0, and sample sizes of 85 and 15. Since $d = (6.0 - 4.8)/2.0 = .6$, Equation 11 yields

$$r = \frac{.6}{\sqrt{(.6)^2 + 4\left(\frac{50}{25.5}\right)}} = .21$$

In an equal-n design, Equation 11 simplifies to one given by Cohen (1988, p. 23) as

$$r = \frac{d}{\sqrt{d^2 + 4}} \qquad (12)$$

Suppose the sample sizes were *inherently unequal,* for example, a comparison of the test scores of patients with a rare disorder to the test scores of patients with common disorders (or test scores of people in general). When sample sizes are inherently unequal, Cohen (1988, p. 24) suggested the following equation for converting d into r:

$$r = \frac{d}{\sqrt{d^2 + \left(\dfrac{1}{PQ}\right)}} \tag{13}$$

where $P =$ the proportion of the overall total sample (N) or population represented by the sample in one group, and $Q = 1 - P$. For example, if the rare disorder occurred in 5% of the population, $P = .05$ and $Q = .95$. When $P = Q$, Equation 13 is equivalent to Equation 12, and, more generally, Equation 13 is an alternative version of Equation 11. The r obtained from Equation 13 or Equation 11 is interpreted as the correlation between the independent variable of group membership (coded, e.g., as treatment $= 1$ and control $= 0$) and the test scores on the dependent variable for sample sizes that are observed to be unequal *and* are assumed on theoretical grounds to be inherently unequal.

HEDGES'S g

A popular unit-free alternative to indexing the difference between two means by d is Larry V. Hedges's g statistic, which transforms the ES into standard score units by dividing $M_1 - M_2$ by the pooled within-sample estimate of the population standard deviation, that is,

$$g = \frac{M_1 - M_2}{S_{\text{within}}} \tag{14}$$

where

$$S_{\text{within}} = \sqrt{\frac{\Sigma(X_1 - M_1)^2 + \Sigma(X_2 - M_2)^2}{df_{\text{within}}}} \tag{15}$$

and X_1 and X_2 are individual scores in samples 1 and 2, respectively (e.g., an experimental and a control group). We note that the denominator of Equation 15 is the df_{within}. In the case of Cohen's d, the analogous denominator would have been N, the total number of independent sampling units.

In the same way that Equation 5 showed that, in an equal-n design, Cohen's d can be obtained from t, we can also obtain Hedges's g from t by

$$g = \frac{2t}{\sqrt{N}} \tag{16}$$

assuming equal sample sizes in the two groups. With unequal sample sizes, we modify this equation to obtain g from t by

$$g = \left(\frac{2t}{\sqrt{N}} \right) \sqrt{\frac{\bar{n}}{n_h}} \tag{17}$$

and, as before, there will be no difference in an equal-n design whether we use Equation 16 or Equation 17.

For example, in the equal-n situation given earlier, where $t(78) = 2.21$ and $d = .50$, we now find (from Eq. 16 or Eq. 17) Hedges's $g = .49$. The slight difference in outcomes is due to the fact that Cohen's d used N for the denominator of the estimated standard deviation, whereas Hedges's g used $N - 1$. The two indices can be converted back and forth, whether the sample sizes are equal or unequal. We convert g into d by

$$d = g \sqrt{\frac{N}{df_{within}}} \tag{18}$$

or d into g by

$$g = d \sqrt{\frac{df_{within}}{N}} \tag{19}$$

Similarly, in an equal-n design, we convert g into r by

$$r = \frac{g}{\sqrt{g^2 + 4 \left(\dfrac{df_{within}}{N} \right)}} \tag{20}$$

but for an unequal-n design, we need the following modification:

$$r = \frac{g}{\sqrt{g^2 + 4 \left(\dfrac{\bar{n}}{n_h} \right) \left(\dfrac{df_{within}}{N} \right)}} \tag{21}$$

For the 95% confidence interval of Hedges's g, we redefine $S_{\text{Cohen's } d}$ in Equation 6 to be $S_{\text{Hedges's } g}$, and since

$$S^2_{\text{Hedges's } g} = \frac{n_1 + n_2}{n_1 n_2} + \frac{g^2}{2(df)} \tag{22}$$

we find

$$S^2_{\text{Hedges's } g} = \left[\frac{40 + 40}{(40)(40)}\right] + \frac{.49^2}{2(78)} = .052$$

and $S_{\text{Hedges's } g} = \sqrt{S^2_{\text{Hedges's } g}} = \sqrt{.052} = .228$. Therefore, the 95% CI $= .49 \pm$ 1.99 (.228) $= .49 \pm. 454$, so the lower and upper limits of Hedges's g in this example are .036 and .944, respectively. Notice that not only was the value of d slightly larger than the value of g, but the CI of d was also slightly wider than that for g. As sample sizes increase, the difference between d and g will diminish. These confidence intervals are based on statistical assumptions of the t distribution, and while t is a robust test, serious violations could jeopardize the accuracy of such estimates. However, when the sampling biases are small, slightly biased samples may provide tolerable estimates of population parameters (Snedecor & Cochran, 1989).

Correlation Indices for Simple Effects

POINT-BISERIAL r

We prefer usually to think of effect sizes in terms of r-type indices, and in this vein, another way of thinking about the relationship in Equation 1 between the size of effect and the size of study is

$$t = \frac{r}{\sqrt{1 - r^2}} \times \sqrt{df} \tag{23}$$

where, in the two-sample case with one dichotomous variable (e.g., assignment to control vs. experimental group) and one continuous variable (scores on the dependent measure), r is the point-biserial correlation, and $df = N - 2$. We suggest the nonsquared ES estimate because squared estimates can mask "small" effects of practical significance (illustrated shortly). Thus, we calculate the point-biserial r from t by

$$r = \sqrt{\frac{t^2}{t^2 + df}} \tag{24}$$

where $df = N - 2$ in the case of two independent groups, and $N = n_1 + n_2$. Suppose we have 40 patients each in the randomly assigned experimental and control conditions, find $t(78) = 3.1$, and so substituting in Equation 24 yields $r = .33$.

Previously we mentioned the $d_{\text{equivalent}}$ statistic as a convenient ES estimate obtained from the total sample size and a p value, and similarly we can estimate $r_{\text{equivalent}}$ from the same basic raw ingredients (Rosenthal & Rubin, 2003). Suppose again we had a Mann-Whitney U test, this time in a study in which four children were taught by a new method (treatment), and five children were taught by an old (control) method. All four treated children were ranked higher than any of the five control children, yielding an exact probability of .008 one-tailed Mann-Whitney U test. With $p = .008$ and $N = 9$, $t(7) = 3.16$, and from Equation 24 we find $r_{equivalent} = .77$, which is analogous to the sample point-biserial r between the treatment indicator (e.g., treatment $= 1$; control $= 0$) and an exactly normally distributed outcome in a two-group design with $N/2$ units in each group and the obtained p. The $r_{equivalent}$ (also $d_{equivalent}$) approach is not a uniformly optimal procedure but is intended for cases in which the actual study is reasonably close in form to the canonical design and where the alternative is to have no ES estimate, or the situation is one in which $r_{equivalent}$ and $d_{equivalent}$ yield estimates that are more accurate than ES estimates computed directly from the data (Rosenthal & Rubin, 2003, p. 496).

INTERVAL ESTIMATES

When the population value of an ES r is not zero (and usually it is not), the distribution of sampled rs is skewed, and the more so, the further the population value of the r falls from zero. Thus, we use the Fisher z-transformed r (i.e., z_r) to obtain the lower and upper limits of a 95% confidence interval around an obtained r, where

$$95\%\text{CI} = z_r \pm 1.96 / \sqrt{N - 3} \tag{25}$$

and then we convert these limits back into units of r. (Tables for these transformations can be found in Rosenthal & Rosnow, 2008, pp. 725–726). For example, for $r = .33$ and $N = 80$, the Fisher $z_r = .34$, so the 95% CI for z_r is given by $.34 \pm 1.96 / \sqrt{N - 3} = .34 \pm .22$, therefore extending from a z_r of .12 to a z_r of .56. Converting z_r values back into r reveals in this case that, with 95% confidence, the population value of r can be estimated to be between .12 and .51.

Some researchers equate their failure to reject the null hypothesis as automatically implying an ES of zero. Inspecting the null-counternull interval can in many cases provide protection against mistaken interpretations (Rosenthal & Rubin, 1994). The counternull value of an obtained ES is the nonnull magnitude of the ES that is supported by exactly the same amount of evidence as is the null value of the ES. To obtain the counternull value of r, we generally work with the symmetrically distributed transformation of r, which again is the Fisher z_r (Rosenthal & Rubin, 1994). When the ES is in the form of a point-biserial r, the following can be used to estimate the counternull value of r from the obtained r:

$$r_{counternull} = \sqrt{\frac{4r^2}{1 + 3r^2}} \tag{26}$$

Suppose $t(16) = 1.25$ and $p = .23$ two-tailed, and from Equation 24 we find $r = .30$. From Equation 26 we find $r_{counternull} = .53$, which forces us to confront the fact that, although it is true that our ES of $r = .30$ did not differ significantly from .00 (the null value in this case), it is no more true than the assertion that our ES of $r = .30$ does not differ significantly from .53. Thus, a conclusion of "no effect" based on $r = .30$ and $p = .23$ two-tailed (or $p = .115$ one-tailed) would be seriously in error, because the counternull value (.53) implies a large ES as the upper limit of our null-counternull interval. We calculate percent coverage of the null-counternull interval by $100(1.00 - p_{two\text{-}tailed})$, which in this example gives a 77% CI. (For Cohen's d or Hedges's g, the counternull value is ordinarily simply twice the value of the d or g, because each is already based on a symmetrical distribution.)

PHI COEFFICIENT

When both variables are scored dichotomously, still another way of representing the relationship in Equation 1 is

$$\chi^2_{(1)} = \phi^2 \times N \tag{27}$$

where $df = 1$ with χ^2 based on a 2×2 table of independent frequencies (i.e., counts), ϕ^2 is the squared Pearson product-moment r between membership in the row category (scored 1 or 0) and membership in the column category (scored 1 or 0), and N is the total number of counts in all four cells. Rearrangement of Equation 27 and solving for ϕ (or r_ϕ) yields

$$r_\phi = \sqrt{\frac{\chi^2_{(1)}}{N}} \tag{28}$$

When sample sizes are small, we often get somewhat more accurate estimates of phi from Fisher's exact test (Rosenthal & Rosnow, 2008, pp. 602–607), which gives the exact one-tailed p for a given table of counts (with row and column totals regarded as fixed). In that case, we go from the df and the exact one-tailed p value to t, and then to Equation 24 to compute phi.

BINOMIAL EFFECT SIZE DISPLAY

Cohen mentioned r^2 as a way of interpreting d, where r^2 (the coefficient of determination) times 100 gives the percent of variance (PV) in one variable that is accounted for by the other variable. For example, a d of .2 (Cohen called it a "small" effect) is associated with a PV of 1% (i.e., $r^2 = .01$). A d of .5 (called a "medium" effect) is associated with a PV of 6% ($r^2 = .059$). A d of .8 (a "large" effect) is associated with a PV of 14% ($r^2 = .138$). Cohen (1988) added: "The only difficulty arising from the use of PV measures lies in the fact that in many, perhaps most, of the areas of behavioral science, they turn out to be so small!" (p. 78). For example, recently it was noted that the average of 322 meta-analyses of social psychological phenomena was $r = .21$ (Richard, Bond, & Stokes-Zoota, 2003), which would account for 4.4% of variance. We suggest two caveats: First, neither experienced psychological researchers nor experienced statisticians seem to have a good intuitive sense of what PV implies in *practical* terms (Rosenthal & Rubin, 1982). Second, sometimes small effects can have profound practical implications. For example, we computed the ES of the landmark 1954 Salk vaccine trial to be $r = .011$, which in PV terms is equivalent to 0%! (Rosnow & Rosenthal, 2003). Yet it is generally accepted that this classic RCT provided convincing evidence of the value of the Salk polio vaccine (Brownlee, 1955). As Cohen (1988) wisely counseled, "the *meaning* of any given ES is, in the final analysis, a function of the context in which it is embedded" (p. 535).

Casting an ES r into a binomial effect size display (BESD) gives us a standardized frame of reference as we ponder the practical meaning of a given value of ES (Rosenthal & Rubin, 1979, 1982). The BESD takes its name from its strategy of casting ES correlations into dichotomous outcomes (such as improved vs. not improved; survived vs. died; success vs. failure; better health vs. worse health) in a 2×2 table with all four of its marginal values *set at 100 each*. The BESD does not require that the raw data be limited to 2×2 tables with uniform margins, and the BESD should not be confused with the raw or empirical data on which the ES r was originally computed (because most actual values in the margins of empirical 2×2 tables are not equal). Setting the marginal values at 100 each is premised on the idea of a theoretical population in which half received the investigational treatment and the other half did not, and with the outcome results split at the median. Say the success (or improvement) rate was higher in the experimental than in the control group, in which case we would compute the BESD-based outcome rate for the experimental group as $100(.50 + r/2)$, and for the BESD rate in the control group, we would calculate $100(.50 - r/2)$. To display a BESD-standardized outcome rate that was higher in the control group (e.g., death rate, recidivism rate, failure rate), we reverse these calculations. In either case, the difference between the BESD outcome rates, divided by 100, will return the value of the r. Thus, a further convenience of the BESD is how easily cell values can be converted to r, and how easily we can go from r to the BESD cell values.

We illustrate this application with the primary results of a more recent biomedical trial of an investigational vaccine, called Gardasil, that was heralded in a front-page story in *The New York Times* (Grady, 2005). The results discussed here refer to the 2-year trial data reported on the Merck Web site (http://www.merck.com) for the vaccine, which was developed for the prevention of cervical cancers linked with human papillomavirus types 16 and 18. There were 10,580 women in this phase of the trial (aged 16–26 from 90 study centers in 13 countries), of whom 5,301 were on a three-dose regimen of the vaccine, and 5,279 received a placebo. Among those who received the vaccine, no cases were reported of the particular cervical precancer or noninvasive cervical cancer, whereas 21 cases were reported for the placebo group. Computing a 1-*df* chi-square on the table of counts for these results, we found $\chi^2 = 21.13$ ($p = 4.3^{-6}$), and from Equation 28, $r = .04$ (rounded from .0447). Casting this r as a BESD, the cancer rate in the placebo group is $100(.50 + .04/2) = 52\%$, and the cancer rate in the vaccine group is $100(.50 - .04/2) = 48\%$. This BESD is shown in Part A of Table 18.1, while Parts B and C show the BESDs for the lower and upper 95% CI limits (Eq. 25). Thus, the r of .04 in Part A implies a 4% difference in cervical cancer from placebo to vaccine groups (i.e., in a theoretical population split into equal halves, with the dependent variable split at the median). Squaring $r = .04$ would, however, lead to the conclusion that the vaccine had no effect ($r^2 = .00$)! That the r was so small reflects the fact that the particular cancer was relatively uncommon in the populations sampled.

One-Sample Effect Sizes

Frequently we find that clinical researchers refer to changes on some dependent variable in a single sample, such as the reduction of symptoms from intake to discharge. However, instead of inspecting the size of the effect, they report a

TABLE 18.1
*BESDs for Obtained Result (r = .04) and for Lower (r = .02)
and Upper Limit (r = .06) of the 95% CI Straddling the
Obtained Result*

	Cancer	No cancer	Σ
A. Obtained r = .04			
Placebo	52	48	100
Vaccine	48	52	100
Σ	100	100	200
B. Lower 95% confidence limit r = .02			
Placebo	51	49	100
Vaccine	49	51	100
Σ	100	100	200
C. Upper 95% confidence limit r = .06			
Placebo	53	47	100
Vaccine	47	53	100
Σ	100	100	200

one-sample significance test and p value. We have described a way of expressing the size of the one-sample effect as a partial point-biserial r (Rosenthal & Rosnow, 2008, pp. 398–400). This r can be estimated from the t test for correlated data by substituting the correlated-t value in Equation 24 with $df = N - 1$. Because the interpretation of this r is not transparent, we refer readers to the detailed discussion in our book cited above. Say we were interested in comparing two effect sizes in the form of r, such as a one-sample r in an experimental group versus that in the control group. Cohen (1988) proposed a procedure that focuses on the difference between Fisher z_r transformed values of each r. This procedure can also be used to compare an obtained one-sample r with a theoretical value of r, where both are expressed in z_r terms. There are also simple meta-analytic procedures for estimating the statistical significance of the difference between ES indices in the form of r (e.g., Rosenthal, 1991).

Later in this chapter we turn to contrasts and r-type indices of ES in multisample trials. We have proposed variants of these procedures for use in a wide variety of designs, including repeated measures designs such as the one-sample case (Rosenthal et al., 2000). Suppose three patients received three applications of an investigational treatment designed to improve cognitive performance. Each patient was measured on four occasions: (a) intake, (b) after Treatment application 1, (c) after Treatment application 2, and (d) after Treatment application 3. Say we hypothesized steady improvement in cognitive performance from intake to treatment application 3. We compute a linear contrast, stating our prediction in simple integers (called *contrast weights,* or *lambda weights*) that sum to zero ($\Sigma\lambda = 0$). Since our prediction is a steady linear increase, we might choose λ weights of -3, -1, $+1$, $+3$, respectively, for the four occasions of measurement. There are alternative ways of computing the contrast and different indicators of ES, but here we illustrate a way of indicating the relative performance of the three patients and a focused significance test and ES for the linear effect in the group as a whole.

Illustrative scores for three patients and the summary ANOVA are shown in Table 18.2. The mean square (MS) for patients is a reflection of how far apart the patients' means were on average. The MS for occasions is a reflection of how far apart the four occasions' means were on average. The MS for the interaction of occasions $\times$ patients is a reflection of the heterogeneity of the patterns or profiles of four scores among the three patients. None of these results specifically addresses the questions of interest. One way to provide clues as to the relative linearity of improvement of performance of patients over time is to correlate each patient's scores on the outcome variable with the respective contrast weights. Correlating Patient 1's scores of 1, 3, 7, and 5 with the corresponding weights of -3, -1, $+1$, and $+3$ yields $r = .80$. Similar correlations for patients 2 and 3 of the repeated measurement scores with their associated λ weights are shown as .40 and 1.00, respectively. Reviewing available records might help to clarify why patient 2's score dropped precipitously (from 6 to 2) at session 2.

TABLE 18.2 (A)
Individual Scores for Three Patients Measured on Four Occasions

Patient	Occasion of measurement				r
	Intake	Session 1	Session 2	Session 3	
1	1	3	7	5	.80
2	0	6	2	4	.40
3	2	4	6	8	1.00
Mean	1.00	4.33	5.00	5.67	$\bar{r} = .73$
S^2	1.00	2.33	7.00	4.33	.0933
λ weights	−3	−1	+1	+3	

TABLE 18.2 (B)
Summary ANOVA for Three Patients Measured on Four Occasions

Source	SS	df	MS	F	p
Between patients	8.00	2	4.00		
Within patients	60.00	9			
Occasions	38.67	3	12.89	3.62	.08
Occasions × patients	21.33	6	3.56		

Because we are also interested in having a focused significance test and ES for the linear prediction, we can calculate a one-sample t on the average r (shown in Table 18.2 as $\bar{r} = .73$) by

$$t = \frac{\bar{r}}{\sqrt{\left(\frac{1}{N}\right)S_r^2}} \tag{29}$$

where N is the number of patients, S_r^2 is the variance of the r values in Part A, and $df = N - 1$. For the data of Table 18.2, we find $t = .73 / \sqrt{(1/3).0933} = 4.14$, $df = 2$, and $p = .027$ one-tailed. The ES is obtained by substituting in Equation 24, with $df = N - 1 = 2$, yielding $r = .95$. The use of "r scores" serves as an example of contrast procedures that can be used with repeated measures designs, but alternative procedures are available and described in Rosenthal et al. (2000, chap. 5).

Indices Specifically for 2 × 2 Contingency Tables

In RCTs for biomedical interventions, the statistical reporting of ratios, rates, and proportions for tables of counts is common. Two popular ratio-type indices are the odds ratio (OR) and relative risk (RR); we now turn to them and another difference-type index, risk difference (RD). Previously we described a way of estimating the ES r (phi) from the 1-df χ^2 by Equation 28. We can also obtain phi directly from

$$\phi = \frac{AD - BC}{\sqrt{(A+B)(C+D)(A+C)(B+D)}} \tag{30}$$

where A, B, C, and D are cell counts defined in Part A of Table 18.3. For the Gardasil data in Part B, we find

$$\phi = \frac{(21)(5,301) - (5,258)(0)}{\sqrt{(5,279)(5,301)(21)(10,559)}} = .04 \text{ (rounded)}$$

and for the Salk vaccine data in Part C, phi = .01 (rounded).

RELATIVE RISK, THE ODDS RATIO, AND RISK DIFFERENCE

With the four cells of the 2×2 contingency table labeled as noted in Table 18.3, relative risk (RR) is computed as

$$RR = \left(\frac{A}{A+B}\right) \bigg/ \left(\frac{C}{C+D}\right) \tag{31}$$

that is, the ratio of the proportion of control patients at risk of a negative outcome to the proportion of treated patients at risk of a negative outcome. Substituting the Gardasil data in Equation 31 yields RR = (21/5,279)/(0/5,301) = ∞, an alarmingly high risk of cancer for the placebo group. For the Salk vaccine data, RR = (115/201,229)/(33/200,745) = 3.48.

The odds ratio (OR) is computed as

$$OR = (A/B)/(C/D) \tag{32}$$

that is, the ratio of control patients with a negative outcome to the control patients with a positive outcome divided by the ratio of treatment patients with a negative outcome to the treatment patients with a positive outcome. For the Gardasil data, substitution in Equation 32 yields OR=(21/5,258)/(0/5,301)=∞. For the Salk vaccine data, Equation 33 yields OR=(115/201,114)/(33/200,712)=3.48.

The risk difference (RD) is computed as

$$RD = \left(\frac{A}{A+B} - \frac{C}{C+D}\right) \tag{33}$$

that is, the difference between the proportion of the control patients at risk of a negative outcome and the proportion of the treated patients at such risk.

TABLE 18.3 (A)
Template With Code Letters

	Negative outcome	Positive outcome	Σ
Control	A	B	A + B
Treatment	C	D	C + D
Σ	A + C	B + D	N

TABLE 18.3 (B)
Outcome Results for High-Grade Cervical Precancers and Noninvasive Cervical Cancers (CIN 2/3 and AIS) Associated With Human Papillomavirus (HPV) Types 16 and 18 in Gardasil RCT

	Cancer	No cancer	Σ
Placebo	21	5,258	5,279
Gardasil	0	5,301	5,301
Σ	21	10,559	10,580

TABLE 18.3 (C)
Outcome Results for Poliomyelitis in Salk Vaccine RCT

	Polio	No polio	Σ
Placebo	115	201,114	201,229
Salk vaccine	33	200,712	200,745
Σ	148	401,826	401,974

Substituting the Gardasil data in Equation 33 yields RD = (21/5,279) − (0/5,301) = .004, far less alarming than the "infinite" OR or RR. For the Salk vaccine data, RD = (115/201,229) − (33/200,745) = .0004, smaller even than the RD of .004 of the Gardasil data.

Table 18.4 provides some further insights into these four indices (RR, OR, RD, and ϕ). Part A shows three sets of study results, with row and column headings noted at the top of the table. Suppose the dependent variable were the mortality rate of patients who receive an investigational treatment or a control treatment. We would pose the following question to the reader: "If I had to be in the control condition, would it matter to me whether I was in Study 1, 2, or 3?" We think most people would answer that, if they were in the control condition, they would prefer to be in Study 1 rather than in Study 2, and surely no control subject would prefer to be in Study 3. Yet, despite the clear phenomeno-

TABLE 18.4 (A)
Original (Nonstandardized) Effect Sizes in Hypothetical 2 ×2 Contingency

	Mortality		Relative risk (Eq. 31)	Odds ratio (Eq. 32)	Risk difference (Eq. 33)	Phi (ϕ) (Eq. 30)
	Died	Alive				
Control	A	B				
Treatment	C	D				
Study 1						
Control	10	990	10.00	10.09	.01	.06
Treatment	1	999				
Study 2						
Control	10	10	10.00	19.00	.45	.50
Treatment	1	19				
Study 3						
Control	10	0	10.00	∞	.90	.90
Treatment	1	9				

TABLE 18.4 (B)
Standardized (BESD-Based) Effect Sizes in Hypothetical 2 ×2 Contingency

	Mortality		BESD-based RR (Eq. 31)	BESD-based OR (Eq. 32)	BESD-based RD (Eq. 33)	BESD-based Phi (ϕ) (Eq. 30)
	Died	Alive				
Control	A	B				
Treatment	C	D				
Study 1						
Control	53	47	1.13	1.27	.06	.06
Treatment	47	53				
Study 2						
Control	75	25	3.00	9.00	.50	.50
Treatment	25	75				
Study 3						
Control	95	5	19.00	361.00	.90	.90
Treatment	5	95				

logical differences among these studies, Part A shows all three relative risks are identical (10.00), which would seem to be a serious limitation to the value and informativeness of the RR index. Notice that the odds ratio behaves more as expected as we go from Study 1 to Study 2 to Study 3, but the infinite OR for Study 3 is disconcerting. The risk differences are never unreasonably far from the value of phi. If we had to choose an all-purpose index from only RR, OR, and RD, we would select RD among these three. But we feel we can do better by a simple BESD adjustment, as described next.

For the BESD adjustment we compute the phi on the raw cell counts (Eq. 30), cast this phi as a BESD (described previously), and then compute the relative risk, odds ratio, and risk difference from the new BESD cell values. Part B of Table 18.4 shows the BESD results for the three studies of Part A and gives the BESD-based RR, OR, and RD calculated from the BESD cell values. We observe the BESD-based RR increasing, as it should, going from Study 1 to Study 2 to Study 3. The BESD-based OR also increases from Study 1 to Study 2 to Study 3, without the "infinity" value of Part A. (A BESD-standardized OR could go to infinity only if phi were 1.0, an unlikely event in behavioral or biomedical research.) The BESD-based RD is shown in Part B to be identical to phi, which means that phi can also be interpreted in terms of the BESD-based RD (also illustrated in Table 18.5 for the Gardasil and Salk vaccine trials).

Effect Sizes in Multisample Trials

In this final discussion we turn briefly to another common design, that in which trials are randomized to more than two independent groups. Imagine a randomized trial with four independent groups, and a declining linear trend in scores from Group 1 to Group 2 to Group 3 to Group 4 was predicted. However, all that was reported was an omnibus F, group means, and the sample sizes. Omnibus F tests (i.e., those with more than 1 df in the numerator) are rarely useful in data analytic work, since they address unfocused questions, yielding only vague answers. However, it is not difficult to test the linear prediction ourselves, employing only the raw ingredients provided. We can also re-create the original ANOVA summary table and show our focused test of the linear prediction carved out of the overall between-group sum of squares ($SS_{between}$). To re-create the overall ANOVA table, we calculate $SS_{between}$ from the group means and sample sizes, and we rearrange the F ratio to solve for MS_{within}. Suppose sample

TABLE 18.5
Summary of Effects for Gardasil RCT and Salk Vaccine RCT

Effect size index	Gardasil RCT	Salk vaccine RCT
Relative risk (RR)	∞	3.48
BESD-based RR	1.08	1.02
Odds ratio (OR)	∞	3.48
BESD-based OR	1.17	1.04
Risk difference (RD)	.004	.0004
BESD-based RD	.04	.01
Phi (φ)	.04	.01

sizes were equal in all four groups ($n = 5$ each), group means were 7.2, 5.2, 2.2, and 1.2, respectively, and the omnibus $F(3, 16) = 54.17$. We find $SS_{between} = 113.75$, and as $df_{between} = 4 - 1 = 3$, $MS_{between} = 37.92$. For the error term, we find $MS_{within} = MS_{between}/F = 37.92/54.17 = .70$.

THE ALERTING *r*

To assess the predicted linear trend, we can compute a contrast F test in four steps. First, we need a set of contrast (λ) weights to represent the predicted trend, and we choose $+3, +1, -1$, and -3 for groups 1, 2, 3, and 4, respectively. Second, we correlate the four contrast weights with the respective four group means, yielding $r = .9845$. We call this correlation between lambdas and group means the "alerting r" ($r_{alerting}$), because it can alert us to a trend of interest and, when squared, reveals the proportion of $SS_{between}$ that can be accounted for by the particular contrast weights. In this case, $r^2_{alerting} = .969$. Third, we multiply the omnibus F value by its numerator df, which gives us the maximum possible value of any contrast F test carved out of $SS_{between}$, or $F(1, 16) = 54.17 \times 3 = 162.51$. The final step is to multiply the squared-alerting r times the maximum-possible-contrast F, or $F(1, 16) = .969 \times 162.51 = 157.5$, the value of F for our contrast. If we also wanted to compute the SS for the contrast, we could do so by multiplying the $r^2_{alerting}$ times $SS_{between}$, which, in our example, yields $SS_{contrast} = .969 \times 113.75 = 110.25$.

THE EFFECT SIZE *r*

We typically want to know not just how well the lambda weights can predict the group means, but how well those weights can predict the individual scores on the dependent variable. This is the purpose of the "effect size r," which is the correlation between λ weights associated with membership in a group (or condition) and scores on the dependent variable. This ES indicator can be obtained by

$$r_{\text{effect size}} = \sqrt{\frac{F_{\text{contrast}}}{F_{\text{contrast}} + F_{\text{noncontrast}}(df_{\text{noncontrast}}) + df_{\text{within}}}} \tag{34}$$

where $F_{contrast} = 157.5$ and $df_{within} = 16$, and we calculate $F_{noncontrast}$ from the leftover $SS_{between}$ (i.e., $SS_{noncontrast} = 113.75 - 110.25 = 3.50$, $df_{noncontrast} = 3 - 1 = 2$, and $MS_{noncontrast} = 3.50/2 = 1.75$, so $F_{noncontrast} = 1.75/.70 = 2.50$), or by

$$F_{\text{noncontrast}} = \frac{F_{\text{between}}(df_{\text{between}}) - F_{\text{contrast}}}{df_{\text{noncontrast}}} \tag{35}$$

with terms as defined above, which finds for our example that

TABLE 18.6
Summary ANOVA Showing Linear Contrast

Source	SS	df	MS	F	p
Between groups	113.75	(3)	37.92	54.17	1.3^{-8}
Linear contrast	110.25	1	110.25	157.50	1.1^{-9}
Leftover noncontrast	3.50	2	1.75	2.50	.11
Within error	11.20	16	.70		

$$F_{\text{noncontrast}} = \frac{54.17(3) - 157.50}{2} = 2.50$$

Table 18.6 shows our summary ANOVA, with the contrast F and noncontrast F carved out of the between-groups SS.

THE CONTRAST r

Sometimes all we have are fewer raw ingredients, and the only ES we can compute is the contrast r (also mentioned in our discussion of one-sample designs). This is a partial correlation between the individual sampling unit scores on the dependent variable and the predicted mean score (represented by the lambda weight) of the group to which the unit scores belong, with other between-group variation removed. This r can be obtained by

$$r_{\text{contrast}} = \sqrt{\frac{F_{\text{contrast}}}{F_{\text{contrast}} + df_{\text{within}}}} \tag{36}$$

which is a variant of Equation 24, since $F_{\text{contrast}} = t^2_{\text{contrast}}$. Substituting in Equation 36, with $F_{\text{contrast}} = 157.50$ and $df_{\text{within}} = 16$, $r_{\text{contrast}} = .953$. Actually, Equations 36 and 24 are both contrast correlations, but because there is no noncontrast variation in the two-group case, $r_{\text{contrast}} = r_{\text{effect size}}$ in the two-group design. In that case, the equal-n contrast r can also be directly obtained by Equation 12, and the unequal-n contrast r can be obtained by Equation 11. When there are more than two groups, it is possible for $r_{\text{effect size}}$ and r_{contrast} to have identical values, but typically r_{contrast} will be larger than $r_{\text{effect size}}$ because all the noncontrast variation is parceled out in the computation of r_{contrast}.

THE BESD r

When there are three or more groups, it is not immediately obvious how to exhibit $r_{\text{effect size}}$ as a BESD. Under the assumption that $SS_{\text{noncontrast}}$ can be considered as random variation, we have presented a way of casting $r_{\text{effect size}}$ as a BESD (Rosenthal et al., 2000). Further discussion is beyond the scope of this chapter but can be found in our book on contrasts and effect sizes (cited earlier), and a brief discussion with calculations can be found in Rosnow, Rosenthal, and Rubin (2000). The premise is that the contrast of interest does, in fact, capture the full predictable relationship between the groups and the outcome variable. In that case, we conceptualize the BESD as reflecting the $r_{\text{effect size}}$ that we would expect to see in a two-group replication with the same total N and the lower-level and upper-level treatment conditions set at lambda levels of $-1\sigma_{\lambda}$ and $+1\sigma_{\lambda}$, respectively.

In sum, r_{alerting} is a way of appraising the predictive power of a contrast and can be used to compute the contrast F from published results when all we have are group means and the omnibus F from an overall ANOVA. The $r_{\text{effect size}}$ indicates the magnitude of the effect on individual scores of participants' assignment to particular groups or conditions. The r_{contrast} (or partial r between the contrast weights and participants' scores after removal of all other between-group variation) is, in some cases, the easiest way of estimating the ES correlation in designs using more than two groups. The r_{BESD} is the value of $r_{\text{effect size}}$ that we would expect to see in a two-group replication under the assumption that our sampling units are the different groups or conditions rather than the individuals found within those groups. There are special adaptations of these indices for use in a variety of contexts from two-group comparison to one-way ANOVA, to factorial designs, to repeated measures designs, and to the case of multiple contrasts (see Rosenthal et al., 2000). Other discussions along the lines of this chapter, or providing different perspectives, can be found in various recent publications (e.g., Grissom & Kim, 2005; Kirk, 2003; Kline, 2004; Rosenthal & Rosnow, 2008; Rosnow & Rosenthal, 2002, 2003; Vacha-Haase & Thompson, 2004).

■ Reporting Effects of Multicenter Trials

There are other issues pertaining to the spirit and substance of data analysis, effect sizes, and the justification of conclusions (e.g., Rosnow & Rosenthal, 1989). However, one further issue that we want to mention concerns the usual reporting of net outcome results in multicenter trials, by which we mean the aggregated or pooled data for all the centers (i.e., rather than the center-by-center results). When a particular outcome is relatively rare in the population studied and the sample size at each center is small, reporting only the aggregate results is frequently seen as a way of improving statistical power. This practice has a long history (Turner, 1997), but it can lead to spurious conclusions because of a statistical irony known as Simpson's paradox (cf. Simpson, 1951). Table 18.7 illustrates an extreme variant in the case of three centers, each with three patients, different levels on the independent (X) and dependent (Y) variables, and effect sizes indicated as the correlations between X and Y. Notice that the correlation of X and Y scores at each center is $r_{xy} = -1.0$.

TABLE 18.7
Hypothetical Results at Three Centers

	Center A			Center B			Center C	
Patient	X	Y	Patient	X	Y	Patient	X	Y
1	10	12	4	100	102	7	1,000	1,002
2	11	11	5	101	101	8	1,001	1,001
3	12	10	6	102	100	9	1,002	1,000
r_{xy}	−1.00			−1.00			−1.00	

However, when we aggregate the nine scores, we find the overall correlation is $r_{xy} = +1.0$. The final point that we want to make is that it is always prudent to report individual center data, if only in an informative display (cf. Hoaglin, Mosteller, & Tukey, 1983), and if there were noteworthy differences associated with individual centers, to explore those differences analytically.

■ References

American Psychological Association. (2001). *Publication manual of the American Psychological Association* (5th ed.). Washington, DC: Author.

Brownlee, K. A. (1955). Statistics of the 1954 polio vaccine trials. *Journal of the American Statistical Association, 272,* 1005–1013.

Cohen, J. (1962). The statistical power of abnormal–social psychological research. *Psychological Bulletin, 66,* 1–29.

Cohen, J. (1969). *Statistical power analysis for the behavioral sciences.* New York: Academic Press.

Cohen, J. (1988). *Statistical power analysis for the behavioral sciences* (2nd ed.). Hillsdale, NJ: Erlbaum.

Cooper, H., & Hedges, L. V. (Eds.). (1994). *The handbook of research synthesis.* New York: Russell Sage Foundation.

Grady, D. (2005, October 7). Vaccine prevents most cervical cancer. *The New York Times,* p. A14.

Grissom, R. J., & Kim, J. J. (2005). *Effect sizes for research: A broad practical approach.* Mahwah, NJ: Erlbaum.

Hoaglin, D. C., Mosteller, F., & Tukey, J. W. (Eds.). (1983). *Understanding robust and exploratory data analysis.* New York: Wiley.

Kirk, R. E. (2003). The importance of effect magnitude. In S. F. Davis (Ed.), *Handbook of research methods in experimental psychology* (pp. 83–105). Malden, MA: Blackwell.

Kline, R. B. (2004). *Beyond significance testing: Reforming data analysis methods in behavioral research.* Washington, DC: American Psychological Association.

Pearl, J. (2000). *Causality: Models, reasoning, and inference.* Cambridge, England: Cambridge University Press.

Richard, F. D., Bond, C. F., Jr., & Stokes-Zoota, J. J. (2003). One hundred years of social psychology quantitatively defined. *Review of General Psychology, 7,* 331–363.

Rosenthal, R. (1991). *Meta-analytic procedures for social research.* Newbury Park, CA.

Rosenthal, R., & Rosnow, R. L. (2008). *Essentials of behavioral research: Methods and data analysis* (3rd ed.). New York: McGraw-Hill.

Rosenthal, R., Rosnow, R. L., & Rubin, D. B. (2000). *Contrasts and effect sizes in behavioral research: A correlational approach.* Cambridge, England: Cambridge University Press.

Rosenthal, R., & Rubin, D. B. (1979). A note on percent variance explained as a measure of the importance of effects. *Journal of Applied Social Psychology, 9,* 395–396.

Rosenthal, R., & Rubin, D. B. (1982). A simple general purpose display of magnitude of experimental effect. *Journal of Educational Psychology, 74,* 166–169.

Rosenthal, R., & Rubin, D. B. (1994). The counternull value of an effect size: A new statistic. *Psychological Science, 5,* 329–334.

Rosenthal, R., & Rubin, D. B. (2003). $r_{equivalent}$: A simple effect size estimator. *Psychological Methods, 8,* 492–496.

Rosnow, R. L., & Rosenthal, R. (1989). Statistical procedures and the justification of knowledge in psychological science. *American Psychologist, 44,* 1276–1284.

Rosnow, R. L., & Rosenthal, R. (2002). Contrasts and correlations in theory assessment. *Journal of Pediatric Psychology, 27,* 59–66.

Rosnow, R. L., & Rosenthal, R. (2003). Effect sizes for experimenting psychologists. *Canadian Journal of Experimental Psychology, 57,* 221–237.

Rosnow, R. L., Rosenthal, R., & Rubin, D. B. (2000). Contrasts and correlations in effect-size estimation. *Psychological Science, 11,* 446–453.

Sedlmeier, P., & Gigerenzer, G. (1989). Do studies of statistical power have an impact on the power of studies? *Psychological Bulletin, 105,* 309–316.

Simpson, E. H. (1951). The interpretation of interaction in contingency tables. *Journal of the Royal Statistical Society, Ser. B13,* 238–241.

Snedecor, G. W., & Cochran, W. G. (1989). *Statistical methods* (8th ed.). Ames: Iowa State University Press.

Turner, S. (1997). Net effects: A short history. In V. R. McKim & S. P. Turner (Eds.), *Causality in crisis? Statistical methods and the search for causal knowledge in the social sciences* (pp. 23–45). Notre Dame, IN: University of Notre Dame Press.

Vacha-Haase, T., & Thompson, B. (2004). How to estimate and interpret various effect sizes. *Journal of Counseling Psychology, 51,* 473–481.

Wilcox, R. R. (2005). New methods for comparing groups: Strategies for increasing the probability of detecting true differences. *New Directions in Psychological Science, 14,* 272–275.

Wilkinson, L., & Task Force on Statistical Inference. (1999). Statistical methods in psychological journals: Guidelines and explanations. *American Psychologist, 54,* 594–604.

SECTION V

SPECIAL TOPICS

19. ETHICAL ISSUES

Michele Galietta and Barbara Stanley

*What was done cannot be undone but we can end the silence. We can
stop turning our heads away. We can look at you in the eye, and
finally say, on behalf of the American people, what the United States
government did was shameful and I am sorry.*
—PRESIDENT BILL CLINTON, MAY 16, 1997, *apologizing to surviving
participants of the Tuskegee syphilis experiment*

In 1997, President Bill Clinton apologized on behalf of the U.S. government
to survivors of the Tuskegee syphilis experiment. The research was conducted
by the U.S. Public Health Service to determine the natural course of syphilis. It was
an egregious example of ethically unsound practices that resulted in severe harm
for many participants. This example, which will be discussed in more detail later,
illustrates the importance of ethical issues in research with human participants.
This chapter is intended to provide a history of the ethical principles underlying
treatment of human subjects in research and to outline contemporary ethical issues relevant to conducting randomized controlled trials (RCTs) for psychosocial
interventions. Tensions between the ethical treatment of participants and research
design issues will be highlighted. This chapter is intended to be aspirational rather
than prescriptive, and readers are encouraged to thoughtfully consider the implications of design choices they make in light of the ethical principles presented.

■ History of Guidelines and Standards for Protection of Research Participants

The catalyst for the development of the first guidelines and standards for human experimentation was the involuntary experimentation on humans by Nazi
scientists during World War II. In response to these atrocities, the judges for the
second Nuremberg Military Tribunal crafted the Nuremberg Code in 1947.
The code outlined a set of directives for the conduct of ethical research with human subjects. First and foremost, the Nuremberg Code established voluntary
and informed consent to be an essential feature of any research with human beings (Nuremberg Code, 1949). The code mandated that designs must be scientifically appropriate, and that researchers be scientifically qualified. The code

405

introduced the notion of weighing risks and benefits involved in the research. In addition, it established that efforts be made to minimize discomfort of participants and that participants should be free to withdraw from participation at their discretion.

In 1964, the World Medical Association established the Declaration of Helsinki (1964), which expanded upon the directives outlined in the Nuremberg Code and established guiding principles for research. The declaration expanded the concept of informed consent to include the need for fully informing research participants of the "aims, methods, anticipated benefits and potential hazards of the study and the discomfort it may entail." In addition, the document identified the ethical issue of dual roles, highlighting the fact that requesting research participation from an individual who is in some way dependent on the investigator has potential to interfere with the autonomy of a decision to decline or participate in research.

By this time, many organizations (both governmental and professional) involved in research had voluntarily established ethical research review procedures based on the Nuremberg Code (Citro, Ilgen, & Marrett, 2003) and the Declaration of Helsinki. Yet, unethical practices continued to emerge (Beecher, 1966). The Tuskegee syphilis study, the Jewish chronic disease hospital study, and the Willowbrook study were three of the most widely publicized and egregious examples of unethical behavior by researchers. In 1932, the Tuskegee syphilis experiment was initiated by the U.S. Public Health Service to determine the natural course of syphilis. Nearly 400 men (mostly poor, black sharecroppers) were enrolled in the study without adequate informed consent; they were simply told they would be treated for "bad blood" (Jones, 1993). They were not told about their diagnosis. They were given free medical treatment and meals, and ironically, free burial insurance.[1] Moreover, although there was no known treatment for syphilis at the start of the study, by the 1940s, penicillin was an established, effective treatment. The study was not discontinued until 1972, when it was publicized and provoked public outrage (Heller, 1972).

The Jewish Chronic Disease Hospital study involved chronically ill patients being injected with live cancer cells without their consent. (For a detailed review of these cases, see Beecher, 1966; Jones, 1993; Katz, 1972; and Brandt, 1978.) The Willowbrook study provides a caution that the presence of procedures for the review of studies does not necessarily ensure adequate protection for participants. Despite being reviewed by an ethics committee, the design of the Willowbrook Study involved injecting intellectually disabled children with a live hepatitis virus (Citro et al., 2003). Although parents signed consent forms for the study, their children could not be admitted or receive treatment at the facility if they did not consent to the study. Thus, the presence of signed consent

1. For more information, visit the Tuskegee survivors Web site at http://www.healthsystem.virginia.edu/internet/library/historical/medical_history/bad_blood/.

forms did not meet ethical requirements, since there was a significant element of coercion involved in the process.

In addition to biomedical research abuses, social science experiments of the time also involved questionable ethical practices, particularly around the issue of deception. In the famous Tearoom Trade studies (Humphreys, 1970), the investigator observed men engaged in sexual acts in public places, then obtained personal information about the individuals through their driver's license numbers, and subsequently contacted and interviewed them without revealing the purpose of the study. In the Milgram obedience study (Milgram, 1963), participants were told they would be participating in a study of learning and memory (instead of a study of obedience to authority). They were told to administer electrical shocks of escalating intensity to individuals tasked with learning word pairs. Many individuals administered what they believed to be lethal shocks to confederates in the experiments. The participants were debriefed after the study, but many experienced lasting distress related to the fact that they behaved inconsistently with their values.

In 1971, the U.S. Department of Health, Education, and Welfare (DHEW) promulgated a guide, called the "Yellow Book," clarifying U.S. policies on the protection of human subjects (Citro et al., 2003). Among other things, the guide reinforced the need to protect participant privacy and confidentiality. Professional organizations began drafting ethical principles with special relevance to human experimentation. The American Psychological Association (1972) was a leader in this regard, developing ethical guidelines based on a "critical incidents" approach. Although most research and professional organizations had established institutional review committees, the DHEW issued comprehensive regulations in 1974 that defined the role of institutional review boards (IRBs) and made it a requirement that all federally funded research be reviewed by an IRB. Also in 1974, Congress passed the National Research Act, which established a national commission charged with investigating the newly established IRB system and making recommendations for additional safeguards for human protections, particularly for participants from vulnerable populations (Citro et al, 2003).

The most significant accomplishment of the commission was the creation of the Belmont Report in 1979. The Belmont Report presented the basic principles underpinning ethical research with human participants; these are respect for persons, beneficence, and justice. Respect for persons is the basis for maximizing the autonomy of individuals to make fully informed decisions consistent with their own personal values. It is also the basis for special protections for those individuals whose autonomy is compromised in some way. Beneficence requires that researchers maximize benefits of participation and minimize potential harms. Justice has most to do with the selection of participants. Researchers are required to balance including all who could potentially benefit from participation with ensuring that the burdens of research are not borne disproportionately by some groups in society.

Governmental regulation of research has expanded, yet the Belmont Report continues to serve as the foundation for such regulations. In 1991, an interagency governmental task force recommended that the 15 governmental departments or agencies that conduct research with human subjects follow consistent procedures with regard to human research; thus a "common rule" was adopted (Citro et al., 2003). Then, in 2002, the Office for Human Research Protections (OHRP) was established for the purpose of overseeing IRBs and providing education and guidance on human research participant protection to both federal and nonfederal bodies and institutions (Citro et al., 2003, p. 76). The OHRP has extremely useful guidelines for practical aspects of research design and implementation. In addition, it offers Web-based education on human research participant protection currently required at most institutions for those conducting or working on research projects (see http://www.nihtraining.com/ohsrsite/index.html).

As concern for the welfare of human participants has increased and regulations guiding the ethical practice of research have proliferated, the challenges involved in conducting sound, ethical research have also increased. Often, good ethical practices make for good research (e.g., excellent record keeping). However, at times ethical obligations can come into conflict with research demands (e.g., the need to recruit adequate numbers of participants and the marginally competent research participant). This chapter is intended to outline ethical issues related to the design and implementation of randomized controlled designs, highlighting areas where tensions are likely to arise. The reader is advised to carefully consider the issues described and to discuss questions and conflicts between research integrity and human subjects considerations with colleagues. The chapter is divided into sections addressing ethical aspects of the following areas: designing studies, obtaining institutional approval, procedures for safeguarding the welfare of participants, and reporting study results.

■ Designing Studies

Competence

Before undertaking any research, psychosocial investigators should consider the area of study they wish to pursue and its relationship to their background, experience, and expertise. The American Psychological Association (2002) has outlined a series of ethical obligations pertaining specifically to the conduct of research (see section 8.1). First and foremost, psychologists engage in research with populations that fall within their range of competence (see APA, 2002, section 2.01). If any significant aspect of the intended research area is beyond one's scope of experience and training, this can often be remedied by collaborating with other researchers or by seeking consultation or supervision. Similarly, one needs to be sensitive to factors that might impact upon one's research, such as age, gender, ethnicity, or socioeconomic status. Study designs must be based on current professional knowledge and data, and must be scientifically sound in order to justify using human subjects. Researchers must maintain current expertise in methodologies, including analysis. Once again, the field is changing so rapidly that most contemporary research involves collaborations between individuals with varying expertise, and often from multiple disciplines.

Other aspects of good scientific practice that also fall within the scope of investigator competence contribute to the ethical soundness of a study. Balancing internal and external validity concerns appropriate to study goals, ensuring adequate power, controlling for threats to internal validity, and correctly interpreting one's data are all part of the ethical obligations of the researcher.

Stage of Research

Clinical trials are typically described in terms of phases that correspond to the stage of research they address (Friedman, Furberg, & DeMets, 1998). The model, derived from biomedical research, is in many ways applicable to psychosocial research, though some differences exist. The most understandable example involves drug studies. In the development and testing of a new drug, Phase I clinical trials are used to test the safety of an intervention and the amount of a drug or intervention needed to produce changes in individuals. Efficacy of the agent is not evaluated at this point. These studies typically involve small numbers of individuals (20 to 80). The purpose of Phase II clinical trials is to determine the degree of effect of the medication in a larger number of individuals (Friedman et al., 1998). These studies may involve within-subject or between-subjects designs and may or may not use randomization. In psychosocial research, phase I research studies are analogous to treatment development research, and phase II trials are analogous to efficacy studies for new treatments. Phase II trials maximize internal validity and are designed to assess the efficacy of a particular treatment compared with a control condition of some type. The choice of comparison group in psychosocial interventions is extremely important and will be discussed in more detail later.

It is important to note that psychosocial research at this phase could be either pilot work (Phase II a) or full-scale RCTs (Phase II b). Some ethical issues related to pilot studies warrant discussion. Pilot studies are frequently conducted to demonstrate substantial evidence that an intervention warrants a large RCT. Such designs typically involve small-scale group designs and random assignment. Researchers have traditionally used such studies to estimate effect sizes for power estimates for the next phase of their research. However, because the standard error of effect sizes is relatively larger in studies with small samples, some have cautioned that they are unable to provide accurate estimates of effect sizes for the use in power calculations (Kraemer, Mintz, Noda, Tinklenberg, & Yesavage, 2006). Thus, interventions with true promise may be ignored and subsequent research avoided. In addition, Kraemer and colleagues (2006) argue that determining power requirements from effect size estimates that are derived from pilot studies often results in underestimation of the actual number of subjects required. So, what is a competent, ethical researcher to do? Kraemer et al. (2006) propose that investigators carefully consider the context in which effect sizes were derived; they suggest attending carefully to the issue of clinical significance and guarding against underestimates of power by not relying on effect sizes derived from small samples. One can see from this example the ethical implications of conducting research with less than the highest standards of competence. Particularly in treatment studies, many hours of participant time could be utilized ineffectively; even worse, truly helpful interventions could be abandoned if the researcher is not cognizant of these methodological issues.

Once efficacy has been established, the next step in psychosocial treatment research is to conduct an effectiveness trial. The purpose of effectiveness trials is to determine whether the intervention can be successful in the community, with patients typically treated in such settings. These studies are analogous to Phase III trials in psychopharmacological research (Hohmann & Parron, cited in Arean & Alvarez, 2002). In such studies, which involve randomization and control or comparison groups, the purpose is to study interventions in larger groups of individuals and compare the interventions with existing treatments. These designs typically emphasize external validity, the generalization of results, to a greater extent than earlier phases of research.

In addition, treatment researchers are often also interested in specific questions related to the successful dissemination of treatments from lab settings to community settings. So, questions like, "How much training does one require to adequately conduct the treatment?" and "What procedures can prevent 'drift' away from the treatment model?" become important. Efficacy and effectiveness studies for psychosocial interventions (equivalent to Phase II and III studies) constitute classic RCTs, and these will be the focus of this chapter. This framework is highly useful because ethical choices in design are often intricately related to the stage of the research one is undertaking. Particular designs that are ethically justifiable at an earlier stage of research may not be ethical at a later stage.

Selection of Study Sample

The ethical principle of justice, established by the Belmont Report (1979), prohibits unfair discrimination against individuals eligible to be research participants. The notion is that both the burdens associated with research and the benefits should be equally borne by all. Particular groups (such as women or children) should not be excluded from research without scientifically based reasons. An example of this is the large number of studies that had been conducted on heart disease in men, despite the fact that heart disease is a leading killer of women as well. Women were originally excluded from these studies on scientific and ethical grounds. With respect to scientific reasons, the differences in female versus male biology were thought to confound study results. With regard to ethical grounds, women of childbearing age were routinely excluded to prevent possible harm to fetuses. There are, of course, times when it is essential to exclude some groups, such as if one is interested in comparing health practices in particular ethnic groups. Inclusion and exclusion criteria for studies need to be clearly outlined, along with a rationale for why one is excluding individuals from a particular group or with a particular characteristic. In early stages of psychosocial intervention research, it is desirable to have a homogeneous group of individuals from the same diagnostic group. In treatment development studies, it would be appropriate to exclude those with significant comorbid conditions. However, this always creates a tension, since doing so limits, to some extent, the generalizability of results. Most treatment outcome experts agree that it is permissible to be restrictive with regard to study population in earlier stages of treatment, and that one should be more inclusive as one moves from efficacy to effectiveness or implementation research.

Research With Special Populations

The corollary to the fact that one must not unfairly exclude individuals or groups from research participation is the fact that one must not use vulnerable populations for convenience (APA, 2002, section 3.01). For instance, studying prisoners to test a new vaccine for the general public might not be ethically advisable. However, studying interventions for violent prisoners who receive frequent disciplinary sanctions offers the chance to significantly improve their quality of life and would be ethically acceptable.

CHILDREN

Researchers are required to obtain written permission from a child's parent or legal guardian (or a designated proxy when permissible by law). In addition, it is a requirement that children provide verbal agreement (*assent*) to participate. In cases where the child does not wish to participate, researchers may not enroll a child, even if the parents have granted permission. Some types of research that may be considered low risk must still receive full IRB review by virtue of the fact that the study involves child participants. Children who are wards of the state may be involved in research provided that that are appointed a special advocate or ombudsman (someone with no interest in the outcome of the research). This could be a member of the IRB, a neutral appointed person, or, in some cases, a legally appointed individual.

PRISONERS

The term *prisoners* in OHRP regulations refers not only to individuals detained in a jail or prison but also to any individuals legally constrained by the criminal justice or, in some cases, mental health system. This would include individuals in prisons, jails, and forensic hospitals, those who are legally committed in civil facilities, and individuals residing in the community who are civilly committed or on probation. Research with such individuals requires that the enticements for participation (e.g., housing, privileges) cannot be so disparate from existing conditions that they would unduly influence decisions to participate. In addition, researchers must ensure that all qualified subjects have an equal opportunity for participation. The risks must be similar to risks that would be reasonable for nonprisoner participants, and participation must not affect their legal status (e.g., parole decisions). Most important, research should be conducted with prisoners if the research concerns that population. Studies that could easily involve general community members should not exclusively use prisoners for convenience. On the other hand, studies of topics addressing particular needs of the population in question are permissible.

INDIVIDUALS DIAGNOSED WITH AIDS/HIV

OHRP regulations emphasize the special need for attention to be focused on confidentiality in studies involving persons diagnosed with HIV or AIDS. Additionally, the guidelines require that new research findings that might affect desire to remain on a trial are communicated to individuals in a timely manner (see http://www.hhs.gov/ohrp/humansubjects/guidance/hsdc84dec.htm).

INDIVIDUALS WITH COGNITIVE IMPAIRMENT

Individuals with cognitive impairment (CI) are at risk, particularly if investigators are operating under an assumption of competence. Of significant concern is their competence to consent. Research has demonstrated considerable capacity-related deficits in individuals with CI (Stanley & Galietta, 2005). Protections focus on ensuring competence to consent through careful attention to informed consent procedures, enhancements to informed consent (when appropriate), and assent and consent by legally authorized guardians where permissible.

DEPRESSED AND SUICIDAL INDIVIDUALS

Many researchers deal with the ethical issues related to individuals with serious depression or suicidality by screening them out of the study through exclusion criteria. This may be appropriate for some studies. It is tremendously important to identify such individuals for safety. However, excluding such individuals is not the only way to provide for their safe, ethical treatment. Designs can be utilized that incorporate sensitive screening and allow for frequent monitoring, and even enhanced treatments (e.g., rescue medications; Oquendo, Stanley, Ellis, & Mann, 2004). The potential advantage to including such individuals in studies, particularly studies of depression or bipolar disorder, is that one avoids decreasing the external validity of the results. Given the high rates of suicidality associated with some disorders, enhanced monitoring and precautions may be preferable to excluding suicidal or severely depressed individuals. Simple alterations in the procedures can enhance the safety of higher risk individuals in trials. These alterations include availability of a 24-hour on-call member of the treatment team, more frequent appointments to assess suicidality, and a detailed safety plan elaborated by the clinician and participant in the event that the participant becomes suicidal.

Selection of Appropriate Comparison Groups

When conducting research with psychiatric and medically ill populations, as opposed to other types of interventions such as health education interventions for the general population, the issue of selecting a control condition becomes considerably more complicated. If a standard of care is established in the community, withholding that treatment (and placing participants in a no-treatment control condition) is not advisable. Control conditions include wait-list, psychosocial placebo, and treatment-as-usual controls. Many have criticized no-treatment controls on a number of fronts, both ethical and methodological (Saks, Jeste, Granholm, Palmer, & Schneiderman, 2002). One must consider the ethical obligation to *do no harm.* In determining what type of control condition to use, one should consider the stage of research. Wait-list conditions or psychosocial placebos are more ethically reasonable in earlier stages of research. Treatment-as-usual (TAU) is a more suitable control in effectiveness trials (Arean & Alvidrez, 2002), whereas efficacy trials might warrant comparators with more experimental control. One caution is that one must be extremely familiar with TAU in the area in which one is conducting research (National Institute of Mental Health, 2005a). Observational research on TAU is advisable. If the existing treatments in the community provide an adequate standard of care, then normal TAU may be acceptable. If, on the other had, existing TAU is significantly poorer than national or established community standards, then TAU may be unethical (Arean & Alvidrez, 2002). In such cases, investigators have two options. One option is to enhance TAU (for instance, TAU plus monitoring). Note that TAU does not have to be the best known treatment, but it is required to meet established community standards. A second option is to use another active treatment as a comparison condition. Although there are certain problems with this approach, this may be a desirable option as well.

Selection of Assessment Instruments

Ethical research requires the use of instruments with adequate psychometric properties. Instruments should have good reliability and validity indicators, and these should be stated in proposals and, eventually, in study results. Researchers should consider the advantages and disadvantages of using new instruments. In cases where there are no existing measures of the construct one is seeking to measure, or if the existing measures are flawed, then using or developing a new instrument is warranted. Of most importance to the issue of ethical design is the issue of construct validity. Are the measures one selects adequately measuring the construct in question? Similarly, even if the construct validity for an instrument is good, one must ensure that the instrument is valid for the population in the proposed study. For instance, in early studies on psychopathy, the construct and predictive validity of the Psychopathy Checklist–Revised (Hare, 2003) was well established. However, neither was established for women or for children. It would not have been sound practice for researchers to use the instrument as a predictor variable in a study, at least not without expressing significant reservations about interpretation of such results. A validation study of the instrument in women would have been a more logical first step.

■ Obtaining Institutional Approval

Once the design is complete, institutional approval must be received before proceeding. The APA ethical guidelines (2002) state, "When institutional approval is required, psychologists provide accurate information about their research proposals and obtain approval prior to conducting research. They conduct research in accordance with the approved research protocol" (section 8.01, p. 11). Virtually all psychosocial intervention research requires institutional approval due to the nature of human subject concerns involved in such research. Researchers are required to know and follow the procedures for obtaining institutional approval in their setting. No aspect of research can commence without prior institutional approval, or a statement from the IRB stating that the protocol is exempt. Researchers need to prepare protocols (i.e., descriptions of study design and procedures) with as much detail as is necessary for the IRB to understand all relevant aspects of the research, to determine the risk-benefit ratio for the study, and to make determination about the safety for participants in the proposed research. It probably goes without saying that one must actually carefully follow the protocol one has presented to the IRB. Once approved, the protocol cannot be deviated from, without an amendment to the approved IRB protocol. So, if one determines that a measure is not likely to provide meaningful data, it is permissible (and desirable) to replace the measure. However, this cannot be done without contacting the IRB administrator and obtaining permission. In addition, the investigator is responsible for reporting any adverse events (to be discussed further later) promptly and accurately. Investigators must also provide reports and renewals to their IRB as requested. Additionally, IRBs may require investigators to obtain certificates of confidentiality (Currie, 2005).

The Department of Health and Human Services (DHH)S has the authority to issue certificates of confidentiality (Currie, 2005). A certificate of confidentiality protects researchers from forced disclosure of identifying information in response to legal requests, including court orders and subpoenas. Anyone conducting sensitive research may apply, whether or not they are receiving federal funding. Sometimes, IRBs will require a researcher to obtain a certificate of confidentiality before approving certain types of research. Although they do not offer absolute protection (courts have requested de-identified data), they do provide additional protection under the law. They may also increase confidence in personal privacy. Certificates of confidentiality are most frequently used in studies involving information about studies that involve questions about sensitive topics or illegal behaviors topics where participants either would refuse to participate or would be unlikely to accurately report the behaviors studied. (e.g., drug use, sexual behaviors). The purpose is twofold: First, it offers additional protections to research participants; second, it makes it possible for researchers to investigate difficult-to-study areas. One consideration in seeking a certificate of confidentiality is the impact on one's ability to conduct research in settings that involve limited confidentiality (e.g., probation, jail, adolescent residential treatment centers). Administrators may be uncomfortable with the notion of a certificate of confidentiality. Researchers who want to conduct research in some of these settings need to clarify what particular information would be shared and what information would be confidential study data. In such cases, researchers may still seek a certificate of confidentiality to ensure the privacy of study data. For detailed instruction on how to apply, see http://grants.nih.gov/grants/policy/coc/appl_extramural.htm.

■ Procedures for Safeguarding the Welfare of Participants

Informed Consent

One of the best safeguards against unethical treatment of human subjects in research is the ethical requirement of informed consent. The doctrine of informed consent has evolved over time. However, there is general agreement that the essential components of informed consent include (a) adequate disclosure of information about the study, including the risks and benefits of participation and available alternatives, (b) competence to understand the information presented and to make a reasoned choice, and (c) voluntariness, or the ability to make the decision free from duress or coercion (Kazdin, 2003; Meisel, Roth, & Lidz, 1977; Melton, Petrila, Poythress, & Slobogin, 1997; Roberts, 2002).

It should be understood that informed consent is a dynamic process between the researcher and potential participant, and that the execution of written agreements merely documents this process. The fact that one has obtained a signature on an informed consent form does not mean that informed consent has taken place. Kazdin (2003) articulately contrasts meeting the letter of the rules versus the spirit of consent.

True informed consent necessitates that the potential participant receive *adequate* information to make an informed decision. In other words, participants must receive all information about the study that might affect their decision to participate or not (Culver & Gert, 1982; Fisher, 2003). Federal regulations dictate that, at a minimum, disclosure should include the following : (a) a description of the purposes, procedures, and duration of the research, including an explicit statement indicating that the project involves research; (b) any foreseeable risks and discomforts; (c) potential benefits to the participant; (d) available alternatives; (e) the limits of confidentiality; (f) the extent of compensation and treatment for injuries; (g) the name of contact persons available to answer questions about the research, the participant's rights as a research subject, and any research-related injuries in case questions or problems arise; and (h) a statement indicating that participation is voluntary and that participants may withdraw at any time without penalty or loss of benefits to which they are otherwise entitled (Citro et al., 2003, p. 82; 45 CFR 46. 116 (a)). This information needs to be presented in simple, nontechnical terminology. Written documentation should be in a language and reading level appropriate for the population being studied. Ample opportunities should be provided for the potential participant to ask questions and have them answered.

COMPETENCY TO CONSENT TO RESEARCH

Competency to consent to research applies to a specific decision at a particular point in time. Competence may fluctuate over time and is also influenced by the complexity of the decision-making demands. Some experts believe that the degree of competence necessary should relate to the degree of risk inherent in the decision (Cassel, 1988; Fellows, 1998). For instance, an individual with some degree of cognitive impairment might be competent to make a relatively simple decision with few alternatives, but might be incompetent to make a more complex decision. Research on competence to consent to research has increased dramatically in recent years. In particular, methods for assessing competence have been formalized. However, there is no universally accepted means for determining competence to consent to research. Professionals may disagree on the degree of competence necessary to make an informed decision. One option is to consider the use of formal screening instruments.

SCREENING FOR INCOMPETENCE TO CONSENT

Researchers should consider base rates of cognitive impairment in the study population. Research involving general populations or college students would not generally require formal screening of competence-related abilities. For high-risk research or research with populations having high rates of cognitive impairment, more formalized screening may be warranted.

It should be noted that competence is believed to be unique to particular situations. Competence to manage one's affairs might require different skills and abilities than competence to provide meaningful consent to a research study. Researchers may wish to consider utilizing a formalized research assessment tool to evaluate prospective participants with regard to their competence to consent to clinical research. The best known such instrument is the MacCAT-CR (Appelbaum & Grisso, 2001), which utilizes a semistructured interview format to evaluate abilities of research participants in the four domains associated with the construct of competence to consent to treatment and research: (a) understanding of information provided by the researcher about the nature of the research study and its procedures, (b) appreciation of the impact of participation or declination of participation for one's particular situation, (c) reasoning abilities—specifically the participant's ability to weigh alternatives and their consequences, and, finally, (d) indicating a choice about whether or not to participate in the research (Appelbaum & Grisso, 2001). The MacCAT-CR is individualized to the unique characteristics of each research protocol. The instrument does not allow for a cut score to determine competence. Rather, it was designed as a tool to assist decision makers in determining competence. It still requires clinical judgment that incorporates elements such as the individual's diagnosis and mental status, as well as the medical and social contexts in which the decision is taking place. There is no total sum score because one serious area of incompetence could render someone incompetent, despite adequate reasoning abilities.

One can make adjustments or enhancements to the manner in which informed consent takes place, thereby increasing the competence of marginally competent individuals. Techniques like frequent reminders of the right to withdraw or to refuse to answer particular questions can enhance competence, as can certain presentation formats for disclosure of information (Barbour & Blumenkrantz, 1978; Benson, Gordon, Mitchell, & Place, 1977; Bruzzese & Fisher, 2003).

Kazdin (2003) has noted the conflict of interest for researchers entailed by the informed consent process. The need to recruit adequate numbers of participants may compromise the adequacy of informed consent. Researchers may be tempted to perform disclosure in a token manner or may discourage questions for fear they will lose participants. Similarly, enrolling individuals who convey a desire to participate, but who lack sufficient capacity to make a well-reasoned choice or those whose decision to participate appears heavily influenced by a treatment provider or family member is not consistent with good ethical practice. Researchers are encouraged to discuss these issues with assistants, especially recruiters, on their studies.

THERAPEUTIC MISCONCEPTION

Research has suggested that the ability of individuals to freely consent to participation in treatment or research may be influenced by the power differential between professionals and patients, the fear of having services withheld, and subtly coercive behavior on the part of professionals (Melton et al., 1997). In particular, experts have identified the issue of "therapeutic misconception." This refers to the tendency of individuals to believe, despite fully adequate disclosure (including information about randomization and blinding in studies) that treatment providers in clinical research studies are acting in their best interests and making treatment decisions (like which treatment an individual will receive) based on their individual treatment needs (Appelbaum, Lidz, & Grisso, 2004). This particular phenomenon should be vigorously screened for and researchers should attempt to disabuse individuals of such notions. This alone may render someone incompetent, despite normal reasoning abilities.

Confidentiality

Ensuring the confidentiality of participants is based on a desire to minimize potential harms and is rooted in the ethical principle of beneficence. Researchers can take many precautions to maximize confidentiality of participants. These include, but are not limited to, storing raw data in locked file cabinets, storing consent forms in a separate location from study data, and using a bridge file (a separate file with subject identifiers and study identification number). The bridge file should also be stored separately and should be destroyed as early as is feasible.

Advances in technology have brought new challenges to maintaining confidentiality. Computers should be protected by passwords. Treatment studies that involve the electronic transfer of medical records are subject to recent the Health Insurance Portability and Accountability Act of 1996 (HIPAA). All researchers should be knowledgeable about the requirements for handling, storing, and transmitting personal health information. In particular, the privacy rule prohibits unauthorized disclosure of information. For more information, see the U.S. DHHS Web site (http://www.hhs.gov/ocr/hipaa). This legislation has had far-reaching effects on the conduct of research. For instance, individual patients may not, in most cases, be blindly approached for recruitment into studies. Similarly, researchers may not have access to general patient files to prescreen for eligibility. Researchers are advised to be familiar with ways in which the privacy rule impacts their studies. In particular, they must ensure that their recruitment procedures do not violate HIPAA legislation.

Safety Protocols and Adverse Events

Researchers should be familiar with ORHP guidelines for safety monitoring, as well as reporting of adverse events. The NIMH (2005b) defines an adverse event as "any unfavorable finding or incidence (e.g., blood level) that does not necessarily need to be related to the intervention." Serious adverse events are defined as follows: "an adverse event that results in any of a number of negative outcomes . . . death, a life-threatening experience, inpatient hospitalization, a persistent or significant disability or incapacitation, or a congenital anomaly or birth defect" (National Institute of Mental Health, 2005b). However, this needs to be contextualized in conjunction with one's local IRB, based on the study sample. For those working with high-risk populations (e.g., chronically suicidal individuals), a suicide attempt during a study would mean something different than a suicide attempt in a study using healthy or mildly psychiatrically impaired individuals. In some populations, a waxing and waning course is part of the illness, and inpatient hospitalization would not necessarily be an adverse event. Although such events need to be reported, considerable work should be done at the outset with the IRB to clarify expectations and develop an acceptable safety-monitoring plan. It is unclear how effective IRBs are at identifying and monitoring these issues (Candilis, Lidz, & Arnold, 2006). It is the responsibility of the researcher to submit a plan along with his or her IRB application.

Researchers should identify anticipated harms to participants, and these should be included in the informed consent process. In addition, researchers conducting government-funded research are required to develop safety- and data-monitoring plans appropriate for the complexity of the study and the level of risk inherent in the study. For most studies, this involves reporting to an independent data- and safety-monitoring board (DSMB). For all Phase III clinical trials, and for some large studies, multisite studies, or high-risk studies, independent DSMBs are required. In some smaller studies or studies with low risk, IRBs may have the investigator serve as the monitor. In such cases, the investigator should develop a safety-monitoring plan and submit it to their IRB as described earlier. It is often helpful to analyze data at several points in the study to identify potential problems early on and, if possible, to correct them. Unanticipated adverse events should be promptly reported to the IRB and OHRP. These conditions ensure that the safety of participants is regularly evaluated and provides a mechanism for determining whether the study should be prematurely terminated.

Reporting Study Results

One significant problem in RCTs is the quality of reporting of the results. Moher, Schultz, and Altman (2001) issued a statement on behalf of an international working group of clinical trialists, statisticians, epidemiologists, and biomedical editors called the Consolidated Standards of Reporting Trials (CONSORT; CONSORT Statement 2001). The statement called for transparency in reporting results of RCTs and provided a checklist for researchers to utilize in preparing publications. The checklist requires detailed information about methods and interventions, as well as research hypotheses and outcome measure. It requires researchers to describe how the sample size was determined, where and how participants were recruited, and how they were randomized. It suggests maintaining flowcharts of participants through each stage of the study. The authors call for information about blinding. Additionally, they advocate reporting adverse events. They state that analyses should be described in full and results explained in the context of existing evidence. Statements about generalizability are also emphasized. The checklist has been adopted by many journal editors.

The checklist is extremely useful and promotes ethics as it decreases the likelihood that results will be misinterpreted or misused. The level of detail specified is particularly useful for psychosocial RCTs, where interventions may be much more complicated than different dosing regimens. Sigmon, Boulard, and Whitcomb-Smith (2002) have added to the discussion by advocating for journal editors to require a checklist of ethical procedures before accepting submissions, although that has not been widely adopted. Additionally, the lack of reporting of negative results has long been a problem. Studies without significant differences are rarely published, yet these may be very important for the field as well. Researchers should consider this and strive to report such findings.

■ Conclusion

The endeavor of conducting RCTs for psychosocial interventions is challenging at times. Regulatory requirements are increasing, and the burdens on researchers are increasing as well. As described, many times sound ethical research practice is consistent with sound research methodology. However, there are times when investigators must balance tensions between competing demands. This chapter has highlighted issues to consider in balancing such tensions and designing and implementing ethical randomized controlled trials involving psychosocial interventions.

■ Acknowledgment

Technical assistance provided by Christina Minervini, MA.

■ References

American Psychological Association. (1972). *Ethical principles in the conduct of research with human participants.* Washington, DC: Author.
American Psychological Association. (2002). *Ethical principles of psychologists and code of conduct.* Retrieved from http://www.apa.org/ethics/code2002.pdf

Appelbaum, P. S., & Grisso, T. (2001). *MacCAT-CR: MacArthur Competence Assessment Tool for Clinical Research.* Sarasota, FL: Professional Resource Press.

Appelbaum, P. S., Lidz, C. W., & Grisso, T. (2004). Therapeutic misconceptions in clinical research: Frequency and risk factors. IRB: *Ethics and Human Research, 26,* 1–8.

Arean, P. A., & Alvidrez, J. (2002). Ethical considerations in psychotherapy effectiveness research: Choosing the comparison group. *Ethics and Behavior, 12,* 63–73.

Barbour, G. L., & Blumenkrantz, M. J. (1978). Videotape aids informed consent decisions. *Journal of the American Medical Association, 240,* 2741–2742.

Beecher, H. K. (1966). Ethics and clinical research. *New England Journal of Medicine, 274,* 1354–1360.

Benson, H., Gordon, L., Mitchell, C., & Place, V. (1977). Patient education and intrauterine contraception: A study of two package inserts. *American Journal of Public Health, 67,* 446–449.

Brandt, A. M. (1978). Racism and research: The case of the Tuskegee syphilis study. *Hastings Center Report, 8,* 21–29.

Bruzzese, J., & Fisher, C. B. (2003). Assessing and enhancing the research consent capacity of children and youth. *Applied Developmental Science, 7,* 13–26.

Candilis, P. J., Lidz, C. W., & Arnold, R. M. (2006). The need to understand IRB deliberations. *IRB: Ethics and Human Research, 28,* 1–5.

Cassel, C. (1988). Ethical issues in the conduct of research in long-term care. *Gerontologist, 28,* 90–96.

Citro, C. F., Ilgen, D. R., & Marrett, C. B. (Eds.). (2003). *Protecting participants and facilitating social and behavioral sciences research.* Washington, DC: National Academy Press.

CONSORT Statement. (2001). The Revised Consort Statement. Retrieved May, 24 2006, from http://www.consort-statement.org/Statement/revisedstatement.htm

CONSORT Statement. (2005). The Consort E-flowchart. Retrieved May, 24 2006, from http://www.consort-statement.org/Downloads/download.htm

Culver, C. M., & Gert, B. (1982). *Philosophy in medicine: Conceptual and ethical issues in medicine and psychiatry.* New York: Oxford University Press.

Currie, P. M. (2005). Balancing privacy protections with efficient research: Institutional review boards and the use of certificates of confidentiality. *IRB: Ethics and Human Research, 27,* 7–13.

Declaration of Helsinki. (1975). Recommendations Guiding Medical Doctors in Biomedical Research Involving Human Subjects. Adopted by the 18th World Medical Assembly, Helsinki, Finland, 1964, and as revised by the 29th World Medical Assembly, Tokyo.

Fellows, L. K. (1998). Competency and consent in dementia. *Journal of the American Geriatrics Society, 46,* 922–926.

Fisher, C. B. (2003). *Decoding the ethics code: A practical guide for psychologists.* Thousand Oaks, CA: Sage.

Friedman, L. M., Furberg, C. D., & DeMets, D. L. (1998). *Fundamentals of clinical trials* (3rd ed.). New York: Springer.

Hare, R. D. (2003). *The Psychopathy Checklist–Revised* (2nd ed.). Toronto: Multi-Health Systems.

Heller, J. (1972, July 26). Syphilis victims in the U.S. study went untreated for 40 years. *The New York Times,* pp. 1, 8.

Humphreys, L. (1970). *Tearoom Trade: Impersonal sex in public places.* Chicago: Aldine Publishing.

Jones, J. H. (1993). *Bad blood: The Tuskegee syphilis experiment.* New York: Free Press.

Katz, J. (1972). *Experimentation with human beings.* New York: Russell Sage Foundation.

Kazdin, A. E. (2003). *Research design in clinical psychology* (4th ed.). New York: Allyn & Bacon.

Kraemer, H. C., Mintz, J., Noda, A., Tinklenberg, J., & Yesavage, J. A. (2006). Caution regarding the use of pilot studies to guide power calculations for study proposals. *Archives of General Psychiatry, 63,* 484–489.

Meisel, A., Roth, L., & Lidz, C. (1977). Towards a model of the legal doctrine of informed consent. *American Journal of Psychiatry, 134,* 285–289.

Melton, G. B., Petrila, J., Poythress, N. G., & Slobogin, C. (1997). *Psychological evaluations for the courts: A handbook for mental health professionals and lawyers* (2nd ed). New York: Guilford.

Milgram, S. (1963). Behavioral study of obedience. *Journal of Abnormal and Social Psychology, 67,* 371–378.

National Commission for the Protection of Human Subjects of Biomedical and Behavioral Research. (1978). *The Belmont Report: Ethical guidelines for the protection of human subjects of research.* Washington, DC: Author.

National Institute of Mental Health. (2005a). Meeting summary; Treatment as usual: Measurement, design and ethics. Retrieved April 21, 2006, from http://www.nimh.nih.gov/scientificmeetings/taunovember02.cfm

National Institute of Mental Health. (2005b). NIMH Policy on Data and Safety Monitoring in Clinical Trials. Retrieved May, 24, 2006, from http://www.nimh.nih.gov/researchfunding/safetymonitoring.cfm

Nuremberg Code. (1949). Trials of War Criminals Before the Nuremberg Military Tribunals Under Control Council Law, *10,* 181–182. Washington, DC: U.S. Government Printing Office.

Oquendo, M. A., Stanley, B., Ellis, S. P., & Mann, J. J. (2004). Protection of human subjects in intervention research for suicidal behavior. *American Journal of Psychiatry, 161,* 1558–1563.

Roberts, L. (2002) Informed consent and the capacity for voluntarism. *American Journal of Psychiatry, 159,* 705–712.

Saks, E. R., Jeste, D. V., Granholm, E., Palmer, B. W., & Schneiderman, L. (2002). Ethical issues in psychological interventions research involving controls. *Ethics and Behavior, 12,* 87–101.

Sigmon, S. T., Boulard, N. E., & Whitcomb-Smith, S. (2002). Reporting ethical practices in journal articles. *Ethics and Behavior, 12*, 261–275.

Stanley, B., & Galietta, M. (2005). Informed consent in treatment and research. In A. Hess & I. Weiner (Eds.), *Handbook of forensic psychology* (3rd ed.). New York: Wiley.

U.S. Department of Health and Human Services. (1984). The Office for Protection from Research Risks: Guidance for institutional review boards for AIDS Studies. Retrieved May, 13, 2006, from http://www.hhs.gov/ohrp/humansubjects/guidance/hsdc84dec.htm

U.S. Department of Health and Human Services. (1993). The Office for Protection from Research Risks: Tips on informed consent. Retrieved May 13, 2006, from http://www.hhs.gov/ohrp/humansubjects/guidance/ictips.htm

U.S. Department of Health and Human Services. (2000a). Office of Human Subjects Research: Criteria for institutional review board (IRB) approval of research involving human subjects. Retrieved May 24, 2006, from http://www.nihtraining.com/ohsrsite/info/sheet3/html

U.S. Department of Health and Human Services. (2000b). Office of Human Subjects Research: Guidelines for NIH intramural investigators and institutional review boards on data and safety monitoring. Retrieved May 24, 2006, from http://www.nihtraining.com/ohsrsite/info/sheet18/html

U.S. Department of Health and Human Services. (2000c). Office of Human Subjects Research: OHRP's compliance oversight procedures for evaluating institutions. Retrieved May 24, 2006, from http://www.hhs.gov/ohrp/compliance/ohrpcomp.html

U.S. Department of Health and Human Services. (YEAR?). Office for Civil Rights—HIPAA: Medical privacy—National standards to protect the privacy of personal health information. Retrieved August 30, 2006, from http://www.hhs.gov/ocr/hipaa.

U.S. Department of Health and Human Services. (2003). Office for Human Research Protections: Guidance on the involvement of prisoners in research. Retrieved May 13, 2006, from http://www.hhs.gov/ohrp/humansubjects/guidance/prisoner.htm1

U.S. Department of Health and Human Services. (2006). Human Research With Children: Answer ID 1011. Retrieved May, 13, 2006, from http://answers.hhs.gov/cgi-bin/hhs.cfg/php/enduser/prnt_adp.php?p_faqid=1011&p_

20. RELEVANCE OF RCTs TO DIVERSE GROUPS

Sopagna Eap and Gordon C. Nagayama Hall

The inclusion of diverse groups should be an integral component to establishing treatment efficacy. Yet in a recent report of the U.S. surgeon general, few randomized controlled trials (RCTs) included an adequate number of ethnic minorities to determine efficacy for groups other than European Americans (U.S. Department of Health and Human Services, 2001). Although randomized controlled trials have become the gold standard in science methodology, their application with ethnic minorities is rare for Asian Americans and Native Americans and somewhat more common for African Americans and Latinos (Miranda et al., 2005). However, the availability of RCTs for all ethnic groups continues to be disproportionately lower than for European Americans. The urgency of including diverse populations in RCT research is especially dire in psychosocial interventions because emotional, behavioral, and psychological factors are more likely to vary than biological factors among different cultural groups.

Currently, ethnic minority groups constitute 30% of the total U.S. population (U.S. Census Bureau, 2000). Ethnic minorities experience psychopathology at an equal or greater rate than European Americans. Because there are few studies that include ethnic minority groups, there is minimal empirical justification to offer current evidence-based treatment to groups other than European Americans. Thus, a large percentage of the population is being underserved and ignored by psychosocial researchers.

■ Inclusion of Diverse Groups in RCTs

Despite the consistent pleas by various researchers for the inclusion of diverse populations in randomized controlled trials (Miranda, Nakamura, & Bernal, 2003; Hall, 2001; S. Sue, 1999), ethnic minorities continue to be underrepresented in evidence-based research. In a recent paper, Miranda et al. (2005) reviewed the available outcome studies with ethnic minority populations. They found that the interventions garnering the most empirical support were cognitive-behavioral therapies (CBTs) and interpersonal therapies (IPTs).

The studies identified by Miranda et al. (2005) had several limitations. First, many included small minority samples. For example, a study by Chambless and Williams (1995) on in vivo exposure for African Americans suffering from panic attacks included a sample of 15 African American subjects. Another study by Spinelli and Endicott (2003) examining the efficacy of IPT group treatment versus parent education of antepartum depression included 13 Latina and 2 African American women.

The majority of the studies reviewed by Miranda et al. (2005) failed to include culturally relevant constructs, such as ethnic identity or acculturation, that may moderate or mediate treatment findings. An individual who identifies more with the majority culture and less with his or her culture of origin may respond similarly to European Americans to treatment. Thus, most researchers were unable to specify a mechanism of action for the effectiveness or ineffectiveness of the treatments. For instance, Jaycox, Reivich, Gilham, and Seligman (1994) and Gillham, Reivich, Jaycox, and Seligman (1995) developed the Optimistic Child Intervention program. Based on the work of Seligman (Seligman et al., 1988), the program aims at increasing optimistic explanatory styles as a means of preventing depression among children. Randomized controlled trials demonstrated that the program was found to be effective at reducing depressive symptoms for mostly middle-class European American children. When it was applied to African American children, however, there were no differences between the experimental and control groups (Miranda et al., 2005). Because the study did not include cultural measures, the researchers could not explain the reason for the lack of effectiveness among African American children.

Finally, many RCTs reviewed by Miranda et al. (2005) were unreplicated. Chambless and Hollon (1998) specified that well-established efficacy studies should include at least two RCTs by at least two different investigators. This criterion is rarely met with ethnic minority populations. For instance, only one RCT attesting to the efficacy of unmodified CBT for depression is available each for Asian Americans (Dai et al., 1999), Latino Americans (Comas-Diaz, 1981), and African Americans (Lichtenberg, Kimbarow, Morris, & Vangel, 1996). Although there are multiple RCT outcome studies of culturally adapted CBT with ethnic minority groups (Miranda, Chung, et al., 2003; Muñoz & Mendelson, 2005; Zhang et al., 2002; Kohn, Oden, Muñoz, Robinson, & Leavitt, 2002), the different variations of CBT are rarely compared with the standard form, and there is seldom more than one study of the culturally adapted treatment by more than one investigator. One exception is the culturally adapted CBT developed by Muñoz and colleagues for ethnic minority clients (Miranda, Chung, et al., 2003; Muñoz & Mendelson, 2005; Kohn et al., 2002).

Clearly, there needs to be an increase in the quality and quantity of RCTs with ethnic minority populations. However, bringing this goal to fruition is more complex than including more ethnic minorities in outcome studies. Typically, ethnic minorities are included in evidence-based outcome research studies for two reasons. First, researchers are concerned with the generalizability of their treatment with ethnic minority populations (Okazaki & Sue, 1996). Empirical support for a specific treatment would be strengthened by research attesting to its widespread efficacy. Second, it is necessary to identify which of the available interventions yield the best outcomes for ethnic minority populations (Miranda, Nakamura, et al., 2003). Treatment of choice may vary by cultural groups.

One purpose of this chapter is to specify culturally relevant issues at each level of the research process for researchers to consider when designing and implementing evidence-based outcome research. A second purpose is to encourage researchers to consider a broader perspective when conducting RCT treatment studies. Multicultural and diversity issues in RCT research should not be limited to merely applying existing treatments to different cultural groups. There are many issues to consider before RCT research can be conceptualized with diverse populations.

■ Culturally Congruent Treatments

Before undertaking RCT research, it is informative to consider how normality is defined, who is likely to benefit from treatment, and how treatment is congruent with the client's cultural context. These questions serve to guide the research process.

Universal and Culture-Specific Psychopathology

To treat ethnic minority populations, it is important to understand how psychopathology is perceived and manifested within the individual's cultural context. Although there can be universal responses to distress, there are also culturally specific reactions, perhaps contributing to the complexity of evaluating treatment outcomes of ethnic minorities. Anxiety and depression are two disorders that have been observed cross-culturally. However, both phenomena have multiple expressions that may influence an individual's response to treatment. In Chinese culture, depression is more often described as "discomfort or distress in the heart" (D. Lee quoted in *Science,* 2006, p. 463). Indeed, for many Asian Americans, emotional distress is often considered a physical problem as opposed to a psychological one. Overemphasis of somatic symptoms is also common among African Americans (Brown, Shulberg, & Madonia, 1996), and Latino Americans (Canino, Rubio-Sripec, Canino, & Escobar, 1992). Researchers should be cognizant of the different idioms of distress that are present among ethnic minority populations because they are relevant for accurate diagnosis and assessment.

Psychosocial stressors may exacerbate symptoms for ethnic minorities. Factors such as discrimination, racism, and poverty affect both psychopathology and perceptions of psychopathology (Simons et al., 2002). Exposure to chronic discrimination can create distrust and anger toward the majority culture, which can be misconstrued as psychopathology. *Healthy paranoia,* a term to describe African Americans' responses to the racism and oppression they experience as a result of their experiences in a predominantly White society, may be responsible for the misdiagnosis of schizophrenia among African Americans (Ridley, 1984). Healthy paranoia may be misinterpreted as a symptom of schizophrenia rather than a reaction to institutionalized racism. Additionally, many mainstream mental health services are not sensitive to the diversity of symptoms that signify distress for ethnic minority clients (S. Sue, Fujino, Hu, Takeuchi, & Zane, 1991).

The stress associated with minority status can be associated with psychopathology (Williams, 2000). Taylor, Henderson, and Jackson (1991) found that life stress and internalized racism were significantly associated with depression among African American women.

These experiences, unique to ethnic minorities, may require adaptations that are often ignored by mainstream therapies. Thus, it is necessary for investigators to consider how the diversity of symptoms and etiology can influence responses to treatment.

Who Is Likely to Benefit Most From Treatment?

Ethnic minorities primarily have access to treatment that has been validated on European Americans for problems relevant to European Americans. Few RCT designs begin with an ethnic minority sample with the intention of addressing the needs of ethnic minority communities. Consequently, most available treatments are aimed at the majority culture. Thus, it is not surprising that European Americans are the primary consumers of mental health services (Zhang, Snowden, & Sue, 1998).

The mere inclusion of ethnic minorities in evidence-based outcome research does not provide sufficient empirical support for its efficacy among diverse cultural groups (Hall, 2001). Separate analyses of ethnic minority subgroups are often not conducted when ethnic minorities are included in outcome research, which leaves unanswered the question of differential efficacy for ethnic minorities. Psychosocial interventions are often based on theoretical underpinnings developed for European Americans. However, research with ethnic minorities often lacks a theoretical basis and instead relies on post hoc analysis of between-group differences (Okazaki & Sue, 1995).

Within-group variation may influence which treatments ethnic minorities may prefer and benefit from. One within-group factor that may moderate treatment outcome is acculturation. Acculturated individuals are more likely to manifest symptoms that are more amenable to Western psychotherapy. Acculturated individuals are less likely to manifest their distress as somatic symptoms (Parker, Chan, Tully, & Eisenbruch, 2005). For this reason, they are more likely to consider psychotherapy as a viable treatment for their problems (Ying & Miller, 1992). Western "talk therapy," however, may not be appealing to less acculturated individuals, who may prefer psychotropic medications to treat symptoms that they interpret as organic.

What Modifications of Existing Treatments Are Needed for Diverse Groups?

Learning the cultural explanations that individuals attach to their psychological distress is an important determinant of evaluating treatment outcomes. These "explanatory models" of illness (Kleinman, 1988) can inform treatment approaches with ethnic minority populations. Research from the National Institute of Mental Health Treatment of Depression Collaborative Research Program found that treatments that were compatible with the patient's cultural explanations resulted in greater patient engagement than treatments that were incompatible (Elkin et al., 1999).

Incorporating cultural etiological explanations into treatment design has resulted in positive outcomes for ethnic minorities in treatment. For example, Latino groups are more likely than European Americans to attribute their psychological distress to contextual variables such as family conflict, acculturative stress, and discrimination (Organista, Dwyer, & Azocar, 1993). Szapocznik and colleagues (1984, 1986, 1989) developed an intervention to reduce family conflict by bridging cultural discrepancies between parents and children. Szapocznik et al. (1989) found that family bicultural effectiveness training increased family functioning and reduced youth problem behavior. Many Asian Americans believe that their emotional distress is due to bad thoughts and a lack of willpower (Murray, 2000; D. Sue, 1996). For Asian Americans, their belief that mental illness is a function of cognitions suggests that cognitive-behavioral interventions, which target maladaptive cognitions, could be effective (S. W. Chen & Davenport, 2005). Indeed, cognitive-behavioral approaches have resulted in decreased depressive symptoms for Asian Americans (Zhao et al., 2002; Dai et al., 1999). These findings help inform which facets of the treatment should be emphasized, and how mental health providers can appeal to their ethnic minority clients.

Cultural values that exist among ethnic minority groups can be generalized to the therapeutic setting to inform culturally relevant treatments. Among ethnic minority groups, there is a strong emphasis on hierarchical relationships and deference to authority figures (Min, 1995; Garrett & Garrett, 1994). Thus, interventions and psychotherapies that are more directive and structured may be more appealing for people who prefer that form of relationship to one that is more collaborative and Socratic. Spirituality and religiosity is another value that is important among many ethnic minority persons (D. Sue, 1996) that may be incorporated in treatment (Boyd-Franklin & Lockwood, 1999). Many African Americans report using religious coping strategies, such as prayer (Broman, 1996) and consulting pastors (Young, Griffith, & Williams, 2003), when experiencing distress, suggesting that ignoring spirituality may alienate many ethnic minority clients. Indeed, a growing body of research is examining the contributions of spirituality and religiosity to healthy psychological functioning (Paloutzian & Park, 2005).

■ Conducting RCTs With Diverse Groups

The majority of psychosocial interventions are developed for the benefit of middle-class European Americans (Dana, 1998). Interventions are grounded in theory developed within a majority culture framework to treat problems reified by Western society. Including ethnic minorities in research designed for the majority culture only serves to enforce this pattern of conducting research. Instead of finding the correct piece to the puzzle, Western culture takes a piece from a different puzzle and forces it to fit. The optimal approach is to find the puzzle piece that belongs. When conceptualizing a research design, investigators should consider the population being studied instead of relying on theories that have not been applied to ethnic minority populations (S. Sue & Sue, 2000). This involves considering issues such as explanatory models of illness, cultural idioms of distress, and expectations for treatment. Formulating a theoretical model requires that researchers first have basic knowledge on the cultural backgrounds and lifestyles of the group being studied.

Collaboration With Diverse Investigators and Community Members

Primary to the research process is the involvement of investigators and community members who belong to the cultural group of interest. It is necessary to include members of diverse cultural groups not only in the research experiment itself but also in the process of research design and implementation (Coleman et al., 1997; Fisher & Ball, 2003). It is common practice for investigators to enter a community to pursue their research agenda only to disavow contact upon study completion (Alvidrez & Arean, 2002). This convention only reinforces the chasm between researchers and participants.

Because it is impossible to have a broad understanding of all cultures, researchers should seek out cultural contacts that may bridge the cultural barrier between the researcher and the participant. These cultural brokers should be involved in the research process from the onset in order to establish a cooperative relationship. Greenwood, Whyte, and Harkavy (1993) suggested an approach they termed *participatory action research* (PAR), which emphasizes the collaborative relationship between the researchers and the community members. Fisher and Ball (2003) incorporated the PAR approach in formulating their tribal participatory research model for research within American Indian and Alaska Native (AIAN) communities. A key theme in the tribal participatory research model is the inclusion of community members at every level of the research process.

Evaluating Standard Versus Culturally Sensitive Treatment

Randomized controlled trials assume that a treatment developed for one group will be relevant for other groups. It is possible, however, that ethnic minorities may prefer more culturally sensitive treatments. There has been a belief among investigators that incorporating culture into treatment precludes it from being considered evidence based. Hall (2001) argued that empirically supported treatments (EST) and culturally sensitive treatments (CST) are compatible and not orthogonal approaches. Indeed, he maintained that CSTs must become ESTs to gain acceptance from both the cultural and scientific communities.

The choice for mental health professionals is in deciding on the relevance of CSTs versus standardized treatments. Even this choice falls along a continuum rather than a dichotomy. There are varying degrees to which treatments can be adjusted to be more culturally appropriate, such as language translation of standard methods or modifying the content of standard methods. The most widely used approach is to provide ethnic minorities treatments that have been developed for European Americans.

Another approach is to provide culturally adapted versions of a standardized treatment. This has been most commonly accomplished with CBT-based interventions. Several cultural iterations of cognitive-behavioral therapy for ethnic minorities have been evaluated in RCTs. Zhang et al. (2002) developed a Taoist CBT that integrates Taoist philosophy into the standard treatment. Evidence suggests that this form of CBT was most efficacious with a Chinese psychiatric population when combined with psychopharmacology. Muñoz and colleagues (Muñoz et al., 1995; Muñoz, 1997) have modified the content and language of CBT to be more culturally appropriate for ethnic minority participants. Martinez and colleagues (Martinez & Eddy, 2005; Castro, Barrera, & Martinez, 2004) have tested a parent management and training program for Latino Americans called Neustras Familias: Andando Entre Culturas (Our Families: Moving Between Cultures) in randomized controlled trials and found positive effects for both parenting and child outcomes. Although some suggest that culture-specific adaptations may jeopardize the efficacy of evidence-based interventions (Elliott & Mihalic, 2004), others suggest that the integrity of these treatments may be enhanced by adapting interventions to specific populations (Martinez & Eddy, 2005).

A less common approach is examining treatments specific to a cultural group. There are fewer examples of a culturally specific treatment that has been evaluated in RCTs for ethnic minorities. Cuento therapy, a treatment that incorporates Puerto Rican folktales and biographies, has been shown to decrease anxiety and phobic symptoms and to increase ethnic identity and self-concept for Puerto Rican children and adolescents (Constantino, Malgady, & Rogler,

1986, 1988; Malgady, Rogler, & Constantino, 1990). Other indigenous treatments that have been used to treat mental illness may warrant further evaluation in RCTs. For instance, countries such as Australia and the United States have centers that provide Naikan and Morita therapies, which were originally developed in Japan (LeVine, 1993; Hedstrom, 1994). Naikan therapy is a structured form of self-reflection in which the individual reflects upon his or her relationship with others. Morita therapy encourages one to accept negative emotions and engage in purposeful action. Morita therapy, specifically, has garnered some preliminary evidence of efficacy in RCTs conducted in China. Chinese researchers have found efficacy for Morita therapy among nonhospitalized neurotic patients (Yun, Li, & Jiang, 2005) and among inpatients with obsessive-compulsive disorder (Zhang, Wu, & Zhang, 2000). Additionally, the efficacy of psychopharmocology may be enhanced when used in conjunction with Morita therapy (Jie, Jian-Qiang, & Qiang, 2005).

Evaluating the appropriateness of the therapies depends on the individual and the context. For acculturated ethnic minority members, standardized treatments may be very suitable and beneficial. Bicultural individuals may benefit most from standardized treatments that include culturally specific elements. Culturally specific treatments may be appealing for ethnic minorities and more mainstream populations. However, the lack of efficacious studies is a barrier for the wider acceptance of non-Western treatments in the scientific community.

Recruitment of Diverse Participants

The most direct reason that ethnic minorities are excluded from outcome studies is that researchers do not recruit a large enough sample size of ethnic minorities to provide statistical power for separate analyses. One reason that researchers face challenges in attempting to recruit a large enough sample size is that academic researchers traditionally utilize college samples, and most ethnic minority groups are underrepresented in college populations (Ward, 2006). Additionally, college samples may differ from community samples in language competency, acculturation, and socioeconomic status (Okazaki & Sue, 1995).

To overcome the limitations of studying college samples, it may be necessary for researchers to recruit participants from ethnic communities and enclaves to obtain more representative ethnic minority samples. Barriers to research participation should be anticipated and addressed. Researchers should be cognizant of the daily realities that their participants experience. Although mundane, issues such as child care, transportation, and financial compensation should be addressed to encourage consistent participation (Chen, Kramer, Chen & Chung, 2005).

Ethnic minorities may be more likely to participate if they perceive the research goals as relevant to them. When ethnic minority participants experience a conflict of interest between themselves and scientists, they may reject all attempts by researchers to work with their community. For instance, the Cree of northern Quebec have rejected almost all attempts by psychological anthropologists to conduct research in their community because of the lack of regard the investigators have shown toward cultural norms and decisions made by local authorities (Darou, Hum, & Kurtness, 1993). The psychosocial intervention should target issues that are relevant to the ethnic minority community. This includes identifying the relevant problems and providing an etiology that resonates with the beliefs of the cultural group. For instance, many Asian immigrants experience family conflict as a result of acculturative differences between family members (Tseng & Fuglini, 2000). If the intervention were to explain the family conflict as a function of cultural conflict between the parent and children, the practitioner is recognizing the struggles of that immigrant family and targeting that particular problem as a relevant and important issue to explore in therapy. If the problem were conceptualized as a communication problem, the Asian American family may be less inclined to trust the mode of psychosocial intervention even if the therapeutic steps were similar.

Random Assignment

There are many ethical issues related to random assignment. The process of assigning individuals to treatment or no-treatment groups may be interpreted negatively by the members of both groups (Alvidrez & Arean, 2002). Participants in the experimental group may interpret their assignment to their own severe pathology or maladjustment rather than as a logistical component of research. Conversely, assignment to the control group may be interpreted as reluctance on the part of the researchers to provide intervention. Historical examples of experimental abuse toward ethnic minorities, such as the Tuskegee syphilis study, have resulted in mistrust among ethnic minority groups. African Americans, American Indians, and Latinos have been reluctant to participate in research studies because of a fear of being harmed for the benefit of science (Harris, Gorelick, Samuels, & Bempong, 1996).

Those who are not assigned to the experimental group may demand inclusion in that group. A common justification for denying treatment to the control group is that the intervention has not been demonstrated to be effective and may not be more beneficial than a no-treatment condition. This argument is less persuasive for ethnic minorities because most interventions have been empirically supported among European Americans before they are transported to other ethnic and cultural groups. Thus, a wait-list condition, rather than a strictly no-treatment condition, may be a more ethical option.

Logistically, the process of random assignment may require creative methodology. For instance, in a tight-knit community, such as among a native tribal group, the community members may be highly enmeshed, making it possible that information can be shared among its members. For those put on a wait-list, information received by other community members may positively or negatively impact perceptions of the psychosocial intervention. Diffusion of information is a common problem in a randomized controlled trial design (Biglan, Ary, & Wagenaar, 2000). Biglan and colleagues suggest an interrupted time series design, or a multiple baseline design, to avoid many of the barriers to conducting community research. For instance, Biglan and colleagues have utilized a system with a set of small communities in which intervention implementation is staggered. Two communities are assigned the intervention. Once a clear intervention effect is achieved, two different communities are given the intervention. This intervention was repeated in another set of four communities. The dependent variable was averaged across the eight communities to measure the effect of the intervention. This research design allows for a control group while also controlling for the possibility of the diffusion of information.

Therapist Characteristics

Therapist characteristics have largely been ignored in randomized clinical trials. One characteristic that may be especially salient to ethnic minorities is the ethnicity of the therapist. Ethnic matching has been shown to positively impact therapy in a number of ways. S. Sue and colleagues (1991) found that ethnic match increased the length of treatment for Asian Americans, African Americans, and Latinos in an outpatient clinic in Los Angeles. However, ethnic match was associated with treatment outcomes for Mexican Americans only. Ethnic match was especially salient for ethnic minorities who did not speak English. However, a meta-analysis by Maramba and Hall (2002) suggests that the effect sizes of many of these studies are small. Thus, there may be variables in addition to ethnic matching that influence treatment outcomes.

Perhaps a better method of understanding therapist characteristics is to examine the context of distal and proximal factors related to therapeutic outcomes (S. Sue & Zane, 1987). Distal factors are further from the therapeutic goals and consequently less associated with outcomes. Proximal factors are closer to therapy goals and may be more informative. Thus, ethnic match may be a distal factor. It may be associated with cultural compatibility and language competency, and thus clients may attribute greater credibility to the therapist. However, ethnic match does not always ensure compatibility between the therapist and client. Proximal factors such as compatibility of cultural values may be more predictive of outcomes. Indeed, in a study by Kim, Ng, and Ahn (2005), 88 Asian American volunteer clients were assigned to a worldview-match condition or a no-match condition with 10 European American counselors and one Hispanic American counselor. Participants assigned to the matched condition reported a stronger working alliance and perceived stronger counselor empathy, even though ethnic match did not occur. Although the study did not examine outcomes, it suggests that therapists' ethnicity may be less of a factor in building a therapeutic alliance than a matching of worldviews.

Treatment Fidelity and Compliance

Treatment fidelity is important in the evaluation and dissemination of psychosocial interventions. The manualization of treatment ensures that the integrity of the treatment is not compromised. Although manuals exist for CBT, parent training, and interpersonal therapy, few of their culturally adapted variants have manuals.

Compliance is also necessary to ensure treatment fidelity. Practitioners and ethnic minority patients, however, may disagree on what constitutes compliance. Roberson (1992) found that rural African Americans would often alter their treatment to fit their lifestyle without informing their doctors. Although their doctors perceived this as noncompliance, the African American patients believed that they were managing their illness successfully. In psychological studies, noncompliance can include missed appointments, nonengagement, not doing homework assigned in therapy, or not practicing skills acquired in therapy. Indeed, evidence suggests that ethnic minorities tend to be more "noncompliant" than European Americans. For instance, although African Americans tended to overutilize outpatient services at a Los Angeles clinic relative to their numbers in the population, they also attended the fewest amount of sessions and were more likely than Asian Americans and Mexican Americans to terminate prematurely (S. Sue et al., 1991). Additionally, ethnic minorities, in general, tend to be less engaged in therapy and attend fewer sessions than European Americans (Atkinson, Lowe, & Matthews, 1995).

Noncompliance may suggest incompatibility between the client and the treatment model or the therapist. For instance, if clients perceive the treatment or the therapist as culturally insensitive, they may not be motivated to engage in the process. As discussed earlier, treatment expectations can impact degree of involvement.

Feedback

An important part of alleviating mistrust is for researchers to provide feedback to participants. Trimble and Lee (1981) emphasized the importance of providing feedback at the conclusion of the research project. Although mandated by the American Psychological Association to be included in all psychological research (Knapp & Vandecreek, 2002), this step is especially crucial when working with minority groups because of past historical abuses perpetrated by researchers in the name of science (Shavers-Hornaday, Lynch, Burmeister, & Tomer, 1997). By providing information, the researchers attenuate the mystique that often shrouds the research process.

Conversely, feedback from participants is also necessary so that researchers can improve their research procedures. Ball and colleagues (personal communication, 2006) discovered during feedback that they had been violating cultural taboos during an observational task with American Indians by allowing a brother and sister to be alone in the same room together. This issue did not surface when they were conceptualizing the research design and was only known after the task was completed.

Relevant Measures and Statistical Analyses

Evaluating the results of the RCT should include an analysis of relevant cultural moderators, mediators, and outcome measures. Examining ethnicity in isolation does little to advance cultural knowledge. Analyzing mean differences between groups does not provide a mechanism for how the intervention operates and does little to inform future research. Developing culturally relevant measures, however, can pose a number of challenges. Okazaki and Sue (1995) have highlighted the methodological and conceptual issues related to the development of culturally relevant assessment measures and provide suggestions for addressing these challenges.

Psychological measures can be important to assess culturally relevant constructs such as cultural values. Specific cultural values may account for differential outcomes among people that are included in the same ethnic category. For instance, loss of face and familism are examples of culturally specific dimensions that have been shown to influence psychopathology and behavior. Loss of face is a value observed in East Asian cultures that involves fulfilling one's social role in order to maintain social harmony. For Asian Americans, a strong concern for loss of face decreases the likelihood of disclosing negative information regarding the self and one's social relationships (Zane & Mak, 2003).

Familism is a value integral to many Latino cultures. It involves a belief that the family is paramount to the individual and that emotional and physical connectedness to the family should be maintained into adulthood (Steidel & Contreras, 2003). The influence of familism on Latino psychopathology has thus far been poorly understood and has yielded mixed results. Some studies suggest that familism may be associated with depression and burden among Hispanic caregivers (Losada et al., 2006), whereas others indicate a protective mechanism of *familism* against psychopathology (Contreras, Lopez, Rivera, Raymond-Smith, & Rothstein, 1999). The complexity in understanding the contribution of cultural values to mental health and well-being underscores the need to investigate these processes in psychosocial interventions.

■ Future Directions

Although efficacy research with diverse groups has progressed over the past decade, it is not progressing fast enough to meet the demands of an increasingly diverse society. RCTs have been embraced by the scientific community but have been slow to be applied to ethnic minority groups. Special considerations need to be taken into account when conducting research with ethnic minorities. Ethnic minorities underutilize mental health resources and are often disengaged when they do utilize resources. Thus, conducting RCT research with diverse populations involves an understanding of the complex interactions between the clients' cultural world and the treatment being offered.

Why has the evolution of psychosocial empiricism been so slow to encompass diversity issues? One reason may be that these issues are perceived as irrelevant by the majority of psychological scientists. The dearth of studies on ethnic minorities in RCTs reflects the marginalization of cultural issues in psychosocial research.

Collaboration between investigators and the ethnic minority community and among research scientists is a necessary component to overcoming structural barriers to ethnic minority research. There are a limited number of diverse investigators and a limited number of resources. In 2001, fewer than 20% of individuals with doctorates in psychology in the United States were ethnic minorities (Bailey, 2004). Overcoming ethnic disparities in RCT research requires that all researchers are engaged and committed to the process. Relying on a select group of investigators to address the mental health needs of ethnic minorities is unrealistic. All researchers and practitioners need to stay current with empirical research and theoretical papers on the topic of diversity, attend meetings that address ethnic minority issues, and have flexibility of thought.

Although this chapter has focused mainly on the applicability of RCT to ethnic minority groups, there are other sources of diversity, such as sexual orientation, religion, and physical disability, that warrant further investigation in RCT research. The ideas discussed thus far are not limited to ethnic minorities but pertain to other marginalized groups as well. Multiculturalism should be embraced and understood on multiple levels. Robinson and James (2003) have edited a book volume that explores the many areas of diversity that characterize human interactions and psychological processes. The needs of nonmainstream groups need not be restricted to ethnic background when applying the principles discussed in this chapter.

The availability of empirically supported research for diverse communities is not just a concern for ethnic minority groups but is a broader societal issue. The indirect costs of ignoring the mental health of minority groups include greater health costs, decreased productivity, and increased crime. Psychological science does society a disservice by neglecting to address the role of diversity and culture in psychosocial research.

■ Acknowledgment

Work on this chapter was supported by National Institute of Mental Health grant R25 MH62575.

■ References

Alvidrez, J., & Arean, P. A. (2002). Psychosocial treatment research with ethnic minority populations: Ethical considerations in conducting clinical trials. *Ethics and Behavior, 12*, 103–116.

Atkinson, D. R., Lowe, S., & Matthews, L. (1995). Asian American acculturation, gender, and willingness to seek counseling. *Journal of Counseling Psychology, 36*, 209–212.

Bailey, D. S. (2004). Number of psychology PhDs declining. *Psychology Monitor, 34*, 18.

Biglan, A., Ary, D., & Wagenaar, A.C. (2000). The value of interrupted time-series experiments for community intervention research. *Prevention Science, 1*, 31–49.

Boyd-Franklin, N., & Lockwood, T. W. (1999). Spirituality and religion: Implications for psychotherapy with African American clients and families. In F. Walsh (Ed.), *Spiritual resources in family therapy* (pp. 90–103). New York: Guilford.

Broman, C. L. (1996). Coping with personal problems. In H. W. Neighbors & J. S. Jackson (Eds.), *Mental health in Black America* (pp. 117–129). Thousand Oaks, CA: Sage.

Brown, C., Shulberg, H. C., & Madonia, M. J. (1996). Clinical presentations of major depression by African Americans and Whites in primary medical care practice. *Journal of Affective Disorders, 41*, 181–191.

Canino, I. A., Rubio-Sripec, M., Canino, G., & Escobar, J. I. (1992). Functional somatic symptoms: A cross-ethnic comparison. *American Journal of Orthopsychiatry, 62*, 605–612.

Castro, F. G., Barrera, M., Jr., & Martinez, C. R., Jr. (2004). The cultural adaptation of prevention interventions: Resolving tensions between fidelity and fit. *Prevention Science, 5*, 41–45.

Chambless, D. L., & Hollon, S. D. (1998). Defining empirically supported therapies. *Journal of Consulting and Clinical Psychology, 66*, 7–18.

Chambless, D. L., & Williams, K. E. (1995). A preliminary study of the effects of exposure in vivo for African Americans with agoraphobia. *Behavior Therapy, 26*, 501–515.

Chen, H., Kramer, E. J., Chen, T., & Chung, H. (2005). Engaging Asian Americans for mental health research: Challenges and solutions. *Journal of Immigrant Health, 7*, 109–116.

Chen, S. W., & Davenport, D. S. (2005). Cognitive-behavioral therapy with Chinese American clients: Cautions and modifications. *Psychotherapy: Theory, Research, Practice, Training, 42*, 101–110.

Coleman, E. A., Tyll, L., La Croix, A. Z., Allen, C., Leveille, S. G., Wallace, J. I., et al. (1997). Recruiting African American older adults for a community-based health promotion intervention: Which strategies are effective? *American Journal of Preventive Medicine, 13,* 51–56.

Comas-Diaz, L. (1981). Effects of cognitive-behavioral group treatment on the depressive symptoms of Puerto Rican women. *Journal of Consulting and Clinical Psychology, 54,* 639–645.

Contreras, J., Lopez, I., Rivera, E., Raymond-Smith, L., & Rothstein, K. (1999). Social support and adjustment among Puerto Rican adolescent mothers: The moderating effect of acculturation. *Journal of Family Psychology, 13,* 228–243.

Costantino, G., Malgady, R. G., & Rogler, L. H. (1986). Cuento therapy: A culturally sensitive modality for Puerto Rican children. *Journal of Consulting and Clinical Psychology, 54,* 639–645.

Costantino, G., Malgady, R. G., & Rogler, L. H. (1988). *TEMAS (Tell-Me-A-Story) manual.* Los Angeles: Western Psychological Services.

Dai, Y., Zhang, S., Yamamoto, J., Ao, M., Belin, T. R., Cheung, F., et al. (1999). Cognitive behavioral therapy of major depressive symptoms in elderly Chinese Americans: A pilot study. *Community Mental Health Journal, 35,* 537–542.

Dana, R. H. (1998). Problems with managed care for multicultural populations. *Psychological Reports, 83,* 283–294.

Darou, W., Hum, A., & Kurtness, J. (1993). An investigation of the impact of psychosocial research on a Native population. *Professional Psychology: Research and Practice, 24,* 325–329.

Elkin, I., Yamaguchi, J. L., Arnkoff, D. B., Glass, C. R., Sotsky, S. M., & Krupnick, J. L. (1999). "Patient-treatment fit" and early engagement in therapy. *Psychotherapy Research, 9,* 437–451.

Elliott, D. S., & Mihalic, S. (2004). Issues in disseminating and replicating effective prevention programs. *Prevention Science, 5,* 47–54.

Fisher, P. A., & Ball, T. J. (2003). Tribal participatory research: Mechanisms of a collaborative model. *American Journal of Community Psychology, 32,* 207–216.

Garrett, J. T., & Garrett, M. W. (1994). The path of good medicine: Understanding and counseling Native American Indians. *Journal of Multicultural Counseling and Development, 22,* 134–144.

Gillham, J. E., Reivich, K. J., Jaycox, L. H., & Seligman, M. E. P. (1995). Prevention of depressive symptoms in schoolchildren: Two year follow-up. *Psychological Science, 6,* 343–351.

Greenwood, D. J., Whyte, W. F., & Harkavy, I. (1993). Participatory action research as a process and as a goal. *Human Relations, 46,* 175–192.

Hall, G. N. (2001). Psychotherapy research with ethnic minorities: Empirical, ethical, and conceptual issues. *Journal of Consulting and Clinical Psychology, 69,* 502–510.

Harris, Y., Gorelick, P. B., Samuels, P., Bempong, S. (1996). Why African Americans may not be participating in clinical trials. *Journal of National Medical Association, 88,* 630–634.

Hedstrom, J. L. (1994). Morita and Naikan therapies: American applications. *Psychotherapy: Theory, Research, Practice, and Training, 31,* 154–160.

Jaycox, L. H., Reivich, K. J., Gilham, J., & Seligman, M. E. P. (1994). Prevention of depressive symptoms in school children. *Behavioral Research and Therapy, 32,* 801–816.

Jie, S., Jian-Qiang, T., & Qiang, Z. (2005). A controlled study of Morita therapy combined with Citalopram in the treatment of obsessive-compulsive disorder. *Chinese Mental Health Journal, 19,* 849–850.

Kim, B. S. K., Ng, G. F., & Ahn, A. J. (2005). Effects of client expectation for counseling success, client counselor world view match, and client adherence to Asian and European cultural values on the counseling process with Asian Americans. *Journal of Counseling Psychology, 52,* 67–76.

Kleinman, A. (1988). *Rethinking psychiatry.* New York: Free Press.

Knapp, S., & Vandecreek, L. (2002). *A guide to the 2002 revision of the American Psychological Association's Ethics Code.*

Kohn, L. P., Oden, T., Muñoz, R. F., Robinson, A., & Leavitt, D. (2002). Adapted cognitive behavioral group therapy for depressed low-income African American women. *Community Mental Health Journal, 38,* 497–504.

LeVine, P. (1993). Morita-based therapy and its use across cultures in treatment of bulimia nervosa. *Journal of Counseling and Development, 72,* 82–90.

Lichtenberg, P. A., Kimbarow, M. L., Morris, P., & Vangel, S. J. (1996). Behavioral treatment of depression in predominantly African American medical patients. *Clinical Gerontology, 17,* 15–33.

Losada, A., Shurgot, R. G., Knight, B. G., Marquez, M., Montorio, I., Izal, M., et al. (2006). Cross-cultural study comparing the association of familism with burden and depressive symptoms in two samples of Hispanic dementia caregivers. *Aging and Mental Health, 10,* 69–76.

Malgady, R. G., Rogler, L. H., & Constantino, G. (1990). Hero/heroine modeling for Puerto Rican adolescents: A preventive mental health intervention. *Journal of Consulting and Clinical Psychology, 58,* 469–474.

Maramba, G. G., & Hall, G. C. N. (2002). Meta-analysis of ethnic match as a predictor of drop-out, utilization, and outcome. *Cultural Diversity and Ethnic Minority Psychology, 8,* 290–297.

Martinez, C. R., & Eddy, J. M. (2005). Effects of culturally adapted parent training on Latino youth behavioral health outcomes. *Journal of Consulting and Clinical Psychology, 73,* 841–851.

Miller, G. (2006). Mental health in developing countries: China—Healing the metaphorical heart. *Science, 311,* 462–463.

Min, P. G. (1995). *Asian Americans: Contemporary trends and issues.* Thousand Oaks, CA: Sage.

Miranda, J., Bernal., G., Lau, A., Kohn, L., Hwang, W., & LaFromboise, T. (2005) State of science on psychosocial interventions for ethnic minorities. *Annual Review of Clinical Psychology, 1,* 113–142.

Miranda, J., Chung, J. Y., Green, B. L., Krupnick, J., Siddique, J., Revicki, D., et al. (2003). Treating depression in predominantly low-income young minority women: A randomized controlled trial. *Journal of the American Medical Association, 54,* 219–225.

Miranda, J., Nakamura, R., & Bernal, G. (2003). Including ethnic minorities in mental health intervention research: A practical approach to a long-standing problem. *Culture, Medicine, and Psychiatry, 27,* 467–486.

Muñoz, R. F. (1997). The San Francisco Depression Prevention Research Project. In G. W. Albee & T. P. Gullota (Eds.), *Primary prevention works* (pp. 380–400). Thousand Oaks, CA: Sage.

Muñoz, R. F., & Mendelson, T. (2005). Toward evidence-based interventions for diverse populations: The San Francisco General Hospital Prevention and Treatment Manuals. *Journal of Consulting and Clinical Psychology, 73,* 790–799.

Muñoz, R. F., Ying, Y. W., Bernal, G., Perez-Stable, E. J., Sorenson, J. L., Hargreaves, W. A., et al. (1995). Prevention of depression with primary care patients: A randomized controlled trial. *American Journal of Community Psychology, 23,* 199–222.

Murray, B. (2000). More assimilated Chinese Americans hold a more Western conception of depression. *Monitor on Psychology, 31,* 15.

Okazaki, S., and Sue, S. (1995). Methodological issues in assessment research with ethnic minorities. *Psychological Assessment, 3,* 367–375.

Organista, K. C., Dwyer, E. V., & Azocar, F. (1993). Cognitive behavioral therapy with Latino outpatients. *Behavior Therapist, 16,* 229–233.

Paloutzian, R. F., & Park, C. L. (2005). *Handbook of the psychology of religion and spirituality.* New York: Guilford.

Parker, G., Chan, B., Tully, L., & Eisenbruch, M. (2005). Depression in the Chinese: The impact of acculturation. *Psychological Medicine, 35,* 1–9.

Ridley, C. R. (1984). Clinical treatment of the nondisclosing Black client: A therapeutic paradox. *American Psychologist, 39,* 1234–1244.

Roberson, M. H. (1992). The meaning of compliance: Patient perspective. *Qualitative Health Research, 2,* 7–26.

Robinson, J. D., & James, L. C. (2003). *Diversity in human interactions: The tapestry of America.* New York: Oxford University Press.

Seligman, M. E. P., Castellon, C., Cacciola, J., Schulman, P., Luborsky, L., Ollove, M. & Downing, R. (1988). Explanatory style change during cognitive therapy for unipolar depression. *Journal of Abnormal Psychology, 97,* 1–6.

Shavers-Hornaday, V. L., Lynch, C. F., Burmeister, L. F., & Tomer, J. C. (1997). Why are African-Americans underrepresented in medical research studies? Impediments to participation. *Ethnicity and Health, 2,* 31–45.

Simons, R. L., Murray, V., McLoyd, V., Lin, K. H., Cutrona, C., & Conger, R. D. (2002). Discrimination, crime, ethnic identity, and parenting as correlates of depressive symptoms among African American children: A multilevel analysis. *Development and Psychopathology, 14,* 371–393.

Spinelli, M. G., & Endicott, J. (2003). Controlled clinical trial of interpersonal psychotherapy versus parenting educational program for depressed pregnant women. *American Journal of Psychiatry, 160,* 555–562.

Steidel, A. G. L., & Contreras, J. M. (2003). A new familism scale for use with Latino populations. *Hispanic Journal of Behavioral Sciences, 25,* 312–330.

Strakowski, S. M., Lonczak, H. S., Sak, K. W., West, S. A., Crist, A., Mehta, R., et al. (1995). The effects of race on misdiagnosis and disposition from a psychiatric emergency service. *Journal of Clinical Psychiatry, 56,* 101–107.

Sue, D. (1996). Asian men in groups. In M. P. Andronico (Ed.), *Men in groups: Insight, interventions and psychoeducational work* (pp. 69–80). Washington, DC: American Psychological Association.

Sue, S. (1999). Science, ethnicity, and bias: Where have we gone wrong? *American Psychologist, 54,* 1070–1077.

Sue, S., Fujino, D. C., Hu, L., Takeuchi, D. T.,& Zane, N. (1991). Community mental health services for ethnic minority groups: A test of the cultural responsiveness hypothesis. *Journal of Consulting and Clinical Psychology, 59,* 533–540.

Sue, S., & Sue, D. W. (2000). Conducting psychological research with the Asian American/Pacific Islander population. In Council of National Psychological Associations for the Advancement of Ethnic Minority Interests (Ed.), *Guidelines for research with ethnic minority communities* (pp. 2–4). Washington, DC: American Psychological Association.

Sue, S., & Zane, N. (1987). The role of culture and cultural techniques in psychotherapy: A critique and reformulation. *American Psychologist, 42,* 37–45.

Szapocnik, J., Kurtines, W. M., Foote, F., Perez-Vidal, A., & Hervis, O. E. (1986). Conjoint versus one person family therapy: The further evidence for the effectiveness of conducting family therapy through one person. *Journal of Consulting and Clinical Psychology, 47,* 623–624.

Szapocznik, J., Santisteban, D., Kurtnines, W. M., Perez-Vidal, A., & Hervis, O. E. (1984). Bicultural effectiveness training (BET): A treatment intervention for enhancing intercultural adjustment. *Hispanic Journal of Behavioral Science, 6,* 317–344.

Szapocnik, J., Santisteban, D., Rio, A., Perez-Vidal, A., & Kurtines, W. M. (1989). Family effectiveness training: An intervention to prevent drug abuse and problem behaviors in Hispanic adolescents. *Hispanic Journal of Behavioral Science, 11,* 4–27.

Taylor, J., Henderson, D., & Jackson, B. B. (1991). A holistic model for understanding and predicting depressive symptoms in African American women. *Journal of Community Psychology, 19,* 306–321.

Trimble, J. E., & Lee, D. J. (1981, April). *Counseling with American Indians: A review of the literature with methodological considerations.* Paper presented at the Annual Meeting of American Educational Research Association, Los Angeles.

Tseng, V., & Fuglini, A. J. (2000). Parent–adolescent language use and relationships among immigrant families with East Asian, Filipino, and Latin American backgrounds. *Journal of Marriage and the Family, 62,* 465–477.

U.S. Census Bureau. (2000). *Census 2000.* Washington, DC: Author.

U.S. Department of Health and Human Services. (2001). *Mental health: Culture, race, and ethnicity. A supplement to Mental Health: A Report of the Surgeon General.* Rockville, MD: Author.

Ward, N. L. (2006). Improving equity and access for low-income and minority youth institutions of higher education. *Urban Education, 41,* 50–70.

Williams, D. R. (2000). Race, stress, and mental health. In C. J. Hogue, M. A. Hargraves, & K. S. Collins (Eds.), *Minority mental health in America: Findings and policy implications from the Commonwealth Fund Minority Health Survey* (pp. 209–243). Baltimore: Johns Hopkins University Press.

Ying, Y., & Miller, M. S. (1992). Help seeking and attitudes of Chinese Americans regarding psychological problems. *American Journal of Community Psychology, 20,* 549–556.

Young, J. L., Griffith, E. E. H., & Williams, D. R. (2003). The integral role of pastoral counseling by African American clergy in community mental health. *Psychiatric Services, 54,* 688–692.

Yun, W. S., Li, J., & Jiang, C. Q. (2005). The effect of non-hospitalized Morita therapy for neurotic patients. *Chinese Journal of Clinical Psychology, 31,* 109–110, 113.

Zane, N., & Mak, W. (2003). Major approaches to the measurement of acculturation among ethnic minority populations: A content analysis and an alternative empirical strategy. In K. M. Chun, P. B. Organista, & G. Marin (Eds.), *Acculturation: Advances in theory, measurement, and applied research* (pp. 39–60). Washington, DC: American Psychological Association.

Zhang, A. Y., Snowden, L. R., & Sue, S. (1998). Differences between Asian and White Americans' help seeking and utilization patterns in the Los Angeles area. *Journal of Community Psychology, 26,* 317–326.

Zhang, X., Wu, G., & Zhang, P. (2000). The modification of Morita therapy in the treatment of obsessive-compulsive disorder and its efficacy. *Chinese Mental Health Journal, 14,* 171–173.

Zhang, Y., Yound, D., Lee, S., Li, L., Zhang, H., Xiao, Z., et al. (2002). Chinese Taoist cognitive psychotherapy in the treatment of generalized anxiety disorder in contemporary China. *Transcultural Psychiatry, 39,* 115–129.

Zhao, J., Chen, Z., Yan, W., Chen, K., Dai, Y., and Chen, Y. (2002). Intervention on depression of the elderly in the community. *Community Mental Health Journal, 16,* 179–180.

21. Multisite Intervention Studies

Olle Jane Z. Sahler and Diane L. Fairclough

■ What Is a Multisite Study?

One of the earliest definitions of a multisite study was provided by Meinert (1986). He stipulated that (a) data must be acquired from two or more distinct, organizationally independent settings, (b) the study must use identical intervention and data collection protocols across all sites, and (c) data must be pooled and then managed and analyzed centrally.

The *organizationally independent settings* stipulation means that, for example, a study involving only the inpatient and outpatient facilities of the same hospital system, or two or more hospitals in the same health care system, would not be considered a multisite study. The *identical protocol* stipulation typically means that the same intervention and control conditions are provided at all sites. However, it is also legitimate for some sites (especially if designated at random) to serve as control sites and the remaining sites to serve as intervention sites as part of the overall plan for the study. *Centralized data management* precludes an arrangement by which data are collected centrally but analysis is performed by individual sites using portions of the entire data set as, for example, comparison data. On the other hand, by mutual agreement, an individual investigator or subgroup of investigators may be granted access to the data set for secondary analysis, typically after papers describing the entire study have been published.

■ Why Multisite Studies?

The three major *advantages* of multisite trials are (a) larger subject pools that can yield larger sample sizes, (b) more rapid accrual, since subjects are recruited simultaneously at each site, resulting in (c) greater power to detect differences (Fuhrer, 2005). Additional related advantages are that geographic distribution and institutional differences in types of patients treated may increase the generalizability of the findings; the study has the potential to examine an infrequently occurring phenomenon in real time because of the higher proportion of the general population being investigated, which, in turn, increases timeliness; and collaborative effort reduces the likelihood that a single investigator's biases will unduly influence either the research design or the interpretation of data (Tate, Findley, Dijkers, Nobunaga, & Karunas, 1999).

These advantages must be weighed against several *disadvantages,* including greater administrative complexity and cost, nonuniform protection of human subjects requirements across institutions, and variable levels of commitment to the project among site principal investigators (PIs). The most important, however, is the possibility of nontrivial site differences in how the study is conducted that have the potential to greatly exceed the inter-interventionist variability that already exists within any single site. This real possibility makes quality assurance and treatment integrity not only critical but also essential components of the overall study design.

Increased complexity and cost result from the typical hierarchical organizational structure of multisite projects in which overall accountability for conduct of the study and authority to allocate resources reside with a single individual at a single site (project PI as distinguished from site PIs, who are responsible for the conduct of the study only at their individual sites). This distribution of responsibility demands excellent communication across the project so that any modifications of the protocol are known quickly and simultaneously throughout the system. Equitable assignment of resources demands that any change in the scope of work at any one site is compensated for by changes in one or more other sites, and that these changes are reflected in how materials and effort are compensated.

The nonuniform protection of human subjects requirements across institutions has become an increasingly important factor in adding to administrative burden and delays in beginning and maintaining the research protocol (Christian et al., 2002). The problem arises in part from problematic local experience that has heightened the sensitivity of a particular site's institutional review board (IRB)—or even the sensitivity of just one board member—to specific issues. Although these issues may or may not be germane to the multisite project under consideration, they nonetheless become the focus of intense scrutiny and, often, very narrow interpretation. Sometimes a local IRB requires modifications in study design that result in changes that must be reflected throughout the entire project. Even if the changes are not substantive, re-reviews at the other sites may be necessary. The development of a central review board and facilitated review process, such as that being experimented with for National Cancer Institute-sponsored studies, could greatly reduce the amount of duplicated effort and inordinate delays currently experienced by the leaders of many multisite projects while still maintaining the integrity of the human protection role for which these boards were actually designed (Christian et al., 2002).

Variable levels of commitment to the project among site principal investigators cannot always be predicted during the process of forming the investigative group and may arise due to unanticipated competing priorities. The most serious consequences are that the site does fulfill its obligations with respect to number of subjects enrolled or quality control of the data submitted. The first problem can sometimes be resolved by altering site requirements with redistribution of resources. The second problem can be compensated for to some degree through the quality control function invested in the central data management facility, which, with the PI, can impose certain additional requirements for data review. Neither situation nor solution is desirable, but if the system as a whole can remain functional with these modifications, they are usually preferred to identifying another site and site PI entirely unless the project is still in its start-up phase.

The most important disadvantage, however, is the possibility of nontrivial site differences in how the study is conducted that have the potential to greatly exceed the inter-interventionist variability that already exists within any single site. This real possibility makes quality assurance and treatment integrity testing not only critical but also essential components of the overall study design. Careful oversight by the site PI is part of the key to treatment integrity. However, systematic error can occur merely because of honest misinterpretation of how, for example, an intervention should be delivered. For this reason, an independent treatment integrity team that reviews, preferably blindly, the operations of all sites is vital. Timely feedback to correct the misinterpretation and review of the proper way to deliver the intervention with both the site PI and the interventionists should be provided. Even with these safeguards, site differences are possible. For instance, in our own experience (see later discussion), one site has had a stable intervention team, composed of regular employees, for the entire time of the project. The other sites have relied on more transient graduate student assistance. A small but significant difference in outcome measures has been found, with the stable team producing better outcomes. This finding raises important issues about delivery of an intervention over time and whether, should an intervention become institutionalized, it might not be even more potent than clinical trials indicate.

In the discussion that follows, we will be drawing many of the examples from a multisite intervention study of problem-solving skills training (PSST) for mothers of children newly diagnosed with cancer in which we have participated for more than a decade. The intervention/data collection sites (large/small, highly urban/urban-suburban, racially and ethnically diverse/racially and ethnically homogeneous) have been relatively stable since the investigation group was first formed and include Childrens Hospital Los Angeles, Cincinnati Children's Hospital, Rambam Medical Center (Israel), San Diego Children's Hospital, St. Jude Children's Research Hospital, University of Oregon Health Sciences Center, University of Pittsburgh Children's Hospital, University of Rochester Medical Center, and UT/MD Anderson Cancer Center. The stability of the participating sites and the site PIs has given us the opportunity to observe the developmental and maturational processes typical of multisite projects over time.

■ Who Needs a Multisite Study?

It is intuitively obvious that multisite studies are of benefit to small programs that have access to few subjects and to the study of conditions that have a low incidence. What about large programs that are studying relatively common conditions? Is it of any benefit to them to become part of a multisite collaboration? The answer is, "It depends."

The following analysis of sites within our own collaboration group was performed to answer the question, "Why do you need so many sites?" when we were reviewed as part of a federal grant application.

The study being proposed focused on problem-solving skills training and included mothers of children newly diagnosed with any form of cancer or brain tumor who (a) understood English sufficiently well to complete questionnaires and participate in the intervention, and (b) lived within 25 miles (i.e., driving distance) of the cancer center where their child was receiving care to optimize their availability for intervention and assessment sessions at the center or at home over a period of 3 months.

Two general facts about childhood cancer provide contextual background. First, approximately 10,000 new cases are diagnosed each year in the United States. This incidence roughly equals that of cancer of the pharynx in adults. Second, there are about 200 sites in the United States that provide cancer care to children. Thus, the average site has about 50 newly diagnosed patients per year.

Several large centers care for 200 to 400 newly diagnosed children each year. It might be assumed that centers this large could conduct studies as single sites. This may be true for certain studies, but certainly not all. As seen in Table 21.1, two very large children's cancer centers (St. Jude Children's Research Hospital [St. Jude] and Childrens Hospital Los Angeles [CHLA]) and one small cancer program (Golisano Children's Hospital at Strong/University of Rochester Medical Center [UR]) from our group are compared regarding expected recruitment from each site, given only the language and distance-from-center eligibility requirements. Note that at each site the recruitment rate is estimated to be 90% and the completion rate is projected at 81%. (These are realistic numbers based on our experience over more than 10 years. In fact, the projected completion rate is an underestimate of our true completion rate of 90%.)

As can be seen, on average, 400 patients are newly diagnosed or treated with induction therapy at St. Jude each year. St. Jude attracts a patient base that is worldwide. Most patients are hospitalized for initial induction therapy, surgery, or radiation treatment and then return to their home institution for continued treatment or return to St. Jude only periodically for the time required for additional specialized treatment. In fact, then, fewer than 20% of the patients treated at St. Jude are from the greater Memphis metropolitan area. If a study, such as ours, requires that the mother be available for meetings at the hospital or at home for 2 to 3 months after diagnosis, recruitment must be lim-

TABLE 21.1
Distribution of Eligible Subjects by Site

	St. Jude Children's Research Hospital	Children's Hospital Los Angeles	University of Rochester
New diagnoses/year	400	300	50
Number of "local" patients	75	175	40
% English-speaking	90%	35%	99%
% participation*	90%	90%	90%
% completion*	81%	81%	81%
Total subjects available for English-language longitudinal intervention/ follow-up	49	45	29

*Based on experience.

ited to individuals within reasonable travel distances. Thus, the eligible population is significantly reduced.

Each year, approximately 300 newly diagnosed childhood cancer patients are treated at CHLA, the primary publicly funded health care provider for most of the immigrant (non-English-speaking) population in the Los Angeles area. When our training program was first instituted, we piloted it only in English, thereby reducing the eligible population at CHLA by 65%.

The UR site treats only about 50 newly diagnosed children annually. Of these, however, about 80% live within reasonable driving distances, and virtually all families speak English.

Thus, discharge to "home" after initial treatment at St. Jude was most likely to mean travel to anywhere in the world except Memphis, making an 8-session in-person intervention rarely possible. Similarly, language spoken was a major barrier to enrollment at Childrens Hospital Los Angeles. (By design, the intervention materials were translated into Mexican Spanish as soon as efficacy was established.)

Thus, despite seemingly robust numbers of new patients at both St. Jude and CHLA, the study parameters precluded participation by large portions of the populations served at these sites, whereas almost all mothers of patients at UR were eligible to participate.

Had the study been a single intervention or one that could be provided over a month or less (typical induction period), virtually all the mothers of patients at St. Jude would have been eligible if they spoke sufficient English, and there would have been little or no need for joining a collaboration. Similarly, if the intervention were available in English and Spanish, virtually all the mothers at CHLA would have been eligible, and there would have been little or no need for joining a collaboration. Regardless of these modifications, however, the UR could not increase its enrollment, and collaboration remained essential.

■ Achieving Generalization

Although our particular collaboration group has recruited subjects in Rochester (New York), Cincinnati, Pittsburgh, Portland (Oregon), Memphis, Houston, San Diego, and Los Angeles in the United States and sites in Israel, the greatest number of subjects have been drawn from Los Angeles, Memphis, and Houston. We have typically relied on these sites to gain access to underrepresented minorities.

Racial/Ethnic Representation

Assuring a percentage of African American participants that reflects the general population has been impossible given that acute lymphoblastic leukemia, the most common form of childhood cancer, has traditionally been relatively rare in non-Caucasian populations (Malcolm, Smith, Gloeckler, James, & Gurney, 2006). In addition, our recruitment and retention of African American mothers as research subjects has been only as successful as recruitment and retention of African American research subjects in the vast majority of studies reported to date (see, e.g., McCaskill-Stevens, McKinney, Whitman, & Minasian, 2005; Moinpour et al., 2000) despite multiple invitations to participate. After our pilot data showed that the PSST intervention was efficacious, we immediately translated the intervention into Mexican Spanish as spoken by the immigrant population most likely to seek care at CHLA, San Diego, MD Anderson, and even the Oregon Health Sciences University in Portland, where northward migration of persons seeking employment has greatly increased the number of Spanish-speaking families. Our goal was to recruit monolingual Spanish-speaking mothers until they constituted 20% of the total subject population.

Two issues surfaced: (a) recruitment and retention among a population that was often composed of illegal immigrants, and (b) whether to merely translate the materials or to transform the intervention to be culturally aligned with the more family-centered approach characteristic of these immigrant families.

Recruitment and Retention

The vast majority of monolingual Spanish-speaking mothers to be recruited at the border centers were from Mexico. Several issues were involved in determining who would and would not be amenable to participation. Illegal status made some mothers wary of becoming involved in our study, since it was clearly not emergency medical treatment or an intervention designed to provide financial resources for care; perhaps they feared that we represented the Immigration and Naturalization Service (INS). Others sought advice from other family members before committing, and their hesitation or suspiciousness, rather than the mother's, led to nonparticipation. Still others did not respond in a timely manner, effectively missing the window of opportunity or failing to keep follow-up appointments for baseline assessments or scheduled intervention sessions. Attempts to facilitate participation by providing additional logistical support, frequent rescheduling of appointments, and providing child care for siblings were only marginally successful. The resulting lower-than-expected participation rate and higher-than-expected noncompletion rate highlight the disorganization and distrust characteristic of people not yet acculturated to life in the United States.

Simple Translation Versus Cultural Realignment

It has become abundantly clear over the past two decades that the "Hispanic" population in the United States is extremely heterogeneous in racial makeup, nationality, heritage, customs, socioeconomic status, and lifestyle. On the one hand, although some similarities exist in religion (predominantly Catholic) and language (variations of Spanish), deeply embedded dissimilarities in background and life experiences make generalizations difficult. On the other hand, most groups maintain a strong affiliation with the family as the final arbiter of behavior and maintain a high level of respect for elders (Ramirez & Suarez, 2006).

Whereas acute medical treatment can be independent of social and cultural mores, the success of chronic care and psychosocial intervention is profoundly affected by ethnic and cultural factors. A dilemma that faced us was whether to simply translate the *Problem-Solving Skills Training Manual* into dialectally appropriate Mexican Spanish or to reorganize the intervention to better align with the social imperatives of the culture as we understood them (see Chapter 20 of this volume regarding multicultural issues in randomized controlled trials). In making this decision, we were fortunate to have had the serendipitous experience of having a collaborator in Israel, where the paradigm had been simply translated into Hebrew and Arabic and provided by bilingual research assistants. In our analyses of site effects, we had found no significant differences in acceptability and efficacy between the sites in the United States and Israel despite a wide spectrum of subjects with highly varied social and cultural norms. This finding led us to believe that the problem-solving approach as we were teaching it might be sufficiently generic to be transcultural. Thus, to explore the empirical question of whether or not PSST would, indeed, be congruent with Mexican culture, we decided on a simple translation into Mexican Spanish as a first trial.

Interestingly, in our study, the effect size for the intervention was even greater among monolingual Spanish-speaking immigrant mothers than it had been among either U.S. citizens regardless of race/ethnicity or Israelis or Arabs living in the Middle East. We are in the process of investigating the mediational effects of PSST in this particular group, but our past studies have shown that there are significant direct effects of the personal intervention model that may be particularly important to the well-being of the less acculturated mothers (i.e., those living in an unfamiliar social environment) with whom we intervened.

Our experience also showed that, although the process was acceptable across cultural lines, the *solutions* the mothers chose to deal with the problems they identified varied according to their social customs. Thus, for example, the solutions to problems such as how to handle decision making within the family, how much assistance the woman could expect from her husband at the hospital, or how to deal with the needs of other children in the family were culture bound.

■ Why a Collaboration Model?

Multisite studies can have a variety of organizational structures. One of the most common is a single PI-dominated model in which a study is conceived and funding is obtained by a single person or small group at one site. Other sites are invited to join after funding is obtained if they meet certain criteria (e.g., adequate subject pool, interest/expertise in the subject being studied). In this model, the protocol has been developed, and participating sites are expected to follow all procedures unless the PI permits some local flexibility or discretion. Typically, however, deviation from the protocol, regardless of the organizational structure of the investigating group, can result in unacceptably low levels of treatment integrity, rendering the findings meaningless.

Strengths of the PI-dominated model include strong leadership in charge of and fully committed to a personally developed investigative plan. The primary role of the site PI is to implement the plan as developed, which can sometimes present logistical dilemmas, since the plan reflects the local resources and biases of the overall project PI. The primary shortcoming of this model is late involvement of the site PIs, with the potential for disagreement with the study plan and frequent requests for modification or discretion.

We adopted a variation on this model almost 20 years ago: a true collaboration with an administrative PI. This model differs from the PI-dominated model by involving all collaborating site PIs in the design and the implementation of the study. All PIs also participate in data analysis, manuscript preparation, and other dissemination strategies.

Strengths of this model include buy-in, the inclusion of different perspectives, and maximal utilization of site PI experience and expertise. We believe that our designs are richer because of close collaboration and that we are able to set realistic goals based on typical past access to subjects meeting eligibility criteria and awareness of potential confounding or competing protocols.

In essence, our collaborations have been designed to accommodate the characteristics of the sites and site PIs involved. In many ways, this model is analogous to the single PI-dominated model except that multiple sites are involved and each site PI takes significant responsibility for the success of the project from the conceptual stage through data analysis and publication.

The major shortcomings of the collaboration model include the amount of negotiation required for agreement on the protocol and the potential for inter-collaborator conflict.

■ Choosing Collaborators Wisely

Investigators decide to join a collaboration for a variety of reasons: scientific or personal curiosity, a sense of being able to contribute, wanting to be at the forefront, or not wanting to be left out. One of the most important tasks of the PI is to determine which of the investigators who might join the group are most likely to contribute effectively to the project either because of particular expertise essential to developing the best experimental design, because of the ability to recruit large numbers of subjects, or because of some personal qualities that are likely to facilitate the group process. This last quality is rarely considered or even known "up front" but becomes invaluable as discussions about methodology become intense. Mediation is less important in the PI-directs-all model, where the design is often set prior to determination of site (and, thus, site PI) but is critical in the collaboration model.

Other, less talked about qualities include the ability to provide uniformly good data in a timely manner (meaning excellent oversight of study personnel) and having the time and interest to participate actively in data analysis and manuscript preparation. Having the world's expert on some topic or other as part of a study group is useful only if that person is willing to commit time and energy to the working of the group. Recruiting less well-known but equally, if not more, thoughtful contributors may be the better choice because they have a reputation to build, and involvement in the collaboration may provide a highly desirable vehicle for accomplishing that goal. In fact, the group then plays a mentoring role in the development of young or more inexperienced investigators, a very worthwhile positive side effect of collaboration.

Another consideration in choosing collaborators is the past history they have with each other regardless of the qualities they may bring to the project. With regard to this issue, the PI needs to make a determination about which collaborator or collaborators are essential to the project and then choose others in consultation. Fortunately, irresolvable conflicts are unusual, but they certainly do occur and need to be avoided from the onset to reduce energy expenditure on non-study-related issues. Avoiding recruiting collaborators who have such irresolvable differences, which typically result from personality conflicts rather than disagreements about science, also enhances the probability that when differences about science do occur, they can be negotiated to consensus.

■ Role of the Principal Investigator

The Science Side

In addition to choosing collaborators wisely, the PI has primary responsibility for organizing the group, administrating its activities, negotiating roles/assignments, and assuring that those roles/assignments are performed appropriately and satisfactorily. By far the best approach to these responsibilities is to adopt a business model with a clearly developed plan of action and a well-defined organizational structure that lists responsibilities and expectations. The expectation report discussed later in the section on logistics is a prime example of public (within the group) notification of where a site PI, for example, stands with regard to fulfilling obligations.

Unfulfilled obligation should lead to either individual (especially if the problem is occurring at only one site) or group problem solving. One role the PI in a collaboration, as opposed to PI-directed research, should never assume is that of problem solver for the group. It is the PI's responsibility to call the problem to attention and to facilitate discussion, but ideas about possible solutions should be generated by the group, and the final solution and who will implement it should be agreed upon by the group.

That being said, it is the responsibility of the PI to run interference in the hope of avoiding full-blown problems. This takes the form of negotiating with funders, holding service providers and suppliers to their contracts, and identifying potential roadblocks to completing the project before they occur.

Finally, the PI must assume final authority over, as well as responsibility for, the scientific conduct of the group. The price for whatever honor and glory may come from being designated the PI is the ability of the group to function effectively in meeting its goals.

The Human Side

As might be expected from the preceding discussion, the three interpersonal roles the PI plays are those of mediator, ego massager, and enforcer. The two personal attributes that will be most helpful to the PI in playing these roles are determination to make the collaboration work and a sense of humor.

Mediation between strong personalities, which collaborators in major multisite projects typically are, is based on mutual respect. As indicated earlier, choosing collaborators who respect each other's integrity, even if they do not agree in their scientific approach or how they have interpreted findings in previous studies, is critical to being able to mediate successfully. In effect, the PI should stack the deck in his or her favor with regard to being able to keep the collaboration functioning effectively toward a common goal.

In our collaboration, heated discussion is the norm. When we have outside consultants, junior investigators, or research assistants join our planning sessions, we repeatedly assure them that we have remained friendly colleagues for years despite the seemingly irreconcilable differences in approach that loom prior to arriving at consensus. We have even weathered the multiple "I told you so" comments that arise when an investigator who was overridden is proved to have been correct on the basis of data analysis or a reviewer's comments.

Fortunately, the ego integrity of each of the collaborators is virtually always strong enough to withstand strong opposition to a point of view. In our early days, however, when we did not know each other as well, occasional flare-ups occurred when comments within the group were interpreted as personal assaults rather than challenges to ideas. The role of the PI is to assure that discussions are maintained at a high conceptual level and that any personal misinterpretations are rectified.

Sometimes cooling off and ego massage are required and should be taken advantage of by all parties. Such instances serve as a reminder that part of the PI's job is to try to anticipate when tempers may flare and attempt to deflect any inappropriate remarks by diverting the conversation or taking a break. Failing that, it is imperative that the PI not take sides. In fact, it is the PI's job to remind everyone that everyone is right. The assumption in joining a collaboration is that all points of view and ideas are equally valued until the time for consensus is reached.

Furthermore, consensus still does not mean that an idea is wrong but that another idea appears as if it will benefit the collaboration's goal more at this point in time. However, as proved by the times "I told you so" has sneaked into our conversations, consensus is not always as correct as it seemed. Regardless of the outcome of the discussion, maintaining genuine openness to dialogue about valid disagreements is a hallmark of the collaborative process.

Having a sense of humor, which includes being able to laugh at oneself, is critical not only for the PI but for the collaborators as well. In addition, being able to let go of an idea without feeling that the idea is integral to one's being is essential. We are serious about the serious work we do, but we each must always try not to take ourselves too seriously while we do it.

■ Logistics of Multisite Studies

Training

By definition, multisite studies involve numerous individuals who will collect and submit data. Ensuring that the methods used are both appropriate and consistent across all sites and throughout the duration of the study requires the development of procedure manuals, training of data collectors, and monitoring of performance over time.

Most investigators anticipate the time and effort needed for initial training, but they often fail to foresee personnel turnover and the need to retrain over time. One way to minimize the burden of meeting ongoing training needs is to develop good procedure manuals that can be easily used as references over the course of the study and for training new personnel. The ease of use is critical. If it is difficult to find the answer to a specific question, the manuals will not be used. A number of short documents on specific topics is preferable to a long document.

It is essential to have a plan for training new personnel. While the initial training session for research assistants across all sites at the beginning of the study may involve bringing them all to a common site, the logistics of location and timing may preclude this approach for new personnel. One option is to have the trainee (a) study the manual(s), (b) observe an experienced research assistant or, if not possible, discuss the logistics of intervention and data collection with an experienced research assistant, and (c) participate in a conference call with the data manager, site PI, and study PI to clarify any outstanding issues. Multiple strategies for ensuring continued quality include careful monitoring of submitted data (not optional), periodic conference calls with data collectors, and site visits (discussed in more detail later).

Randomization

A critical decision is whether to have centralized or decentralized randomization and data entry. Decentralized randomization is accomplished independently at each site according to a standard, study-specific formula. Centralized randomization allows for more careful monitoring and control of the procedure, but it requires more resources. Options include electronic methods using phone- or Internet-based programs and person-to-person contact using phone, e-mail, or fax. Electronic methods allow for rapid randomization at any time, including nights and weekends. However, they require initial programming and continued access to technical expertise to deal with problems such as server crashes and changes in software version. Person-to-person contact methods require less technical resources, but they have limitations. Randomization by phone is restricted to hours when the phone is staffed. Communication via e-mail or fax may involve lags of up to 24 hours (72 hours over weekends). A critical issue with all these methods is ensuring confidentiality by using de-identified personal information whenever possible and encryption of communications if this is not feasible (see later discussion).

Data Entry

Options for data entry include manual entry and scanning and may occur at a data management center or locally at each site. Primary factors in the choice of where data are entered include who provides the data (research personnel or the subject) and the media used for collection. Many psychosocial interventions rely heavily on paper questionnaires completed by the subjects. Although these questionnaires can be converted to scannable forms, it is more difficult and time-consuming for many individuals to complete these and thus increases the patient burden. The programming resources are cost-effective only for very large studies, and the data management resources to deal with scanning errors often negate any time savings. Centralized data entry of questionnaire data is generally more efficient than local data entry because forms can be batched (combined with questionnaires from other subjects) and entered by an individual with rapid typing skills. For the limited amount of demographic and clinical data that is generally provided by research personnel, the choices between paper and electronic forms will depend on such issues as how rapidly information needs to be accessed, the availability of computers at the data collection sites, and the benefit of having a single data collection medium.

Study Monitoring

Problems in a multisite study, such as lagging accrual or submission of incomplete data, can emerge quickly but may be difficult to detect early without careful monitoring. We have developed several strategies for keeping abreast of the pace of a study. The first is a monthly "expectation report" that is circulated to all study personnel. This report contains a summary of overall and site-specific accrual relative to planned rates that clearly communicates whether each site and the study as a whole are ahead of target, on target, or behind target.

Figure 21.1 illustrates one method of displaying this information. As a result of the less-than-expected rate of accrual in the study depicted, early interventions to increase accrual and budgetary plans to lengthen the study 1 year through a no-cost extension were implemented.

The second part of the expectation report indicates what data have been received and what data are pending or expected. Figure 21.2 illustrates how adherence for a study with three assessments over time can be monitored. Note that target dates for future assessments as well as cutoff dates for obtaining those assessments are specified and serve as reminders to the data collectors to schedule and follow up on assessments. A site that is lagging can be identified easily and steps taken to address the problem, such as having the site PI redistribute research assistant effort. The PI typically discusses serious problems privately with the site PI beforehand, but during our periodic PI/RA conference calls, we draw attention to these problems, brainstorm solutions, and follow up shortly afterward to assess success. Although our examples focus on recruitment and data submission, the expectation report can also include information on any other time-sensitive aspects of a given study.

The second strategy is site visits that combine a formal audit with problem-solving sessions and training refreshers. The audit may include verification of

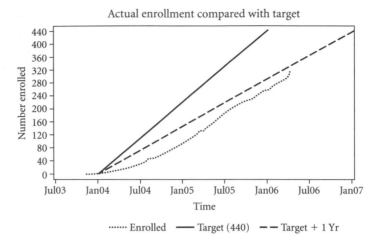

FIGURE 21.1. Actual and expected accrual. The solid line indicates the expected rate of accrual, and the dashed line indicates the rate necessary to complete the study with a 1-year, no-cost extension to the grant. The series of dots indicate the actual enrollment.

consent and Health Insurance Portability and Accountability Act (HIPAA) forms (if copies of these are not sent to a central location), verification of clinical information in local medical records that is used to determine eligibility, ready access to current procedure manuals, and completeness of clinical notes appropriate to the intervention. Problem solving may include issues such as recruitment, follow-up, and completeness and timely submission of data.

Data Management

The practical aspects of good data management are never formally taught and are generally learned through experience. Most investigators initially underestimate the time required and the need to establish clear procedures. With multiple sites, we have found that it is important to have a system for tracking data submission.

One of the strategies that has proved useful is a method for acknowledging receipt of data by the data management center (DMC). Prior to implementing such a system, we experienced frequent claims that data had been sent but were never received. We now include a cover sheet with all data submission packages that indicates who sent the material, when it was sent, the carrier, and a listing of the contents. When the package is received at the DMC, the contents are checked, and a copy of the sheet is sent back to the site as an acknowledgment. If the package is not received, the sender can track the package through the carrier or resend the materials. At the DMC, an inventory of data submitted is kept in an electronic database and is used in the monthly expectation report described earlier.

Expectation Report for Site D

ID	Rand Date	Status T1	Target for T2	End of T2 window	Status T2	Target for T3	End of T3 window	Status T3
1	31May05	Completed	23Aug05	04Oct05	Completed	29Nov05	31Jan06	Completed
2	14Jun05	Completed	06Sep05	18Oct05	Completed	13Dec05	14Feb06	Completed
3	05Jul05	Completed	27Sep05	08Nov05	Completed	03Jan06	07Mar06	Refused
4	03Aug05	Completed	26Oct05	07Dec05	Completed	01Feb06	05Apr06	Completed
5	26Aug05	Completed	18Nov05	30Dec05	Completed	24Feb06	28Apr06	Expected
6	27Sep05	Completed	20Dec05	31Jan06	Refused	28Mar06	30May06	Expected
7	07Oct05	Completed	30Dec05	10Feb06	Completed	07Apr06	09Jun06	Expected
8	02Nov05	Completed	25Jan06	08Mar06	Withdrawn	03May06	05Jul06	Withdrawn
9	15Nov05	Completed	07Feb06	21Mar06	Late	16May06	18Jul06	Pending
10	16Dec05	Completed	10Mar06	21Apr06	Expected	16Jun06	18Aug06	Pending
11	24Jan06	Completed	18Apr06	30May06	Expected	25Jul06	26Sep06	Too early
12	03Feb05	Completed	28Apr06	09Jun06	Pending	04Aug06	06Oct06	Too early
13	03Mar06	QUERY	26May06	07Jul06	Pending	01Sep06	03Nov06	Too early
14	19Apr05	Expected	12Jul06	23Aug06	Too early	18Oct06	20Dec06	Too early

FIGURE 21.2. Example of an expectation report for a study with three assessments. Assessments are scheduled just prior to randomization (T1), between 8 and 12 weeks (T2), and between 6 and 8 months (T3). There is one late report (T2 for ID no. 9) and one outstanding query (T1 for ID no. 13). One subject withdrew from the study for reasons unrelated to the intervention (ID no. 8), and two subjects refused to complete one of the assessments (T2 for ID no. 6 and T3 for ID no. 3).

The second strategy that has proved critical is timely data checking and queries. With early detection, it is often possible to retrieve missing information or resolve problems that it is rarely possible to do at the end of the study due to elapsed time or changes in personnel (e.g., the responsible research assistant is no longer employed by the study). Upon receipt of the data, we immediately check the clarity of the copies and the completeness of the data, paying special attention to dates. Most of the obvious and critical errors in dates occur in recording the year. Typical errors are recording the current year in a birth date or the previous year during the first months of a new year. When missing or inconsistent information that is key to the study and potentially recoverable is identified, queries are generated and tracked to resolution.

Subject Confidentiality (HIPAA)

Maintaining the confidentiality of sensitive information about subjects has always been a critical part of ethical research practice. When studies involve multiple sites, HIPAA regulations have created the need for formalized procedures to ensure confidentiality. Several steps can facilitate the maintenance of confidentiality when information is transferred between sites. First, since randomization is the first time that information is likely to be transferred, we carefully identify enough information about a subject to allow randomization, but we omit information that could identify an individual to nonstudy personnel. For example, we include only characteristics that are used in the stratification (site and language) by subjects' initials in addition to passwords to access the program. The second transfer is the submission of data. We have carefully organized the data and forms so that there are three types. The first has clearly identifying information, specifically full name and contact information, but no information that will be used in the analysis of the study. Because there is no need in this study for the DMC to have this information, clear instructions on the form state that it is not to be sent to the data management center. However, in other studies such as mailed educational materials or phone surveys, this information may be needed to conduct the intervention or assessments. In this case, electronic transmissions of explicit contact information should be encrypted and the information stored in separate databases with limited access. The second type of form contains information that could be potentially used to identify the subject, but would require great effort. This includes dates of birth, diagnosis, treatment, and other characteristics that are rare. Determining what degree of detail is really necessary can minimize potential problems with this type of data. For example, it may not be necessary to have the exact date of birth when only the year (or month and year) is necessary to compute age. The third type are forms that contain no identifying information at all except a unique study identification number. Questionnaires often fall into this group. If these are completely de-identified, data entry can be performed by outside organizations or temporary help without formal training in confidentiality.

Statistical Considerations

In intervention studies involving multiple sites, there is the possibility of variation in the characteristics of the subjects, the usual care all subjects may experience, and the intensity of delivery of the intervention. We mitigate the impact of the first two factors by stratifying randomization by site. Consistent delivery of the intervention is facilitated by the development of good procedure manuals, careful training, and ongoing monitoring. With adequate sample sizes, these factors will be balanced across the intervention arms. In the analysis phase, variation among sites may be addressed by including site as a fixed or random effect. Theoretically, we would include site as a random effect if we believed that the sites were a random selection of all possible sites and we wanted to extend the inference to all possible sites. In practice, the sites are not randomly selected (or typical of the broad spectrum of sites), and the number of sites is typically small, so they are included in the model as fixed effects.

■ Authorship and Giving Credit

A final issue that bridges the scientific and interpersonal workings of any collaborative effort is authorship in publications. At the outset of the collaboration, we devised a *written* agreement signed by all senior investigators indicating that the body of data obtained exists as a common pool for potential use by each and all of us, collectively or separately, by mutual agreement of all the members of the collaboration. By common agreement, papers describing the overall project findings were the responsibility of the project PI and project biostatistician to prepare in a timely fashion. The order of authorship beyond that would be determined by who, within the group, took the most active roles in preparing the manuscript. However, each collaborator would review the paper and sign a copyright statement indicating review and agreement with what had been written. All principal collaborators would be listed on all manuscript publications and all platform and poster publications. In those instances where the entire listing is not possible, remaining group members are to be identified in the acknowledgment section. We believe that group integrity should determine who is listed as an author and not an arbitrary rule made by the editor of a given publication (Flanagin, Fontanarosa, & DeAngelis, 2002; Serwint, Feigelman, & Dumont-Driscoll, 2003).

The agreement includes a clause whereby any principal collaborator or site PI could submit a concept proposal for a specific data analysis (e.g., comparison of effect on subgroups) to the project PI. This proposal would then be distributed to all collaborators for review, discussion and acceptance, modification, or rejection. Authorship would be based on the same criteria as for papers prepared by the PI with the exception that authorship could be limited. Principal collaborators not listed as authors in these secondary analyses were to be acknowledged for their contribution to the database, if samples other than those obtained solely at the author's or authors' institution(s) were used.

A final clause stipulates that if a collaborator requesting permission to do a secondary analysis is unable to complete the proposed analysis, any other collaborator could request group permission to take over the project. This agreement has worked well over the years, and site PI participation in developing, editing, and reviewing manuscripts has been outstanding.

■ Summary

A multisite study is defined as a study that is conducted at two or more organizationally independent institutions that gather data for central analysis using identical methodologies. Advantages include access to large subject pools representing diverse populations from wide geographic areas. As a result, the time required to enroll a critical N to detect even modest, but important, differences can be substantially reduced. Disadvantages, aside from the increased cost inherent in maintaining excellent communication, are primarily logistic and center around investigator buy-in at the various sites, ensuring treatment integrity across sites, and rigorous monitoring of subject accrual, data completeness and accuracy, and the equitable division of labor and authorship credit in reporting results.

Whether the multisite study is based on the more hierarchical principal investigator–initiated model or the collaborated model where site PIs help design and take greater responsibility for the conduct of the study, a strong central administrator and a stringent data manager are essential to successful implementation.

■ References

Christian, M. C., Goldberg, J. L., Killen, J., Abrams, J. S., McCabe, M. S., Mauer, J. K., et al. (2002). A central institutional review board for multi-institutional trials. *New England Journal of Medicine, 346,* 1405–1408.

Flanagin, A., Fontanarosa, P., & DeAngelis, C. (2002). Authorship for research groups. *Journal of the American Medical Association, 288,* 3168.

Fuhrer, M. J. (2005). Conducting multi-site clinical trials in medical rehabilitation research. *American Journal of Physical Medicine and Rehabilitation, 84,* 823–831.

Malcolm, A., Smith, L. A., Gloeckler, R., James, G., & Gurney, J. R. (2006). *Leukemia.* National Cancer Institute, SEER Pediatric Monograph. Retrieved [DATE, YEAR] from http://www.nci.gov

McCaskill-Stevens, W., McKinney, M. M., Whitman, C. G., & Minasian, L. M. (2005). Increasing minority participation in cancer clinical trials: The minority-based community clinical oncology program experience. *Journal of Clinical Oncology, 23,* 5247–5254.

Meinert, C. L. (1986). *Clinical trials: Design, conduct, and analysis.* New York: Oxford University Press.

Moinpour, C. M., Atkinson, J. O., Thomas, S. M., Underwood, S. M., Harvey, C., Parzuchowski, J., et al. (2000). Minority recruitment in the prostate cancer prevention trial. *Annals of Epidemiology, 10,* S85–S91.

Ramirez, A. G., & Suarez, L. (2006). Hispanic cultures. Retrieved [May 14, 2007] from http://www.healthline.com/galecontent/hispanic-cultures

Serwint, J. R., Feigelman, S., & Dumont-Driscoll, M. (2003). Listing contributions of investigators in research groups. *Journal of the American Medical Association, 289*, 2212.

Tate, D. G., Findley, T., Dijkers, M., Nobunaga, A. I., & Karunas, R. B. (1999). Randomized clinical trials in medical rehabilitation research. *American Journal of Physical Medicine and Rehabilitation, 78*, 486–499.

INDEX